1999
YEAR BOOK OF
GASTROENTEROLOGY™

Statement of Purpose

The YEAR BOOK Service

The YEAR BOOK series was devised in 1901 by practicing health professionals who observed that the literature of medicine and related disciplines had become so voluminous that no one individual could read and place in perspective every potential advance in a major specialty. In the final decade of the 20th century, this recognition is more acutely true than it was in 1901.

More than merely a series of books, YEAR BOOK volumes are the tangible results of a unique service designed to accomplish the following:

- to *survey* a wide range of journals of proven value
- to *select* from those journals papers representing significant advances and statements of important clinical principles
- to provide *abstracts* of those articles that are readable, convenient summaries of their key points
- to provide *commentary* about those articles to place them in perspective

These publications grow out of a unique process that calls on the talents of outstanding authorities in clinical and fundamental disciplines, trained literature specialists, and professional writers, all supported by the resources of Mosby, the world's preeminent publisher for the health professions.

The Literature Base

Mosby and its editors survey approximately 500 journals published worldwide, covering the full range of the health professions. On an annual basis, the publisher examines usage patterns and polls its expert authorities to add new journals to the literature base and to delete journals that are no longer useful as potential YEAR BOOK sources.

The Literature Survey

The publisher's team of literature specialists, all of whom are trained and experienced health professionals, examines every original, peer-reviewed article in each journal issue. More than 250,000 articles per year are scanned systematically, including title, text, illustrations, tables, and references. Each scan is compared, article by article, to the search strategies that the publisher has developed in consultation with the 270 outside experts who form the pool of YEAR BOOK editors. A given article may be reviewed by any number of editors, from one to a dozen or more, regardless of the discipline for which the paper was originally published. In turn, each editor who receives the article reviews it to determine whether the article should be included in the YEAR BOOK. This decision is based on the article's inherent quality, its probable usefulness to readers of that YEAR BOOK, and the editor's goal to represent a balanced picture of a given field in each volume of the YEAR BOOK. In addition, the editor indicates when to include figures and tables from the article to help the YEAR BOOK reader better understand the information.

Of the quarter million articles scanned each year, only 5% are selected for detailed analysis within the YEAR BOOK series, thereby assuring readers of the high value of every selection.

The Abstract

The publisher's abstracting staff is headed by a seasoned medical professional and includes individuals with training in the life sciences, medicine, and other areas, plus extensive experience in writing for the health professions and related industries. Each selected article is assigned to a specific writer on this abstracting staff. The abstracter, guided in many cases by notations supplied by the expert editor, writes a structured, condensed summary designed so that the reader can rapidly acquire the essential information contained in the article.

The Commentary

The YEAR BOOK editorial boards, sometimes assisted by guest commentators, write comments that place each article in perspective for the reader. This provides the reader with the equivalent of a personal consultation with a leading international authority—an opportunity to better understand the value of the article and to benefit from the authority's thought processes in assessing the article.

Additional Editorial Features

The editorial boards of each YEAR BOOK organize the abstracts and comments to provide a logical and satisfying sequence of information. To enhance the organization, editors also provide introductions to sections or individual chapters, comments linking a number of abstracts, citations to additional literature, and other features.

The published YEAR BOOK contains enhanced bibliographic citations for each selected article, including extended listings of multiple authors and identification of author affiliations. Each YEAR BOOK contains a Table of Contents specific to that year's volume. From year to year, the Table of Contents for a given YEAR BOOK will vary depending on developments within the field.

Every YEAR BOOK contains a list of the journals from which papers have been selected. This list represents a subset of approximately 500 journals surveyed by the publisher and occasionally reflects a particularly pertinent article from a journal that is not surveyed on a routine basis.

Finally, each volume contains a comprehensive subject index and an index to authors of each selected paper.

The 1999 Year Book Series

Year Book of Allergy, Asthma, and Clinical Immunology: Drs. Rosenwasser, Boguniewicz, Borish, Routes, Spahn, and Weber

Year Book of Anesthesiology and Pain Management®: Drs. Tinker, Abram, Chestnut, Roizen, Rothenberg, and Wood

Year Book of Cardiology®: Drs. Schlant, Collins, Gersh, Graham, Kaplan, and Waldo

Year Book of Chiropractic®: Dr. Lawrence

Year Book of Critical Care Medicine®: Drs. Parrillo, Balk, Calvin, Franklin, and Shapiro

Year Book of Dentistry®: Drs. Meskin, Berry, Jeffcoat, Leinfelder, Roser, Summitt, and Zakariasen

Year Book of Dermatology and Dermatologic Surgery™: Drs. Thiers and Lang

Year Book of Diagnostic Radiology®: Drs. Osborn, Birdwell, Dalinka, Groskin, Maynard, Pentecost, Ros, Smirniotopoulos, and Young

Year Book of Emergency Medicine®: Drs. Wagner, Dronen, Davidson, King, Niemann, and Hamilton

Year Book of Endocrinology®: Drs. Bagdade, Braverman, Fitzpatrick, Horton, Kannan, Landsberg, Molitch, Morley, Odell, Poehlman, and Rogol

Year Book of Family Practice®: Drs. Berg, Bowman, Davidson, Dexter, and Scherger

Year Book of Gastroenterology: Drs. Aliperti and Fleshman

Year Book of Hand Surgery®: Drs. Amadio and Hentz

Year Book of Medicine®: Drs. Klahr, Frishman, Malawista, Mandell, Jett, Young, Barkin, and Bagdade

Year Book of Neonatal and Perinatal Medicine®: Drs. Fanaroff, Maisels, and Stevenson

Year Book of Nephrology, Hypertension, and Mineral Metabolism: Drs. Schwab, Bennett, Emmett, Hostetter, and Moe

Year Book of Neurology and Neurosurgery®: Drs. Bradley and Gibbs

Year Book of Nuclear Medicine®: Drs. Gottschalk, Blaufox, Coleman, Strauss, and Zubal

Year Book of Obstetrics, Gynecology, and Women's Health®: Drs. Mishell, Herbst, and Kirschbaum

Year Book of Oncology®: Drs. Ozols, Eisenberg, Glatstein, Loehrer, and Urba

Year Book of Ophthalmology®: Drs. Wilson, Augsburger, Cohen, Eagle, Grossman, Laibson, Maguire, Nelson, Penne, Rapuano, Sergott, Spaeth, Tipperman, Ms. Gosfield, and Ms. Salmon

Year Book of Orthopedics®: Drs. Morrey, Beauchamp, Currier, Tolo, Trigg, and Swiontkowski

Year Book of Otolaryngology–Head and Neck Surgery®: Drs. Paparella, Holt, and Otto

Year Book of Pathology and Laboratory Medicine®: Drs. Raab, Cohen, Dabbs, Olson, and Stanley

Year Book of Pediatrics®: Dr. Stockman

Year Book of Plastic, Reconstructive, and Aesthetic Surgery®: Drs. Miller, Bartlett, Garner, McKinney, Ruberg, Salisbury, and Smith

Year Book of Psychiatry and Applied Mental Health®: Drs. Talbott, Ballenger, Frances, Lydiard, Meltzer, Jensen, and Tasman

Year Book of Pulmonary Disease®: Drs. Jett, Castro, Maurer, Peters, Phillips, and Ryu

Year Book of Rheumatology, Arthritis, and Musculoskeletal Disease™: Drs. Panush, Hadler, Hellmann, LeRoy, Pisetsky, and Simon

Year Book of Sports Medicine®: Drs. Shephard, Drinkwater, Eichner, Torg, Alexander, and Mr. George

Year Book of Surgery®: Drs. Copeland, Bland, Deitch, Eberlein, Howard, Luce, Seeger, Souba, and Sugarbaker

Year Book of Urology®: Drs. Andriole and Coplen

Year Book of Vascular Surgery®: Dr. Porter

1999

The Year Book of GASTROENTEROLOGY™

Editor-in-Chief

Giuseppe Aliperti, M.D.

Associate Professor of Medicine, Washington University School of Medicine, Barnes-Jewish Hospital, St. Louis, Missouri

Mosby

St. Louis Baltimore Boston Carlsbad Naples New York Philadelphia Portland London
Madrid Mexico City Singapore Sydney Tokyo Toronto Wiesbaden

Mosby
Dedicated to Publishing Excellence

Publisher: Cheryl A. Smart
Developmental Editors: Laura C. Berendson and Colleen Cook
Manager, Periodical Editing: Kirk Swearingen
Manuscript Editor: Pat Costigan
Project Supervisor, Production: Joy Moore
Production Assistant: Laura Bayless
Manager, Literature Services: Idelle L. Winer
Illustrations and Permissions Specialist: Steve Ramay

1999 EDITION

Printed in the United States of America
Composition by Reed Technology and Information Services, Inc.
Printing/binding by Maple–Vail

Editorial Office:
Mosby, Inc.
11830 Westline Industrial Drive
St. Louis, MO 63146

International Standard Serial Number: 0739–5930
International Standard Book Number: 0-8151–9620-2

Associate Editor

James W. Fleshman, Jr., M.D.

Associate Professor of Surgery, Chief, Section of Colon and Rectal Surgery, Washington University School of Medicine, Barnes-Jewish Hospital, St. Louis, Missouri

Contributing Editors

Jamie S. Barkin, M.D.

Professor of Medicine, University of Miami, Miami, Florida; Chief, Division of Gastroenterology, Mount Sinai Medical Center, Miami Beach, Florida

Marc J. Bernstein, M.D.

Assistant Professor of Medicine, Division of Gastroenterology, Washington University School of Medicine; Attending Physician, Barnes-Jewish Hospital, St. Louis, Missouri

Elisa H. Birnbaum, M.D.

Assistant Professor, Washington University School of Medicine; Attending Physician, Barnes-Jewish Hospital, St. Louis, Missouri

William W. Dexter, M.D.

Director, Sports Medicine; Assistant Director, Family Practice Residency, Maine Medical Center, Portland, Maine; Assistant Professor, Department of Family Medicine, University of Vermont, Burlington, Vermont

Jeffrey A. Drebin, M.D., Ph.D.

Assistant Professor of Surgery, Washington University School of Medicine; Assistant Professor of Surgery, Barnes-Jewish Hospital, St. Louis, Missouri

Thomas E. Read, M.D.

Assistant Professor of Surgery, Washington University School of Medicine, Barnes-Jewish Hospital, St. Louis, Missouri

Jeff R. Willis, M.D.

Instructor of Medicine, Washington University School of Medicine, St. Louis, Missouri

Table of Contents

Journals Represented

Mosby and its editors survey approximately 500 journals for its abstract and commentary publications. From these journals, the editors select the articles to be abstracted. Journals represented in this YEAR BOOK are listed below.

Abdominal Imaging
American Journal of Epidemiology
American Journal of Gastroenterology
American Journal of Medicine
American Journal of Roentgenology
American Journal of Surgery
American Surgeon
Annals of Internal Medicine
Annals of Surgery
Annals of Thoracic Surgery
Archives of Internal Medicine
Archives of Surgery
Australasian Radiology
British Journal of Surgery
British Medical Journal
Cancer
Clinical Infectious Diseases
Digestive Diseases and Sciences
Diseases of the Colon and Rectum
Endoscopy
European Journal of Surgery
Gastroenterology
Gut
Hepatology
International Journal of Cancer
International Journal of Radiation, Oncology, Biology, and Physics
Journal of Clinical Oncology
Journal of Family Practice
Journal of General Internal Medicine
Journal of Pediatric Gastroenterology and Nutrition
Journal of the American Board of Family Practice
Journal of the American College of Surgeons
Journal of the Royal College of Surgeons of Edinburgh
Lancet
Mayo Clinic Proceedings
Medical Care
New England Journal of Medicine
Postgraduate Medical Journal
Psychological Medicine
Radiology
Radiotherapy and Oncology
Southern Medical Journal
Surgery
Transplantation
World Journal of Surgery

Standard Abbreviations

The following terms are abbreviated in this edition: acquired immunodeficiency syndrome (AIDS), cardiopulmonary resuscitation (CPR), central nervous system (CNS), cerebrospinal fluid (CSF), computed tomography (CT), deoxyribonucleic acid (DNA), electrocardiography (ECG), health maintenance organization (HMO), human immunodeficiency virus (HIV), intensive care unit (ICU), intramuscular (IM), intravenous (IV), magnetic resonance (MR) imaging (MRI), ribonucleic acid (RNA), and ultrasound (US).

Note

The Year Book of Gastroenterology is a literature survey service providing abstracts of articles published in the professional literature. Every effort is made to assure the accuracy of the information presented in these pages. Neither the editors nor the publisher of the Year Book of Gastroenterology can be responsible for errors in the original materials. The editors' comments are their own opinions. Mention of specific products within this publication does not constitute endorsement.

To facilitate the use of the Year Book of Gastroenterology as a reference tool, all illustrations and tables included in this publication are now identified as they appear in the original article. This change is meant to help the reader recognize that any illustration or table appearing in the Year Book of Gastroenterology may be only one of many in the original article. For this reason, figure and table numbers will often appear to be out of sequence within the Year Book of Gastroenterology.

1 The Esophagus

General

Effect of Large Fundal Varices on Changes in Gastric Mucosal Hemodynamics After Endoscopic Variceal Ligation

Tayama C, Iwao T, Oho K, et al (Kurume Univ, Japan)

Endoscopy 30:25-31, 1998 1–1

Background.—Portal hypertensive gastropathy (PHG) causes bleeding in patients with cirrhosis. These patients can also have bleeding from esophageal varices. Endoscopic variceal ligation (EVL) has been developed to treat esophageal variceal bleeding, but its effect on PHG has not been documented. Changes in gastric mucosal hemodynamics after EVL were compared in patients with cirrhosis with and without large fundal varices.

Study Design.—Between November 1995 and August 1996, 8 patients with large fundal varices and 19 patients without large fundal varices were enrolled in this study. Baseline assessments of gastric mucosal hemoglobin content (IHB) and gastric mucosal oxygen saturation (ISO_2), as well as PHG, were recorded at the antrum and the corpus. EVL was performed with an endoscopic ligating device at 1-week intervals until all varices were destroyed. Gastric mucosal hemodynamic assessments were repeated 3 days after the initial EVL and 7 days after the final EVL.

Findings.—Neither PHG nor gastric mucosal hemodynamic parameters were modified at the antrum by EVL in patients with or without large fundal varices. At the corpus, PHG and IHB significantly increased and ISO_2 significantly decreased after EVL in those patients without large fundal varices. These parameters did not change significantly in patients with large fundal varices.

Conclusions.—The aggravation of PHG after EVL is caused by congestion of gastric mucosal circulation. Large fundal varices are protective by reducing this congestion. Patients without large fundal varices are at risk for development of EVL-associated PHG. Propranolol reduces PHG-associated bleeding. Whether propranolol administration can prevent EVL-induced PHG aggravation, especially in patients without large fundal varices, remains to be determined.

► This article describes the use of advanced endoscopic research tools to measure gastric mucosal hemodynamics. The focus of the study was PHG and its response to endoscopic ligation of esophageal varices. The objective data obtained from laser-Doppler velocimetry and reflectance spectrophotometric measurements was interpreted alongside more apparent endoscopic findings such as the presence and size of gastric varices, as well as the visible severity of portal gastropathy.

From the data, the authors demonstrated that variceal ligation, like sclerotherapy, can worsen congestion of the gastric mucosal circulation. This can result in worsened portal gastropathy. Fundic varices seemingly served as a decompressing reservoir and decreased the risk of worsened gastropathy after the endoscopic treatment of esophageal varices. This paper provides useful insights into the pathogenesis of PHG and identifies a group of patients who may be expected to be at high risk for this complication.

M.J. Bernstein, M.D.

The Clinical and Economic Value of a Short Course of Omeprazole in Patients With Noncardiac Chest Pain

Fass R, Fennerty MB, Ofman JJ, et al (Tucson VA Med Ctr, Ariz; Arizona Health Sciences Ctr, Tucson; Oregon Health Sciences Univ, Portland; et al)
Gastroenterology 115:42-49, 1998 1–2

Background.—Assessing new patients with noncardiac chest pain (NCCP) can involve a variety of costly tests. The efficacy of the omeprazole test (OT) in diagnosing gastroesophageal reflux disease (GERD) in patients with NCCP was determined, and the potential cost savings were estimated.

Methods.—Thirty-nine patients were randomly assigned to omeprazole or placebo for 7 days. Patients were then crossed over to the opposite treatment after a washout period, and baseline symptom assessment was repeated. Before randomization, the patients had 24-hour esophageal pH monitoring and upper endoscopy.

Findings.—Of the 37 patients completing the study, 23 were considered to have GERD-positive (62.2%) results, and 14 were considered to have GERD-negative results. Seventy-eight percent of the patients with GERD-positive results and 14% of patients with GERD-negative results had positive findings on the OT, which yielded a sensitivity and specificity of 78.3% and 85.7%, respectively. The OT resulted in an average cost savings of $573 per patient assessed. It also enabled a 59% reduction in the number of diagnostic procedures.

Conclusions.—The OT is a sensitive and specific method for diagnosing GERD in patients with NCCP. The use of this strategy enables significant cost savings and reduces the number of diagnostic tests done.

The Acid Suppression Test for Unexplained Chest Pain

Castell DO, Katz PO (Allegheny Univ, Philadelphia)

Gastroenterology 115:222-224, 1998 1–3

Background.—Most patients with unexplained or noncardiac chest pain remain without diagnoses. In 1982, DeMeester et al. demonstrated that 46% of patients discharged from a coronary care unit with a diagnosis of noncardiac chest pain had abnormal gastroesophageal reflux (GER). A recently published study by Fass et al. describes an innovation in the diagnosis of and therapy for potential GER-related noncardiac chest pain.

The Acid Suppression Test for Unexplained Chest Pain.—Fass et al. (Abstract 1–2) tested the hypothesis that high-dose omeprazole administered for 1 week would provide an effective, accurate, cost-effective approach to the treatment of patients with frequently recurring (at least 3 times a week for 3 months) chest pain. In the 37 patients studied, coronary artery disease had been excluded. The results showed that 62.2% of the patients had evidence of reflux disease, including 7 patients with abnormal esophageal acid exposure by pH testing only, 8 with erosive esophagitis only, and 8 with both. Seventy-eight percent of the patients with GER-positive fndings and 14% of the patients with GER-negative findings had a positive result on the omeprazole test (at least a 50% decrease in chest pain frequency during the treatment period). A positive result on the omeprazole test had a sensitivity of 78.3% and a specificity of 85.7%. However, these findings cannot necessarily be extrapolated to the large population of patients with unexplained chest pain. The research subjects in the Fass et al. study were 36 men and only 1 woman; however, unexplained chest pain occurs in almost twice as many women as men. Women and men differ in esophageal sensation to various stimuli. In women, esophageal pain thresholds to balloon distension are lower. Despite this limitation, the results of the Fass et al. study suggest that clinicians may initiate an appropriate trial of acid-suppression therapy in patients with unexplained chest pain after coronary artery disease has been excluded.

▶ Intermittent chest pain of a noncardiac source is a frequent and frustrating clinical problem. Obviously, intrinsic to our approach to this problem is exclusion of a cardiac source. Once this is accomplished, we need to consider GERD, as it is a frequent source of NCCP. Extensive testing has usually been required to suggest this etiology. These tests include 24-hour ambulatory extraesophageal pH monitoring and endoscopy. Abstract 1–2 shows the value of a trial of a high-dose proton pump inhibitor (omeprazole at 40 mg AM and 20 mg PM) to presumably treat GERD and suppress chest pain.

Use of this therapeutic trial as opposed to diagnostic testing resulted in significant cost savings ($573.00 per patient) and a 59% reduction in diagnostic procedures.

In summary, simple is better!

J.S. Barkin, M.D.

Laryngeal Manifestations of Gastroesophageal Reflux Before and After Treatment With Omeprazole

Shaw GY, Searl JP (Univ of Kansas Med Ctr, Kansas City)

South Med J 90:1115-1122, 1997 1–4

Background.—Laryngeal manifestations of gastroesophageal reflux disease (GERD) are believed to be prevalent. The diagnosis is based mainly on symptoms. Additional testing has traditionally included laryngoscopy, the intake of barium, manometry, and single- and double-probe pH monitoring. In the current study, the common symptoms associated with GERD were identified, and a standard scale was used to objectively describe the laryngoscopic findings.

Methods.—Ninety-six patients with symptoms suggesting reflux laryngitis were assessed. Surveys to grade patients' symptoms were administered. Standardized videolaryngostroboscopic examination and computerized acoustic analysis were also performed. Patients were then given a uniform regimen of dietary restriction and omeprazole for 12 weeks, and assessments were repeated.

Findings.—This regimen resulted in a significant improvement in all symptoms except granulomas. Patients with hoarseness before treatment showed a significant improvement on acoustic measures of jitter, shimmer, habitual frequency, and frequency range.

Conclusions.—In patients with symptomatic reflux laryngitis, standardized videolaryngoscopy and acoustic analysis are useful methods for diagnosis and treatment monitoring. Antireflux treatment with omeprazole is effective, as demonstrated by objective measures.

Comorbid Occurrence of Laryngeal or Pulmonary Disease With Esophagitis in United States Military Veterans

El-Serag HB, Sonnenberg A (Dept of Veterans Affairs Med Ctr, Albuquerque, NM; Univ of New Mexico, Albuquerque)

Gastroenterology 113:755-760, 1997 1–5

Background.—Gastroesophageal reflux disease (GERD) may be a risk factor for the occurrence of extraesophageal complications. The co-morbid occurrence of sinus, laryngeal, and pulmonary diseases was studied in individuals with and without reflux esophagitis.

Methods.—Data were obtained on 101,366 patients with erosive esophagitis or esophageal stricture discharged from veterans hospitals between 1981 and 1994. An equal number of control research subjects without these conditions comprised a control group.

Findings.—Erosive esophagitis and esophageal stricture were associated with sinusitis (odds ratio [OR], 1.6), pharyngitis (OR, 1.48), aphonia (OR, 1.81), laryngitis (OR, 2.01), and laryngeal stenosis (OR, 2.02). The disorders were also associated with chronic bronchitis (OR, 1.28), asthma (OR, 1.51), chronic obstructive pulmonary disease (OR, 1.22), pulmonary fibrosis (OR, 1.36), bronchiectasis (OR, 1.26), pulmonary collapse (OR, 1.31), and pneumonia (OR, 1.15).

Conclusions.—Erosive esophagitis and esophageal strictures appear to be associated with a large variety of extraesophageal diseases involving the sinuses, pharynx, larynx, and lungs. The risks for these clinically relevant complications ranged from 1.2-fold to 2-fold.

▶ GERD may be complicated by extraesophageal conditions that may occur even with the lack of symptoms of heartburn. These include sinusitis, pharyngitis, aphonia, laryngitis, laryngeal stenoses, chronic bronchitis, asthma, chronic obstruction, lung disease, pulmonary fibrosis and collapse, bronchiectasis, and pneumonia.

Shaw and Searl (Abstract 1–4) reported objective evidence of laryngeal manifestation healing, except granulomas, by omeprazole—a proton pump inhibitor. Therefore, we must search for GERD in patients with a wide spectrum of laryngeal or pulmonary diseases, even in those without a history of GERD, and realize that acid suppression is the approach to their successful treatment.

J.S. Barkin, M.D.

Esophagogastroduodenoscopy Performed by a Family Physician: A Case Series of 793 Procedures

Pierzchajlo RPJ, Ackermann RJ, Vogel RL, et al (Tifon, Ga; Mercer Univ, Macon, Ga)

J Fam Pract 46:41-46, 1998 1–6

Introduction.—Flexible sigmoidoscopy is performed by up to 29% to 57% of U.S. family physicians and 42% of general internists. Primary care physicians perform esophagogastroduodenoscopy (EGD) substantially less often than flexible sigmoidoscopy. Up to 1% of some U.S. populations have endoscopy each year. Access to this technology can be problematic, particularly in rural areas. A large series of EGDs performed by a family physician in a solo rural practice is reviewed.

Methods.—Medical records were retrospectively reviewed for data regarding demographics, indications for EGD, endoscopic and pathologic findings, and complications for all EGDs performed by the family physician over 7 years.

Results.—Six hundred two patients underwent 793 EGDs. Mean age of 421 women and 181 men was 51.8 years. The second portion of the duodenum was intubated in 99% of EGDs. The most frequent indications for EGD were 60.5%, abdominal pain; 23.0%, gastrointestinal bleeding; 11.6%, dysphagia; and 10.7%, heartburn. Of 451 biopsies obtained in 385 procedures, 38% were taken from the distal esophagus and 38% were taken from the gastric antrum. The most frequent endoscopic diagnoses were 54%, gastritis; 25%, esophagitis; and 15%, normal findings. Two malignancies were found: 1 gastric lymphoma and 1 carcinoma metastatic to the stomach. There was 1 minor complication: 1 patient had an immediate urticarial rash after administration of IV meperidine.

Conclusion.—This is the largest reported series of EGDs by a single primary care physician. The complication rate compares favorably with the largest series in gastrointestinal literature. The physician in this series gained all of his endoscopic skills after residency.

▶ This article really caught my attention. Many of us perform flexible sigmoidoscopies, few perform esophagogastroduodenoscopies. I included this case series report simply in the hope that this might also pique your interest, and, perhaps, to motivate you, as it has me, to investigate the possibility of acquiring this skill. This is a service that family doctors can perform, and, as the author of this study has, perform expertly and safely in a busy practice setting.

W.W. Dexter, M.D.

Gastroesophageal Reflux Disease

Cost Effectiveness of Treatment for Gastro-oesophageal Reflux Disease in Clinical Practice: A Clinical Database Analysis

Eggleston A, Wigerinck A, Huijghebaert S, et al (Janssen Research Found, Beerse, Belgium; Univ of Liverpool, England)
Gut 42:13-16, 1998 1–7

Background.—Health care expenditures for gastrointestinal disease continue to increase. Patients with gastroesophageal reflux disease (GORD), a chronic condition, tend to require long-term care. The cost-effectiveness of treatment of uncomplicated GORD with cisapride (CIS), ranitidine (RAN), and omeprazole (OME) was examined to determine the most cost-effective treatment strategy.

Study Design.—Patients seen by primary care physicians during 1995 with a first episode of uncomplicated GORD were identified from the MediPlus United Kingdom (UK) database. The 257 patients identified were retrospectively divided into 3 groups on the basis of initial treatment: 80 treated with CIS, 90 with RAN, and 87 with OME. These 3 groups were comparable with respect to age, gender, co-morbidity, and other types of gastrointestinal disease. All health resources consumed in the 6 months after diagnosis were assessed, including prescriptions, physician consultations, hospitalizations, and diagnostic tests. All costs were expressed in British pounds (£) at 1996 value.

Findings.—The average cost for the initial 6 months of treatment was £136 for CIS, £177 for RAN, and £189 for OME per patient. The most important cost variables were cost and quantity of medication. The average number of 1-month prescriptions during this period was 1.85 (£49) for CIS, 2.57 (£67) for RAN, and 2.96 (£105) for OME therapy. Antacid use was higher in the CIS and RAN groups, but their contribution to cost per patient during this period was not significant. The number of visits to general practitioners in this period was 2.4 for CIS (£60.31), 2.9 for RAN

(£73.06), and 2.6 for OME (£65.52). The average number of nondrug interventions per patient was 0.34 in the RAN group (£23.80), compared with less than 0.2 in the CIS (£9.60) and OME (£11.10) groups.

Conclusions.—This analysis indicated that for patients experiencing a first episode of uncomplicated GORD, most of the cost of therapy was attributable to primary care consultations and antireflux medication. These results indicate that a stepped approach to patient management, starting therapy with a prokinetic or H_2 receptor antagonist and reserving more potent and expensive antireflux medication for cases in which adequate symptom control was not achieved, was the most cost-effective.

► The study by Eggleston et al. is a retrospective database analysis of the cost-effectiveness of alternative treatment for patients with uncomplicated GORD in the primary care setting. The major costs for treating patients with GORD in the primary care setting are for consultations with a specialist and antireflux medication use. The results of this study indicate that for initial treatment in patients with uncomplicated GORD, the initial approach should be the use of H_2 receptor antagonists or a prokinetic agent. This results in significant cost savings. They go on to conclude that the use of more potent acid-suppressant medications, such as proton pump inhibitors, or referral to subspecialists should be reserved for patients who fail to respond to an adequate trial of this initial approach. In the primary care setting, using H_2 receptor antagonists or prokinetic agents is certainly reasonable in the subset of younger patients with uncomplicated reflux without alarm features. This strategy may result in some cost savings. However, GORD is a chronic disease, and many of the patients eventually require the more potent acid suppression with the more expensive proton pump inhibitors. These patients, at some point, may require referral to a specialist for investigation. Therefore good clinical follow-up remains important.

G. Aliperti, M.D.

Empirical Therapy Versus Diagnostic Tests in Gastroesophageal Reflux Disease: A Medical Decision Analysis

Sonnenberg A, Delcò F, El-Serag HB (Univ of New Mexico, Albuquerque)

Dig Dis Sci 43:1001-1008, 1998 1–8

Objective.—With the variety of diagnostic tests and pharmacologic and surgical armamentaria for treating gastroesophageal reflux disease (GERD), it is difficult for physicians to decide how to manage patients efficiently and cost-effectively.

Methods.—A decision tree for GERD management was developed to calculate the threshold probability of GERD for which empirical therapy was more cost-effective than diagnostic testing. Bayes' formula was used to transform sensitivity and specificity data of various symptoms into probability for GERD in a specific patient. Medication costs were estimated from average wholesale prices.

Results.—The threshold probability for empirical therapy depended on the costs of the diagnostic procedure vs. the costs of a missed diagnosis, the length and costs of GERD therapy, and the costs of treating patients who received a misdiagnosis of GERD. For the most part, the cost savings of a diagnostic procedure outweighed the occasional cost of treating a patient who received a misdiagnosis of GERD. The highest cost was associated with erroneous empirical treatment of a peptic ulcer patient.

Conclusion.—In general, empirical therapy is warranted for patients who have multiple symptoms of GERD, but it is not warranted when peptic ulcer disease is an important alternative diagnosis.

▶ Sonnenberg, in this decision and analytic model, looks at the question of whether to choose empirical therapy first or a diagnostic testing first in patients who present with GERD. The results of this analysis indicate that patients with multiple symptoms from which the commission can commonly diagnose GERD would be good candidates for empirical therapy. This approach would not be warranted in patients who might be considering surgery or needing long-term antisecretory therapy. A subset of patients who present with classic GERD symptoms and who are younger, without any alarm features, certainly would be good candidates for initial empirical therapy. However, often symptoms may be suggestive of peptic ulcer disease as well as GERD, and these patients need to have further diagnostic workup. Furthermore, it is important to remember that these patients require good follow-up. In patients who require long-term therapy, further investigation is probably warranted.

G. Aliperti, M.D.

The Utility of Endoscopy in the Management of Patients With Gastroesophageal Reflux Symptoms

Blustein PK, Beck PL, Meddings JB, et al (Universities of Calgary and Alberta, Canada)

Am J Gastroenterol 93:2508-2512, 1998 1–9

Background.—The value of endoscopy in the treatment of patients with symptoms of gastroesophageal reflux disease (GERD) has not been established. The effects of endoscopy on subsequent management of patients with uncomplicated reflux symptoms were investigated.

Methods.—Seven hundred forty-two patients with GERD symptoms underwent endoscopy. Endoscopists recorded treatment before endoscopy, endoscopic findings, and their treatment recommendations after endoscopy.

Findings.—Patients undergoing endoscopy because of failed therapy or because of GERD symptoms alone did not differ in pre-endoscopy treatment or esophagitis grade. For patients receiving omeprazole, the most common recommendation after endoscopy was to maintain or increase the dose. For patients receiving an H_2 blocker, the most common postendoscopy recommendation was to switch to omeprazole therapy, independent of esophagitis grade. The incidence of Barrett's esophagus was low. No cases of esophageal cancer were identified.

Conclusions.—Most patients in this series were switched to omeprazole therapy after endoscopy for GERD symptoms, regardless of the endoscopic findings. Thus, a trial of a proton pump inhibitor for patients receiving H_2-blocker therapy should be considered before endoscopy.

▶ The value of routine endoscopy in patients with classic symptoms of GERD has been assessed in this article. In only 26% of the patients was marked esophagitis detected by endoscopy. The values are consistent with prior studies. In general, endoscopy for the assessment of uncomplicated GERD had a low yield and did not significantly modify therapy. In fact, regardless of the endoscopic findings, patients with symptoms were switched from an H_2 blocker to a proton pump inhibitor; if they were using a proton pump inhibitor before the endoscopy, the dose was increased. In this study of 742 patients, no cancer was found and the incidence of Barrett's esophagus was low (6.3%). The authors conclude that a trial of a proton pump inhibitor before endoscopy should be considered and that endoscopy itself did not change the management of patients treated with H_2 blockers. This approach is already widely used on the basis of the clinical observation of experienced gastroenterologists.

G. Aliperti, M.D.

Meal Type Affects Heartburn Severity

Rodriguez S, Miner P, Robinson M, et al (Univ of Oklahoma, Oklahoma City; Glaxo Wellcome Inc, Research Triangle Park, NC)

Dig Dis Sci 43:485-490, 1998 1–10

Background.—Fat, chocolate, peppermint, and onions are thought to cause heartburn by reducing lower esophageal sphincter pressure (LESP) or increasing transient LES relaxations. Coffee, orange juice, tomato products, and capsaicin have been reported to be direct irritants to the esophagus. Heartburn severity, number of episodes, and changes in esophageal pH induced by 3 meals were compared.

Methods.—Twelve symptomatic volunteers were enrolled in the study. On different occasions, the participants ate a McDonald's Quarter Pounder, french fries, and a chocolate shake; McDonald's Sausage Biscuit with Egg, cheese, raw onion, and chocolate milk; and Wendy's Chili and red wine.

Findings.—The increase in the number of reflux episodes over baseline for the hamburger meal was a mean of 28.8; for the sausage biscuit meal, it was a mean of 36; and for the chili meal, it was a mean of 43.7. The sausage biscuit and chili meals increased reflux compared with the hamburger meal, but the chili and sausage biscuit meals did not differ from one another. Onset and peak heartburn times for the hamburger meals were 45 and 90 minutes, respectively. Onset and peak heartburn times for the sausage biscuit meal were 30 and 120 minutes, respectively. Onset and peak heartburn times for the chili meal were 15 and 150 minutes.

Conclusions.—Despite the lower fat content, chili and red wine produced more reflux and heartburn pain than the other meals. Thus, high-fat meals are apparently not preferable in provocative meal studies. Factors such as pH, volume, chemical content, and individual food ingredients must also be considered when choosing meals for clinical studies.

Effect of Increasing the Fat Content But Not the Energy Load of a Meal on Gastro-oesophageal Reflux and Lower Oesophageal Sphincter Motor Function

Penagini R, Mangano M, Bianchi PA (Univ of Milan, Italy)
Gut 42:330-333, 1998 1–11

Background.—Fatty foods are generally thought to be harmful for patients with reflux disease. However, there are no objective data to substantiate this belief. The effect of fat on gastroesophageal reflux and lower esophageal sphincter (LES) motor activity was investigated.

Methods.—Fourteen patients with reflux disease and 13 healthy individuals were given a high-fat (52% fat) and a balanced (24% fat) meal on 2 different occasions. For 180 minutes after each meal, esophageal pH, LES, and esophageal pressures were recorded. Seven patients and 8 control research subjects were in the recumbent position during recording, and the others were sitting.

Findings.—The percentage of time at a pH value of less than 4 and the reflux episode rate were higher in the patients than in the control research subjects. Patients also had an increased percentage of transient LES relaxations associated with reflux. Eating the high-fat meal did not increase the reflux episode rate or exposure to esophageal acid in either group, regardless of body posture. Also, the high-fat meal did not affect the rate of transient LES relaxations, their association with reflux, or basal LES pressure.

Conclusions.—Gastroesophageal reflux is not increased after consumption of fatty foods, at least for the first 3 hours after the meal. The relationship between fat and the induction of heartburn in reflux disease appears to be more complex than is commonly believed.

▶ Numerous foods and beverages can induce heartburn; however, their physiologic mechanisms differ. Fatty foods have been assumed to induce heartburn, but when a high-fat meal was compared with an equal-energy balanced meal, it did not affect transient LES relaxation or basal LESP. Rodriguez et al. (Abstract 1–10) reinforced these data when they found that the meal they administered with the lowest fat content induced the greatest number of reflux episodes. However, we need to realize that other meal-related factors may predispose to heartburn, including ingestion of chocolate, peppermint, onions, coffee, orange juice, and tomato products. We therefore need to focus on eliminating certain foods from the diets of patients with gastroesophageal reflux disease.

J.S. Barkin, M.D.

Cholecystectomy-induced Gastroesophageal Reflux: Is It Reduced by the Laparoscopic Approach?

Rothwell JF, Lawlor P, Byrne PJ, et al (St James's Hosp, Dublin)
Am J Gastroenterol 92:1351-1354, 1997 1–12

Background.—Cholecystectomy is the most common elective abdominal procedure done in the Western Hemisphere. Twenty percent to 50% of patients continue to report symptoms after this procedure, including flatulent dyspepsia, pain in the upper abdomen, nausea, and vomiting. Such symptoms may be attributed to persistent biliary abnormalities or coexistent gastrointestinal conditions erroneously thought to result from asymptomatic gallstones preoperatively. These symptoms may result from the effects of gallbladder removal. The effect of laparoscopic cholecystectomy on the indices of gastroesophageal reflux was studied.

Methods.—Twenty-eight patients undergoing open cholecystectomy and 22 patients undergoing laparoscopic cholecystectomy were included in the prospective study. Twenty-four–hour pH studies and manometry were done before and 3 months after surgery.

Findings.—The mean DeMeester acid score rose from 14.8 to 34 after open cholecystectomy and from 13.9 to 28.9 after laparoscopic cholecystectomy. In both groups, the reduction in mean lower esophageal sphincter pressure was nonsignificant.

Conclusions.—In patients undergoing open or laparoscopic cholecystectomy, the incidence of gastroesophageal reflux significantly increases within 3 months of surgery. Although laparoscopic cholecystectomy is less invasive, the surgery type did not affect the extent of esophageal dysfunction in these patients.

▶ Cholecystectomy is the most common elective abdominal operation performed in the Western Hemisphere. Postoperatively, patients may complain of upper abdominal discomfort, the so-called postcholecystectomy syndrome. Rothwell et al. emphasize that an increased incidence of gastroesophageal reflux occurs after cholecystectomy, regardless of the surgical approach (open or laparoscopic). Therefore, gastroesophageal reflux disease, with its wide spectrum of manifestations, must be considered as a treatable cause of the postcholecystectomy syndrome.

J.S. Barkin, M.D.

Omeprazole as a Diagnostic Tool in Gastroesophageal Reflux Disease

Schenk BE, Kuipers EJ, Klinkenberg-Knol EC, et al (Free Univ Hosp, Amsterdam; 't Lange Land Hosp, Zoetermeer, The Netherlands; Bronovo Hosp Den Haag, The Netherlands)

Am J Gastroenterol 92:1997-2000, 1997 1–13

Introduction.—A reliable and simple method for detecting gastroesophageal reflux disease (GERD) is needed. Symptoms of GERD can be alleviated within 2 to 4 weeks by the profound inhibition of gastric acid secretion with 20 to 40 mg of omeprazole. It is not likely that retrosternal complaints of non-GERD origin will respond to this therapy. The diagnostic value of empirical treatment of GERD with omeprazole was assessed in patients with symptoms suggestive of GERD.

Methods.—Upper gastrointestinal endoscopy and 24-hour esophageal pH monitoring were performed in 85 patients with symptoms suggestive of GERD, especially heartburn, regurgitation, or dysphagia. Patients with reflux esophagitis grade 0 or 1 were randomized in double-blind fashion to either 40 mg of omeprazole or placebo daily. The effect of treatment was assessed after 1 to 2 weeks by a symptom questionnaire scored on a 4-grade Likert scale and by symptomatic response outcome. These reports were compared with findings of 24-hour pH-metry.

Results.—Of 85 eligible patients, 54 had no signs of esophagitis at endoscopy and 31 had esophagitis grade 1. The pH registration revealed pathologic gastroesophageal reflux in 47 patients (55%). Forty-one and 44 patients, respectively, were randomized to treatment with omeprazole or placebo. There was a significant association between pH registration and response to omeprazole, but not to placebo. Using pH-metry as the gold standard, the positive and negative predictive values of pH monitoring were 68% and 63%, respectively. Similar sensitivity was observed when pH-metry was compared with the presence of esophagitis.

Conclusion.—Symptom response to 40 mg of omeprazole for 14 days in patients with symptoms indicative of GERD is a simple and inexpensive method for diagnosing GERD. The sensitivity and specificity of this approach were comparable to that of 24-hour pH monitoring.

► Confirming diagnosis and screening for Barrett's esophagus have been 2 important reasons for having patients with GERD undergo esophagogastroduodenoscopy (EGD). Two articles (Abstracts 1–13 and 1–16) put this practice in a different light. The latter, by Macdonald, Wicks, and Playford, reports on a very large series of endoscopies over a lengthy period with a very low incidence of Barrett's esophagus. Frankly, I was astounded at the number of EGDs performed by the 3 authors: about 900 per year per author! Basically, their methodology was simply to report the results of their own endoscopic findings. Even so, I think their conclusions regarding screening patients with Barrett's are reasonable. For me, the bigger concern raised by their data regards the widespread use of EGD for diagnosis. I draw no conclusions for or against; I am just intrigued by their data.

This article also speaks to this issue. Schenk et al. present data that, in a fairly robust manner, support what probably is already a common practice: an empirical trial of omeprazole for presumed GERD. If such a trial is successful, an EGD is probably not warranted, certainly not to screen for Barrett's. A caveat: Note that the dose of omeprazole used was 40 mg once daily. The authors report other studies using anywhere from 20 to 80 mg. I favor 40 mg, either once daily or in 2 divided doses.

W.W. Dexter, M.D.

Barrett's Esophagus

Barrett's Esophagus and the Presence of *Helicobacter pylori*

Henihan RDJ, Stuart RC, Nolan N, et al (St James's Hosp, Dublin; The Meath Hosp, Dublin)

Am J Gastroenterol 93:542-546, 1998 1–14

Objective.—Some investigations have indicated a possible association between *Helicobacter pylori* and Barrett's esophagus. The prevalence of *H. pylori* in reflux esophagitis, Barrett's esophagus, and adenocarcinoma of the esophagus was determined, and the presence or absence of *H. pylori* was correlated with the severity and type of inflammation, and with metaplasia, dysplasia, and their complications in a retrospective study.

Methods.—Biopsy specimens from 82 patients with Barrett's esophagus, 19 patients with adenocarcinoma of the esophagus, and 40 patients with reflux esophagitis without columnar metaplasia were examined for *H. pylori.*

Results.—*H. pylori* was found in 23.2% of patients with Barrett's esophagus only. All these patients had gastric metaplasia and 43 had intestinal metaplasia (Table 2). *H. pylori* was significantly associated with

TABLE 2.—Distal Esophageal Biopsies From 82 Patients With Barrett's Esophagus

	Number of Patients	*H. pylori*-positive	Percentage	
Inflammation				
Acute: present	49	13	26.5	p = NS
absent	33	6	18.2	
Chronic: present	65	19	29.2	$p < 0.01$
absent	17	0	0	
Type of metaplastic epithelium				
Gastric only	39	11	28.2	p = NS
Gastric and Intestinal	43	8	18.6	
Complications*				
Present	45	11	24.4	p = NS
Absent	37	8	21.6	

*Stricture or ulceration (Reprinted by permission of the publisher from Henihan RDJ, Stuart RC, Nolan N, et al: Barrett's esophagus and the presence of *Helicobacter pylori. Am J Gastroenterol* 93:542-546. Copyright 1998 by Elsevier Science Inc.)

severity of chronic and acute inflammation in patients with Barrett's esophagus.

Conclusion.—Although most patients with Barrett's esophagus do not have *H. pylori*, those with the gastric type of columnar epithelium are at significantly higher risk of infection. When present, *H. pylori* was significantly associated with severity of chronic and acute inflammation in patients with Barrett's esophagus.

▶ The role, if any, of *Helicobacter pylori* infection in esophageal disease remains unclear. Some investigators have postulated a role for *H. pylori* in gastroesophageal reflux disease, Barrett's esophagus, and adenocarcinoma of the esophagus. In this retrospective study, Henihan et al. attempt to define a possible role for *H. pylori* in 82 patients with Barrett's esophagus, 19 patients with adenocarcinoma of the esophagus, and 40 patients with gastroesophageal reflux disease without Barrett's esophagus. *H. pylori* infection was found in 23% of the patients with Barrett's esophagus, but in none of the patients with adenocarcinoma of the esophagus or with gastroesophageal reflux disease. Of the patients with *H. pylori* infection and Barrett's esophagus, all were found to have gastric metaplasia. None of the *H. pylori*–infected patients with Barrett's esophagus had evidence for dysplasia, either. The exact role of *H. pylori* infection in patients with Barrett's esophagus is uncertain. However, 45 patients in the Barrett's esophagus group had complications, including structural alteration. Twenty-four percent of these patients were *H. pylori* positive, compared to 21% of the patients without complications. This study suggests that *H. pylori* infection has little influence in patients with gastroesophageal reflux disease and adenocarcinoma of the esophagus. *H. pylori* infection is associated with Barrett's esophagus and gastric metaplasia and its exact role is uncertain, but it may contribute to complications such as strictures or ulcerations.

G. Aliperti, M.D.

Esophageal Manometry and Ambulatory 24-Hour pH Monitoring in Patients With Short and Long Segment Barrett's Esophagus

Loughney T, Maydonovitch CL, Wong RKH (Walter Reed Army Med Ctr, Washington, DC)

Am J Gastroenterol 93:916-919, 1998 1–15

Objective.—Whether short-segment Barrett's esophagus (SSBE) is an early or mild form of long-segment Barrett's esophagus (LSBE) or a different disorder is unclear. The esophageal manometric characteristics and 24-hour pH profiles of patients with SSBE were prospectively assessed and compared with those of a cohort of patients with LSBE.

Methods.—Upper endoscopy and 2 mucosal biopsies distal to the squamocolumnar junction were performed in 203 consecutive patients. SSBE was diagnosed in 28 patients, 22 of whom underwent esophageal manometry and ambulatory 24-hour pH monitoring. Results were compared with

TABLE 1.—Demographics and Manometric Data

	SSBE (n = 21)	LSBE (n = 18)	Control (n = 15)	p Value
Age	61.6 ± 2.6*	53.7 ± 3.8*	35.9 ± 3.6	0.0001
Gender, M:F	14:7	17:1	9:6	NS
LESp	12.3 ± 1.6*†	5.1 ± 1.0*	16.9 ± 1.5	0.0000
Esophageal Amplitude	77.6 ± 6.2	54.8 ± 13.4*	94.5 ± 8.7	0.0264

*P < 0.05 vs. control subjects.
†P < 0.05 SSBE vs. LSBE.
Abbreviations: SSBE, short-segment Barrett's esophagus patients; *LSBE,* long-segment Barrett's esophagus patients; *LESp,* lower esophageal sphincter pressure.
(Reprinted by permission of the publisher from Loughney T, Maydonovitch CL, Wong RKH: Esophageal manometry and ambulatory 24-hour pH monitoring in patients with short and long segment Barrett's esophagus. *Am J Gastroenterol* 93:916-919. Copyright 1998 by Elsevier Science Inc.)

those of 18 patients with LSBE and of 15 control patients with normal 24-hour pH studies.

Results.—Control patients were significantly younger than SSBE and LSBE patients (35.9 vs. 61.6 vs. 53.7). Lower esophageal sphincter pressure and esophageal amplitude were significantly higher in SSBE patients than in LSBE patients (Table 1). Johnson-DeMeester 24-hour pH monitoring data, measured 5 and 10 cm above the lower esophageal sphincter, and the percent total, upright, and supine reflux, measured 5 and 10 cm above the lower esophageal sphincter, were significantly higher in LSBE patients than in SSBE patients.

Conclusion.—The severity and length of acid exposure are important factors in the development of Barrett's esophagus. Severity of disease may be related to the degree of lower esophageal sphincter competence.

► Loughney et al. compared the results of esophageal manometry and 24-hour dual pH monitoring in 22 patients with SSBE to results in 18 patients with LSBE. There were also, in a control group, 15 patients with normal 24-hour pH study. The results show that lower esophageal sphincter pressures were higher in the SSBE patients than in the LSBE. On 24-hour pH manometry, the LSBE patients had higher Johnson-DeMeester scores, as well as a significantly greater percentage of time with upright reflux and supine reflux, compared to patients with short-segment esophagus. These data indicate that both the degree and length of acid exposure determine the extent of the development of Barrett's esophagus.

G. Aliperti, M.D.

Ten Years' Experience of Screening Patients With Barrett's Oesophagus in a University Teaching Hospital

Macdonald CE, Wicks AC, Playford RJ (Leicester Gen Hosp, England)

Gut 41:303-307, 1997 1–16

Introduction.—There is a strong link between gastroesophageal reflux disease and Barrett's metaplasia, yet the natural history of Barrett's esophagus is not well understood. Symptom severity is not a good indicator of macroscopic damage, thus symptomatology should not be used to select patients at increased risk of Barrett's metaplasia. Findings of annual screenings in 409 patients with Barrett's metaplasia were reported.

Methods.—Medical records of all patients with the suggestion of Barrett's esophagus were reviewed for data regarding age, sex, evidence of any previous endoscopy performed elsewhere, and any additional illnesses. Patients were considered to have Barrett's esophagus if there was an area of biopsy-confirmed columnar metaplasia extending over a region of 3 cm or greater. The benefit of performing annual screening in patients with Barrett's esophagus was explored.

Results.—Of 29,374 upper gastrointestinal endoscopies performed from 1984 to 1994, Barrett's esophagus was detected for the first time in 409 patients (1.4%). The sex distribution of these findings was about equal; most patients were aged 50 years or older. Thirty-five percent of patients were considered appropriate for annual screening. Throughout screening, the length of the esophagus did not vary over time. Of 379 patients in whom yearly endoscopies were performed for screening purposes, carcinoma was detected in only 1 patient as a result of annual screening. Carcinoma was discovered as a result of progressive dysphagia in 2 additional patients. All 3 of these patients had "long-segment" regions of Barrett's metaplasia longer than 8 cm, with a stricture that was observed on initial endoscopy.

Conclusion.—Annual screening of all patients with Barrett's metaplasia detected on initial endoscopic examination has a poor yield. Resources need to be focused on patients who have findings of ulceration or stricture in addition to Barrett's metaplasia.

▶ Confirming diagnosis and screening for Barrett's esophagus have been 2 important reasons for having patients with GERD undergo esophagogastroduodenoscopy (EGD). Two articles put this practice in a different light. This one, by Macdonald, Wicks, and Playford, reports on a very large series of endoscopies over a lengthy period with a very low incidence of Barrett's esophagus. Frankly, I was astounded at the number of EGDs performed by the 3 authors: about 900 per year per author! Basically, their methodology was simply to report the results of their own endoscopic findings. Even so, I think their conclusions regarding screening patients with Barrett's are reasonable. For me, the bigger concern raised by their data regards the widespread use of EGD for diagnosis. I draw no conclusions for or against; I am just intrigued by their data.

An article in the previous section also speaks to this issue. Schenk et al. (Abstract 1–13) present data that, in a fairly robust manner, support what probably is already a common practice: an empirical trial of omeprazole for presumed GERD. If such a trial is successful, an EGD is probably not warranted, certainly not to screen for Barrett's. A caveat: Note that the dose of omeprazole used was 40 mg once daily. The authors report other studies using anywhere from 20 to 80 mg. I favor 40 mg, either once daily or in 2 divided doses.

W.W. Dexter, M.D.

Esophageal Carcinoma

Esophageal Carcinoma: Depth of Tumor Invasion Is Predictive of Regional Lymph Node Status

Rice TW, Zuccaro G Jr, Adelstein DJ, et al (Cleveland Clinic Found, Ohio)
Ann Thorac Surg 65:787-792, 1998 1–17

Objective.—The relationship between depth of tumor invasion and regional lymph node status of esophageal cancer and whether depth of tumor invasion is a predictor of regional lymph node metastasis (N1) were retrospectively determined.

Methods.—Records of all 359 consecutive patients (83.8% male) with esophageal cancer who underwent esophagectomy at The Cleveland Clinic Foundation between January 1, 1983, and August 1, 1997, were reviewed for T and N stage. Esophageal resection, lymphadenectomy, and reconstruction were performed. Resection specimens were examined pathologically.

Results.—There were 295 (82%) patients with adenocarcinoma, 55 (15%) with squamous cell carcinoma, and 9 (3%) with adenosquamous carcinoma. There were 65 patients with T1, 37 with T2, 219 with T3, and 9 with T4 tumors. There were 161 patients with N0 tumors and 198 with N1 tumors. There were 327 patients with M0 tumors and 32 with M1 tumors. There were 29 patients with stage 0, 58 with stage I, 70 with stage IIA, 22 with stage IIB, 148 with stage III, and 32 with stage IV disease. The likelihood of N1 disease increased significantly with increasing T status. The percentage of patients with N1 disease was 0% for Tis, 10.8% for T1, 43.2% for T2, 77.2% for T3, and 66.7% for T4 status. This increased prevalence was true for patients with adenocarcinoma and with squamous cell carcinoma. Longitudinal tumor growth in the lymphatic-rich submucosa may be the best predictor of regional lymph node metastases. Increasing T status, adenocarcinoma, and poor differentiation were predictive of N1 disease according to multivariate analysis.

Conclusion.—Esophageal cancer patients with higher T status, adenocarcinoma, and poorly differentiated tumors are at increased risk of N1 disease.

► This article examines the linkage between tumor size and nodal metastases in patients undergoing surgical resection for esophageal carcinoma.

Patients with both adenocarcinoma and squamous carcinoma are included in this series, and the results do not differ for these 2 tumor types. Importantly, patients with tumor size greater than T1 lesion, that is, disease confined to the esophageal wall, underwent a blunt, transhiatal-type esophagectomy, but all other patients underwent an esophagectomy with thoracotomy and extensive lymphadenectomy. Thus, lymphatic retrieval would be biased away from T1 patients and toward more extensive lymph node retrieval in patients with larger tumors. Interestingly, however, the authors find that as tumors progress from T2 through T4, there is a progressive increase in the patients having positive lymph nodes. While it is not entirely surprising that larger tumors have more commonly spread to lymphatics at the time of surgery, this does point out that in stratifying patients for studies of therapy, it will be important to include tumor size. Particularly since the transhiatal approach may offer a more limited lymphadenectomy than more extended thoracic approaches, the frequency of nodal disease in patients undergoing a transhiatal approach may be inaccurately determined, and this study suggests that if lymphadenectomy will benefit any patients, it is likely to benefit those with a larger and more bulky disease. However, the true merit of extended mediastinal lymphadenectomy in patients with carcinoma of the esophagus remains controversial.

J.A. Drebin, M.D., Ph.D.

Nissen Fundoplication

Oesophageal Dysmotility Is Not Associated With Poor Outcome After Laparoscopic Nissen Fundoplication

Beckingham IJ, Cariem AK, Bornman PC, et al (Queen's Med Centre, Nottingham, England; Univ of Cape Town, South Africa)

Br J Surg 85:1290-1293, 1998 1–18

Objective.—It has been suggested that fundoplication should be avoided or modified in patients with severe motility disorders because they are at high risk of postoperative dysphagia. The outcome of patients with normal and abnormal esophageal body motility after laparoscopic Nissen fundoplication was prospectively compared.

Methods.—Manometry was performed in 81 consecutive patients (46 men), aged 15 to 69 years, with long-standing gastroesophageal reflux disease. Patients had fundoplication and were monitored for 1 year. The main outcome measure was dysphagia.

Results.—Five patients were converted to an open procedure. Reflux-related symptoms improved in all patients regardless of motility status. Manometry revealed that 48 patients had normal motility and 33 had abnormal motility. Fourteen patients with normal motility and 15 with abnormal motility had dysphagia before surgery. Three months after surgery, 13 patients with normal motility and 4 with abnormal motility had new or more severe dysphagia, requiring dilatation in 5 and 2, respectively. At 1 year, 6 patients with normal motility and 5 patients with abnormal motility had dysphagia.

Conclusion.—Manometric assessment prior to fundoplication was not predictive of dysphagia after surgery.

► This article addresses the outcomes in patients undergoing Nissen fundoplication who have a preoperative diagnosis of an esophageal motility disorder. This group of patients presents a dilemma to the surgeon because it has been thought that the procedures done for reflux may themselves result in negative effects on esophageal motility with resulting increases in dysphagia. Indeed, many surgeons perform partial wraps in patients with documented esophageal motility disorders using a procedure such as a Toupet or Dorr rather than a 360° Nissen fundoplication. The studies presented here demonstrated that this may not, in fact, be necessary. Although there was a significant incidence of dysphagia after Nissen fundoplication in patients with esophageal dysmotility, this was not significantly different from the rate seen in patients with normal esophageal function based on preoperative testing. Indeed, the long-term outcomes were equivalent in the normal and in the dysmotility groups, and there was some manometric evidence of improvement of esophageal function in patients undergoing Nissen fundoplication. Collectively, these results suggest that preoperative esophageal manometry may not be required in all patients prior to Nissen fundoplication and that a more selective approach to manometry could result in equivalent outcomes. However, given the relatively excellent short-term results seen with partial fundoplication–type approaches, I suspect many surgeons will still feel uncomfortable performing 360° Nissen-type fundoplications on patients with documented dysmotility. The availability of long-term follow-up studies demonstrating the equivalence or lack of equivalence between Nissen fundoplications and the partial wrap–type fundoplications will potentially lead to alterations in surgical practice.

J.A. Drebin, M.D., Ph.D.

The Treatment of Gastroesophageal Reflux Disease With Laparoscopic Nissen Fundoplication: Prospective Evaluation of 100 Patients With "Typical" Symptoms

Peters JH, DeMeester TR, Crookes P, et al (Univ of Southern California, Los Angeles)

Ann Surg 228:40-50, 1998 1–19

Objective.—Laparoscopic Nissen fundoplication, offering success rates exceeding 90%, is becoming the new standard of surgical treatment for gastroesophageal reflux disease (GERD). As a result of this less invasive technique, a growing number of patients are being referred for surgical treatment. The "typical" symptoms of GERD, such as heartburn, regurgitation, and dysphagia, are easily related to the problem of reflux. The postoperative response of atypical symptoms—such as cough, hoarseness, or wheezing—is less reliable. The results of laparoscopic Nissen fundoplication in 100 patients with typical symptoms of GERD were reported.

Technique.—The authors describe their technique of laparoscopic Nissen fundoplication, with modifications such as incorporation of the posterior vagus nerve in the fundoplication, extension of the dissection posterior to the gastroesophageal junction and the degree of fundic mobilization, and attention to the geometry of the fundoplication. After hiatal and crural dissection, the esophagus is retracted and the crura approximated using 3 or 4 interrupted 0 silk sutures. A large needle is passed down the left upper 10-mm port to ensure a durable closure. In fundic mobilization, an anterior to posterior orientation is preferred. The posterior pancreaticogastric branches are divided posterior to the upper stomach, continuing until the right crus and caudate lobe are visible from the left side. To create the fundoplication, a Babcock clamp passed through the left lower port is used to grasp the midportion of the posterior fundus, which is passed left to right behind the esophagus. The anterior fundus wall is then brought over the anterior esophageal wall, above the supporting Penrose drain. The anterior and posterior fundic lips are folded around the fundus to meet at the 9-o'clock position and envelop the esophagus without twisting the fundus. The fundoplication is fixed with a U-stitch and 2 anchoring sutures of 2-0 silk placed above and below. After the operation has been completed, the stomach should be in its original plane, with the fundoplication suture line facing right anterior and the greater curvature in the left posterior direction.

Results.—This procedure achieved relief of the patients' primary symptoms in 96% of cases. Eighty-three percent of patients considered themselves cured. There were few complications and no deaths. The length of hospital stay decreased from 6.3 days for the first 10 patients to 2.3 days for the last 10 patients.

Conclusions.—Laparoscopic Nissen fundoplication is safe and highly effective in relieving the typical symptoms of GERD. Antireflux surgery may be considered for patients who do not have esophagitis but are dependent on proton pump inhibitors to remain free of symptoms, particularly younger patients and those at risk of severe disease. Routine crural closure avoids migration of the fundoplication into the chest.

▶ This article from the esophageal surgery group at the University of Southern California presents the results of laparoscopic Nissen fundoplication in a series of 100 patients. This series documents not only excellent clinical outcomes in reducing symptoms of GERD but also correlative physiology: both pH probe and lower esophageal manometry returned to normal in the vast majority of patients. Complications and side effects of the surgery were themselves quite limited, and the vast majority of patients had a very satisfactory outcome with modest discomfort. It is important to note that this study was carried out in patients with "typical" symptoms. Patients underwent pH probe and lower esophageal manometry documenting reflux and abnormalities of the lower esophageal sphincter. With appropriate patient selection and meticulous attention to technical details, the authors have set the standard for outcomes in surgery for reflux disease. Failure to thoroughly work up patients may result in performing fundoplication for problems other than reflux disease, with an obvious lack of patient improvement. Similarly, lack of meticulous technique can be associated with fairly disastrous outcomes at the gastroesophageal junction. A sizable fraction of the population has symptomatic reflux. The ability of laparoscopic surgical treatment to eradicate symptoms in such patients suggests that the application of this procedure will continue to grow in the coming years.

J.A. Drebin, M.D., Ph.D.

2 The Stomach and Duodenum

Helicobacter pylori

A Prospective Randomized Trial Comparing the Use of Omeprazole-based Dual and Triple Therapy for Eradication of *Helicobacter pylori*

Chu K-M, Choi H-K, Tuen HH, et al (Univ of Hong Kong, China)

Am J Gastroenterol 93:1436-1442, 1998 2–1

Background.—*Helicobacter pylori* is an important cause of peptic ulcer disease. The development of therapies that effectively eliminate *H. pylori* infection has been challenging. Dual and triple omeprazole-based therapies for the elimination of *H. pylori* infection were compared in a prospective randomized single-center clinical trial.

Study Design.—All adult patients with endoscopically confirmed acid-peptic disease and *H. pylori* infection seen at Queen Mary Hospital, Hong Kong, were eligible to participate in this study. Between June 1995 and March 1997, 1,000 consecutive patients were prospectively randomized to receive either a 2-week course of 20-mg omeprazole and 1-g amoxicillin twice daily (OA) or a 1-week course of 20-mg omeprazole once daily, clarithromycin 500 mg twice daily, and metronidazole 400 mg twice daily (OCM). Patients were followed up each month for 3 months, then every 2 to 3 months, at the outpatient clinic. Endoscopy was performed at 6 to 8 weeks, and antral mucosal biopsy specimens were obtained. Patients were evaluated with both an intent-to-treat (ITT) and per-protocol (PP) analysis.

Results.—Side effects occurred in 29.6% of patients in the OCM group and 10.6% in the OA group. The only significant difference in side effects was taste disturbance. One patient in the OA group and 4 in the OCM group could not tolerate their medication. Seven patients in the OA group and 13 in the OCM group refused follow-up endoscopy. In the remaining 975 patients, positive endoscopic findings were significantly more common in the OA group than in the OCM group. The overall *H. pylori* elimination rates were 73.6% for OA and 92% for OCM by ITT analysis. The overall elimination rates were 74.8% for OA and 95.2% for OCM by PP analysis.

Conclusions.—Cure of *H. pylori* infection leads to long-term remission from peptic ulcer disease. A 1-week course of omeprazole, clarithromycin, and metronidazole is a safe, well-tolerated, and cost-effective treatment for the elimination of *H. pylori* infection in patients with peptic ulcer disease.

Triple Versus Dual Therapy for Eradicating *Helicobacter pylori* and Preventing Ulcer Recurrence: A Randomized, Double-blind, Multicenter Study of Lansoprazole, Clarithromycin, and/or Amoxicillin in Different Dosing Regimens

Schwartz H, Krause R, Sahba B, et al (Baptist Hosp, Miami, Fla; Parkridge Hosp, Chattanooga, Tenn; California Research Found, San Diego, Calif; et al)

Am J Gastroenterol 93:584-590, 1998 2–2

Objective.—Although *Helicobacter pylori* eradication therapy can prevent recurrence of peptic ulcer disease, the optimal therapeutic regimen has not been established. A double-blind, randomized, multicenter study compared the ability of lansoprazole, clarithromycin, and amoxicillin with that of lansoprazole and either clarithromycin or amoxicillin, and with lansoprazole alone, to eradicate *H. pylori* and prevent ulcer recurrence.

Methods.—Patients with active or historical peptic ulcer disease were randomly allocated to receive lansoprazole (30 mg twice daily), clarithromycin (500 mg twice daily), and amoxicillin (1 g twice daily) (n = 64); lansoprazole (30 mg twice daily) and clarithromycin (500 mg twice daily) (n = 66); lansoprazole (30 mg twice daily) and clarithromycin (500 mg 3 times a day) (n = 66); lansoprazole (30 mg twice daily) and amoxicillin (1 g 3 times a day) (n = 66); lansoprazole (30 mg 3 times a day) and amoxicillin (1 g 3 times a day) (n = 65); or lansoprazole (30 mg 3 times a day) (n = 69) for 2 weeks. Endoscopy and biopsy were performed at baseline, week 6, 3 months, and 6 months. Outcome measures were *H. pylori* eradication and ulcer recurrence. Safety was assessed in all patients.

Results.—Triple therapy eradicated *H. pylori* in significantly more patients than did the other regimens (Table 2). The ulcer recurrence rates at 6 months were 7% (2 of 30) for triple therapy, 22% (5 of 23) for lansoprazole (30 mg twice daily) and clarithromycin (500 mg twice daily), 15% for lansoprazole (30 mg twice daily) and clarithromycin (500 mg 3 times a day), 23% for lansoprazole (30 mg twice daily) and amoxicillin (1 g 3 times a day), 13% for lansoprazole (30 mg 3 times a day) and amoxicillin (1 g 3 times a day), and 69% for lansoprazole (30 mg 3 times a day). Patients with eradicated infection at 6 weeks were less likely to have an ulcer recurrence than patients with infection (11% vs. 47%). Adverse events were reported by 23% to 33% of patients receiving any combination of lansoprazole and clarithromycin and by 13% to 26% of patients on the other regimens.

TABLE 2.—*Helicobacter pylori* Eradication at 4 to 6 Weeks Posttreatment, by Treatment Group

	Lansoprazole + Clarithromycin + Amoxicillin	Lansoprazole *b.i.d.* + Clarithromycin *b.i.d.*	Lansoprazole *b.i.d.* + Clarithromycin *t.i.d.*	Lansoprazole *b.i.d.* + Amoxicillin *t.i.d.*	Lansoprazole *t.i.d.* + Amoxicillin *t.i.d.*	Lansoprazole
% (n/N)	94% (44/47)†	57% (28/49)	75% (36/48)	53% (26/49)	77% (39/51)‡	2% (1/53)§
95% CI*	82.5, 98.7	42.2, 71.2	60.4, 86.4	38.3, 67.5	62.5, 87.2	0.0, 10.1

*95% confidence interval.
†*P* 1 ≤ to 0.006, vs. dual therapy groups.
‡*P* equals 0.01, between dual therapy treatment groups with amoxicillin.
§*P* ≤ to 0.001, vs. dual therapy group.
(Reprinted by permission of the publisher from Schwartz H, Krause R, Sahba B, et al: Triple versus dual therapy for eradicating *Helicobacter pylori* and preventing ulcer recurrence: A randomized, double-blind, multicenter study of lansoprazole, clarithromycin, and/or amoxicillin in different dosing regimens. *Am J Gastroenterol* 93:584-590. Copyright 1998 by Elsevier Science Inc.)

Conclusion.—Triple therapy was significantly more effective than double therapy or monotherapy in eradicating *H. pylori* infection.

▶ These 2 studies (Abstracts 2–1 and 2–2) look at the optimal treatment regimen for eradication of *Helicobacter pylori* infection. The first study by Chu et al. looks at omeprazole-based dual and triple therapy, while the other study by Schwartz et al. looks at lansoprazole-based dual and triple therapy. These articles confirm that recommended therapy for *H. pylori* infection is a proton pump inhibitor based triple therapy consisting of omeprazole or lansoprazole combined with clarithromycin and amoxicillin or metronidazole. Generally, the proton pump inhibitor based dual therapy is not recommended as initial treatment for *H. pylori* infection, because of lower eradication rates. Although some studies have supported a 1-week course of treatment, at this time a 10 to 14-week course is standard.

G. Aliperti, M.D.

Has the Impact of *Helicobacter pylori* Therapy on Ulcer Recurrence in the United States Been Overstated? A Meta-analysis of Rigorously Designed Trials

Laine L, Hopkins RJ, Girardi LS (USC School of Medicine, Los Angeles; Division of Anti-Infective Drug Products, Rockville, Md)

Am J Gastroenterol 93:1409-1415, 1998 2–3

Objective.—Although *Helicobacter pylori* is known to cause peptic ulcer disease, reported rates of ulcer healing and eradication vary depending on whether the studies were conducted overseas or in the United States. The effect of *H. pylori* eradication on ulcer recurrence in North American duodenal ulcer patients was assessed by examining treatment studies that met rigorous methodologic criteria.

Methods.—A meta-analysis was performed on double-blind, randomized trials with outcome measures of target populations of non–NSAID-using patients with endoscopically documented duodenal ulcers and biopsy confirmed *H. pylori* infections. Studies had to include scheduled follow-up examinations for 6 months or more and eradication documented 4 weeks or more after completion of treatment. Potential treatment differences were identified and studies with placebo arms were analyzed separately. A subgroup analysis was performed on complete studies vs. abstracts or unpublished results.

Results.—Seven studies met inclusion criteria, and corroborative, corrective, or missing information was obtained. There was 100% agreement among reviewers. Recurrence rates ranged from 8% to 40% for *H. pylori*-negative patients and from 43% to 65% for *H. pylori*-positive patients, but the common odds ratio for ulcer recurrence in patients who were cured was 0.20. This odds ratio, combined with a recurrence rate of 56%, means that 2.8 patients would have to be treated to prevent 1 recurrence at 6 months. If no patients lost to follow-up who had eradication had a recurrence, the pooled recurrence rate would be 16% rather than 20%.

Conclusion.—Meta-analysis shows that eradication of *H. pylori* infection significantly decreases the odds of ulcer recurrence. Nonetheless, 20% of this group will have ulcer recurrence within 6 months.

► There are many studies expressing the effect of *Helicobacter pylori* eradication of peptic ulcer disease. The quality and the results of many of these studies differ. In this article, Loren Laine has attempted to study the effects of *H. pylori* on ulcer recurrence, specifically in North America, by examining studies that meet rigorous design criteria. Seven studies were identified and their data were analyzed. The result confirmed that eradication of *H. pylori* in patients with duodenal ulcer disease decreases the chance of recurrence, with an odds ratio of 0.20. Another finding was that 20% of patients had recurrent ulcers within 6 months, despite eradication of *H. pylori* and even when the patients denied use of nonsteroidal anti-inflammatory agents (NSAIDs). This observation confirms the finding that there is a subset of patients with peptic ulcer disease that is not caused by *H. pylori* infection or NSAIDs. This confirms reports, by many gastroenterologists in certain areas of the country, of a high proportion of patient with non- *H. pylori*, non–NSAID-induced peptic ulcer disease.

G. Aliperti, M.D.

Helicobacter pylori Infection and Gastric Neoplasia: Correlations With Histological Gastritis and Tumor Histology

Komoto K, Haruma K, Kamada T, et al (Hiroshima Univ, Japan; Univ of Sydney, Australia)

Am J Gastroenterol 93:1271-1276, 1998 2–4

Objective.—Although some studies have found an association between *Helicobacter pylori* infection and gastric carcinoma, some studies have ruled out the relationship. The relationships between *H. pylori* infection and gastric carcinoma and histologic gastritis and between gastric neoplastic diseases and demographic and familial risk factors were investigated.

Methods.—Patients who received a diagnosis of gastric carcinoma (n = 105, 78% men) or adenoma (n = 36, 78% men) between 1991 and 1996 and 105 age- and sex-matched controls with dyspepsia or mass survey for gastric carcinoma were evaluated for *H. pylori* infection by Giemsa staining and IgG serology. Mucosal inflammation, atrophy, and IM were graded on a 0 to 3 scale on which 0=none and 3=severe. Gastric carcinoma was categorized as intestinal or diffuse. *H. pylori* infection was classified as cardia (the area in the stomach within 20 mm of the esophagogastric junction) or noncardia.

Results.—The prevalence of *H. pylori* infection was higher in gastric carcinoma and adenoma patients than in controls (Table 1). The odds ratio for *H. pylori* positivity increased with age in control patients but decreased with age in cancer patients, with patients aged less than 60 years having an

TABLE 1.—Comparison of the Measured Parameters Among Patients With Gastric Carcinoma, Adenoma, and Control Subjects

Diseases	Carcinoma	Adenoma	Control
No.	105	36	105
M/F	82/23	28/8	82/23
Mean age	64.9 ± 1.2	65.5 ± 1.8	62.4 ± 1.1
Hp-Antibody positive rate (%)	93.3*	94.4*	71.4
Odds ratio	5.60	6.80	1.00
95% CI	2.33-13.45	1.54-30.10	
Hp-Giemsa stain positive rate (%)	96.2*†	77.8	73.3

*$P <$ than 0.05 as compared with control subjects.
†$P < 0.05$ as compared with adenoma.
(Reprinted by permission of the publisher from Komoto K, Haruma K, Kamada T, et al: *Helicobacter pylori* infection and gastric neoplasia: Correlations with histological gastritis and tumor histology. *Am J Gastroenterol* 93:1271-1276. Copyright 1998 by Elsevier Science Inc.)

odds ratio of 19.38, patients aged 60 to 69 years having an odds ratio of 4.49, and patients aged more than 69 years having an odds ratio of 2.14. *H. pylori* positivity was significantly more common in patients with noncardia than in patients with cardia (odds ratio, 5.67 vs. 5.20). Histologic tumor type, stage and macroscopic type did not affect the prevalence of *H. pylori* infection, nor did coffee use, blood group A status, or family history of gastric cancer. Intestinal-type gastric cancer patients with gastric carcinoma and adenoma had significantly higher atrophy and IM scores in both pyloric and fundic mucosa than did patients with diffuse-type gastric carcinoma or *H. pylori*-positive controls. Smoking was related to intestinal-type gastric carcinoma (odds ratio, 6.56) and adenoma (odds ratio, 7.50) in men. The prevalence of *H. pylori* infection was similar for patients with early and advanced tumor stages (odds ratio, 6.60 vs. 4.27).

Conclusion.—There is a significant association between *H. pylori* infection and gastric carcinoma. *H. pylori* is a significant risk factor for gastric adenoma. Smoking was significantly correlated with intestinal-type gastric carcinoma and adenoma in men.

▶ *Helicobacter pylori* is recognized as one of the major causes of peptic ulcer disease, chronic gastritis, mucosa-associated lymphoid tissue lymphoma, and gastric adenocarcinoma. This histologic study by Komoto et al. looked at the relationship between *H. pylori* infection and gastric neoplastic disease. The authors compared 105 patients with gastric carcinoma to 105 age- and sex-matched control subjects. The results showed that there was a significantly increased prevalence of *H. pylori* infection among patients with gastric carcinoma and adenoma, compared to age- and sex-matched controls. The authors also looked at other risk factors and found an association with smoking, but not with alcohol.

G. Aliperti, M.D.

Symptomatic Benefit From Eradicating *Helicobacter Pylori* Infection in Patients With Nonulcer Dyspepsia

McColl K, Murray L, El-Omar E, et al (Western Infirmary, Glasgow, Scotland; Victoria Infirmary, Glasgow, Scotland; Univ of Glasgow, Scotland)

N Engl J Med 339:1869-1874, 1998 2–5

Introduction.—The management of dyspepsia is unsatisfactory. Few trials have demonstrated that active treatment is superior to placebo in this disorder that affects up to 40% of the Western world. Elimination of *Helicobacter pylori* infection is helpful in patients with gastric or duodenal ulcers; it is not known if this is helpful in patients with dyspepsia who have no evidence of ulcer disease. The effect of eradicating *H. pylori* was assessed in patients with nonulcer dyspepsia in a large, randomized, placebo-controlled trial.

Methods.—The efficacy of 2 weeks of treatment of 20 mg of omeprazole orally twice daily, 500 mg of amoxicillin 3 times daily (substitution of 500 mg tetracycline 3 times daily in patients allergic to penicillin), and 400 mg of metronidazole 3 times daily was assessed in 160 patients and compared with treatment with omeprazole alone in 158 patients. All patients had symptoms of dyspepsia and no evidence of ulcer disease on upper gastrointestinal endoscopy. Symptoms were assessed at baseline and 1-year follow-up using the Glasgow Dyspepsia Severity Score. Resolution of symp-

TABLE 2.—Outcomes of the Patients at 1 Year

Characteristic	Omeprazole and Antibiotics (N = 154)	Omeprazole Alone (N = 154)	P Value
Resolution of symptoms (%)	21	7	<0.001
Glasgow Dyspepsia Severity Score†			
Mean ±SD	5.4 ± 4.0	6.2 ± 3.6	0.07
Range	0-14	0-16	
Quality-of-life score‡			
Mean ±SD	566 ± 179	556 ± 175	0.61
Range	50-786	113-776	
H. pylori-negative (%)	85	12	<0.001
Medication prescribed in past 6 mo (%)	43	53	0.09
Histamine H_2-receptor antagonists	25	28	
Proton-pump inhibitors	16	22	
Both	1	3	
Medication prescribed for >3 of the past 6 mo (%)	20	30	0.05
Eradication therapy prescribed during follow-up (no.)	3	9	0.08

*Ten patients were lost to follow-up: 6 patients in the group assigned to omeprazole and antibiotics and 4 patients in the group assigned to omeprazole alone.

†Total scores can range from 0 (no symptoms or limitations) to 20 (severe symptoms most days, requiring regular medication).

‡Quality of life was measured with the SF-36; scores can range from 0 (worst) to 800 (best).

toms was considered a score of 0 or 1 (maximum score, 20) in the preceding 6 months.

Results.—At 1 month after completion of treatment with omeprazole and antibiotics, 132 of 150 patients (88%) had a negative test for *H. pylori*, vs. 7 of 152 (5%) of patients assigned to receive omeprazole alone. At 1-year follow-up, 21% of patients in the omeprazole and antibiotic group and 7% of patients in the omeprazole alone group had resolution of dyspepsia (Table 2). In the combination treatment group, symptoms resolved in 27% of those who had symptoms for 5 years or less and in 12% of patients who had symptoms for over 5 years.

Conclusion.—Treatment with omeprazole and antibiotics for eradication of *H. pylori* infection in patients with nonulcer or functional dyspepsia is more likely to resolve symptoms than is treatment with omeprazole alone.

▶ Chronic abdominal pain or discomfort, referred to as dyspepsia, is a common medical problem. When the diagnostic work-up fails to define a cause such as peptic ulcer disease or gastroesophageal reflux disease, this entity is referred to as nonulcer dyspepsia. The etiology of nonulcer dyspepsia remains unknown and treatment is often unsatisfactory and costly. Recently, the American Gastroenterological Association has advocated new management guidelines, including noninvasive testing and treatment of *Helicobacter pylori* infection, rather than endoscopy, in young dyspeptic patients without alarm features. Two commonly recommended treatments for patients with nonulcer dyspepsia have been empiric acid suppression, often with a proton pump inhibitor and a trial of therapy for *H. pylori* infection. McColl performed a randomized placebo controlled trial evaluating the efficacy of these 2 management strategies. In this study, 160 patients with nonulcer dyspepsia received omeprazole 20 mg twice a day in combination with 500 mg of amoxicillin 3 times a day and metronidazole 400 mg twice a day and 158 patients received omeprazole 20 mg twice a day, alone. These patients were examined over 1 year. Their results indicate that at 1 year, dyspepsia had resolved in 21% of the patients given the combination of omeprazole and antibiotics, as compared to 7% of the patients given to omeprazole alone. The authors' conclusion was that in patients with *H. pylori* infection and nonulcer dyspepsia, treatment with omeprazole and antibiotics to eradicate infection is more likely to resolve symptoms than treatment with omeprazole alone. This study provides evidence in support of the strategy of noninvasive testing of young patients with dyspeptic symptoms without alarm features and of treating *H. pylori* infection.

J. Willis, M.D.

Cost Savings in Duodenal Ulcer Therapy Through *Helicobacter pylori* Eradication Compared With Conventional Therapies: Results of a Randomized, Double-blind, Multicenter Trial

Sonnenberg A, for the Gastrointestinal Utilization Trial Study Group (Univ of New Mexico, Albuquerque; et al)

Arch Intern Med 158:852-860, 1998 2–6

Background.—Treatment of duodenal ulcer disease with antibiotic therapy directed toward *Helicobacter pylori* infection may be more cost-effective than antisecretory therapy. This possibility was investigated in a randomized, double-blind, multicenter clinical trial.

Methods.—Seven hundred twenty-seven patients received 500 mg of clarithromycin 3 times a day plus 40 mg of omeprazole daily for 14 days, followed by 20 mg of omeprazole daily for another 14 days (group 1); 20 mg of omeprazole daily for 28 days (group 2); or 150 mg of ranitidine twice daily for 28 days (group 3). Clinical success was determined 4 to 6 weeks and 1 year after the end of treatment. In addition, the use of health care resources for ulcer-related problems was documented every month for 1 year after treatment.

Findings.—Patients in group 1 used fewer health care resources for ulcer-related problems in the year after treatment than did patients in group 2 or 3. In group 1, fewer endoscopies were performed, fewer patients received drugs to treat an ulcer, and fewer clinic visits were made. In addition, none of the group 1 patients was admitted to the hospital, compared with 5 and 6 in groups 2 and 3, respectively. When ulcer-related costs were defined as the outcome variable in a multivariate linear regression analysis, therapy significantly influenced costs. Clinical success rates and cure of *H. pylori* infection were significantly better in group 1 than in the other 2 groups.

Conclusions.—Combined clarithromycin and omeprazole therapy is associated with significantly fewer uses of health care resources for ulcer-related problems and a significant cost savings during the year after treatment. Patients who received this combination treatment also had significantly better clinical outcomes than patients who received only omeprazole or ranitidine.

► The discovery of *H. pylori* as the agent responsible for duodenal ulcers has radically modified the approach to therapy for this disease. Intuitively, it makes sense that eradication of the organism would result in improved outcomes as determined by reduced frequency of recurrences and lower morbidity attributable to complications.

This second study assesses the economic impact of the eradication of *H. pylori* with combination therapy compared with traditional therapy with H_2 antagonists. The sample size is adequate and includes three groups. In the first, antibiotic therapy was combined with a proton pump inhibitor, the second group was treated with proton pump inhibitor alone, and the third group was treated with H_2 antagonists. The patients were interviewed regularly for one year. The author concluded that eradication of *H. pylori* resulted in significant cost savings in the first group, compared with the other two control groups. This is not surprising, because the rate of ulcer recurrence after eradication therapy should be much lower than recurrence after conventional therapy. Probably additional economic advantages would be expected to occur if the analysis were extended to a longer period. Indirect costs associated with loss of work and quality of life might also be significantly impacted, although indirect costs were not considered in the present study.

G. Aliperti, M.D.

Molecular Analysis of the Progression From *Helicobacter pylori*-Associated Chronic Gastritis to Mucosa-Associated Lymphoid-Tissue Lymphoma of the Stomach

Zucca E, Bertoni F, Roggero E, et al (Ospedale San Giovanni, Bellinzona, Switzerland; Ospedale San Gerardo, Monza, Italy; Istituto Cantonale di Patologia, Locarno, Switzerland)
N Engl J Med 338:804-810, 1998 2–7

Background.—Evidence suggests an association between chronic gastritis from *Helicobacter pylori* and mucosa-associated lymphoid-tissue lymphoma of the stomach. Presented are the cases of two patients in whom lymphomas developed years after the diagnosis of chronic gastritis.

> *Case Studies.*—The patients were a man and a woman who underwent gastric biopsies in 1981 and 1984, respectively, at the ages of 36 and 48 years. These samples were obtained years before the onset of the lymphomas in both patients. The samples were analyzed using a patient-specific polymerase chain reaction (PCR) approach. Analysis revealed that the lymphomas arose from a B-cell clone at the site of the chronic gastritis in both patients.

Conclusions.—Each B cell contains immunoglobulin heavy chain genes in a novel configuration, which provides a marker for small populations of monoclonal B cells that can be identified by PCR in pathologic specimens. Analysis of B-cell clonality by PCR may facilitate treatment of *H. pylori*, especially in patients with lymphoid infiltrates suggestive of cancer at histologic evaluation. Because the presence of such a B-cell population may represent an early, reversible step in the process of lymphomagenesis, antibiotic treatment of gastritis should be considered in patients with a monoclonal B-cell population to decrease the risk of a lymphoma.

Helicobacter pylori Infection Induces Gastric Cancer in Mongolian Gerbils

Watanabe T, Tada M, Nagai H, et al (Takeda Chemical Industries Ltd, Osaka, Japan)
Gastroenterology 115:642-648, 1998 2–8

Background.—Although epidemiologic studies suggest that *Helicobacter pylori* infection plays an important role in gastric carcinogenesis, no direct proof of the association between *H. pylori* infection and gastric carcinogenesis has been presented. The relationship between *H. pylori* infection and gastric carcinogenesis was further investigated in an animal model of long-term *H. pylori* infection.

Methods.—Mongolian gerbils were inoculated orally with *H. pylori*. Sequential morphological changes in the stomach were studied for up to 62 weeks.

Findings.—At week 26, infected gerbils showed signs of severe active chronic gastritis, ulcers, and intestinal metaplasia. By week 62, adenocarcinomas had developed in the pyloric region of 37% of the infected animals. All tumors were composed of well-differentiated intestinal-type epithelium. The development of these tumors appeared to be closely associated with intestinal metaplasia.

Conclusions.—In this animal model, long-term *H. pylori* infection induced adenocarcinomas. These data suggest that *H. pylori* infection is involved in gastric carcinomas in humans.

▶ *H. pylori* may be the most common infection worldwide. It has a causal role in peptic ulcer disease, and there is an epidemiologic association with mucosa-associated lymphoid tissue (MALT) lymphoma and gastric cancer. The 2 patients that Zucca et al. (Abstract 2–7) reported lend further credence to the suggested progression from *H. pylori*-associated chronic gastritis to overt MALT lymphoma, from a B-cell clone at the site of chronic gastritis.

While *H. pylori* has been classified by the World Health Organization as a group I carcinogen in humans, we have lacked a direct demonstration that *H. pylori* is actually associated with gastric carcinogenesis. This has now been successfully demonstrated in the gerbil model by Watanabe et al. (Abstract 2–8). These 2 studies emphasize the importance of *H. pylori* as a cause of MALT lymphoma and gastric cancer, underscoring that, when found, *H. pylori* infection should be treated.

J.S. Barkin, M.D.

Pharmacologic Considerations

Omeprazole and Ranitidine in Long-term Treatment of Duodenal Ulcer: A Double-blind Comparison of Length of Time in Remission

Díaz de Rojas F, Berenguer J, Rodrigo L, et al (Schering-Plough, Madrid; Hosp La Fe, Madrid; Hosp Central de Asturias, Madrid; et al)

Dig Dis Sci 43:1964-1969, 1998 2–9

Objective.—Duodenal ulcers (DUs) can be healed with H_2-receptor antagonists or omeprazole, but lack of prophylactic treatment or eradication therapy results in a relapse rate of 70% to 100% during the first year. To discover whether 20 mg omeprazole daily would keep patients in remission for a longer time than standard ranitidine therapy does, a double-blind multicenter study compared the length of time in remission.

Methods.—A total of 472 patients were given 20 mg daily omeprazole for 4 or 8 weeks until healing was confirmed endoscopically. The patients were randomly allocated to receive either omeprazole 20 mg in the morning and a ranitidine placebo in the evening or ranitidine 150 mg in the

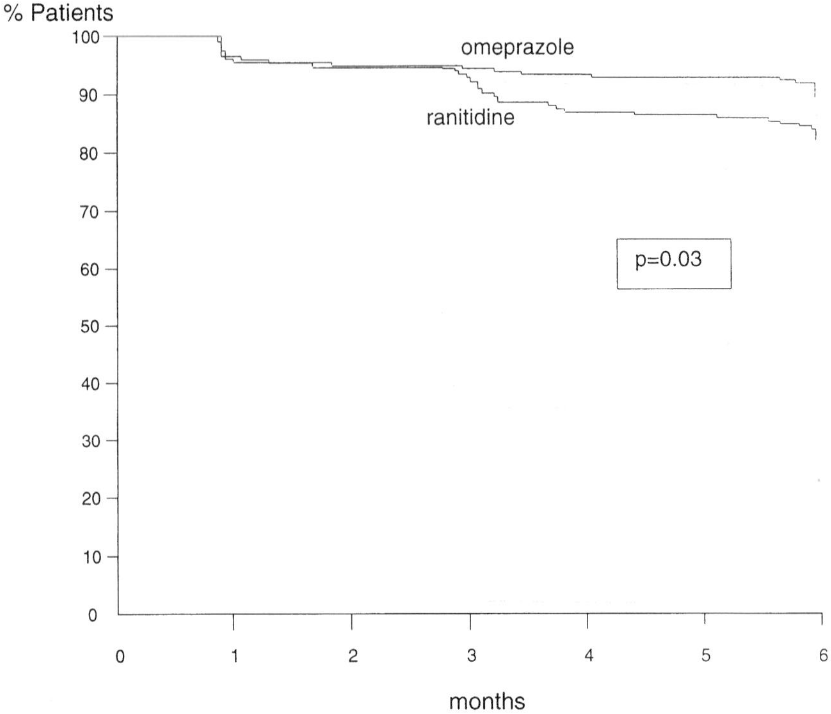

FIGURE 2.—Kaplan-Meier survival curves for the proportion of patients in remission. Intention to treat approach. (Courtesy of Díaz de Rojas F, Berenguer J, Rodrigo L, et al: Omeprazole and ranitidine in long-term treatment of duodenal ulcer: A double-blind comparison of length of time in remission. *Dig Dis Sci* 43:1964-1969, 1998. Plenum Publishing Corporation.)

morning and an omeprazole placebo in the morning for 24 weeks. Endoscopy was performed monthly until healing occurred and then at 1, 3, and 6 months during maintenance therapy. The outcome measure was healing status.

Results.—The healing status was 87% at 4 weeks and 93% at 8 weeks. Original ulcer size and smoking status were significantly related to healing at 4 weeks. Twenty omeprazole patients and 36 ranitidine patients relapsed. The remission rates at 6 months were significantly higher for omeprazole patients (90%) than for ranitidine patients (82%) (Fig 2). Patients with a shorter history of DU disease and those with fewer ulcer episodes had a lower risk of relapse than their counterparts. The incidence of adverse events was similar in the 2 groups.

Conclusion.—Significantly fewer DU patients maintained on omeprazole than patients maintained on ranitidine relapsed.

► The aim of this multicenter study of 472 patients with duodenal ulcer disease was to assess which maintenance therapy, omeprazole 20 mg per day or ranitidine 150 mg, better sustained remission after healing of their ulcers. The end point of the study was recurrence of duodenal ulcer verified by endoscopy, with or without symptoms, at the end of the study period of 6 months. The results showed that an estimated remission rate at 6 months was 90% for omeprazole and 82% for ranitidine. The authors' conclusion was that there was a slight advantage to omeprazole at 20 mg per day for maintenance treatment of patients with duodenal ulcers. This study lends support to previous evidence that duodenal ulcer recurrence ranges from 20% to 30% on H2 receptor antagonists maintenance therapy vs. 10% on omeprazole. However, this study has a major drawback, in that the authors did not assess *H. pylori* status in these patients; the results need to be taken in that context.

G. Aliperti, M.D.

One-Week Antibiotics Versus Maintenance Acid Suppression Therapy for *Helicobacter pylori*-Associated Peptic Ulcer Bleeding

Sung JJY, Leung WK, Suen R, et al (Chinese Univ of Hong Kong)

Dig Dis Sci 42:2524-2528, 1997 2–10

Objective.—Eradication of *Helicobacter pylori* is known to reduce recurrence of peptic ulcer, but clinicians are reluctant to treat only the infection when bleeding occurs. Both nonrandomized and prospective randomized studies have shown that patients with recurrent peptic ulcer bleeding, treated with antibiotics rather than acid suppression, do not have recurrent bleeding. The efficacy of antibiotic therapy was compared with that of maintenance acid suppression therapy in preventing recurrent ulcer bleeding in patients infected with *H. pylori*.

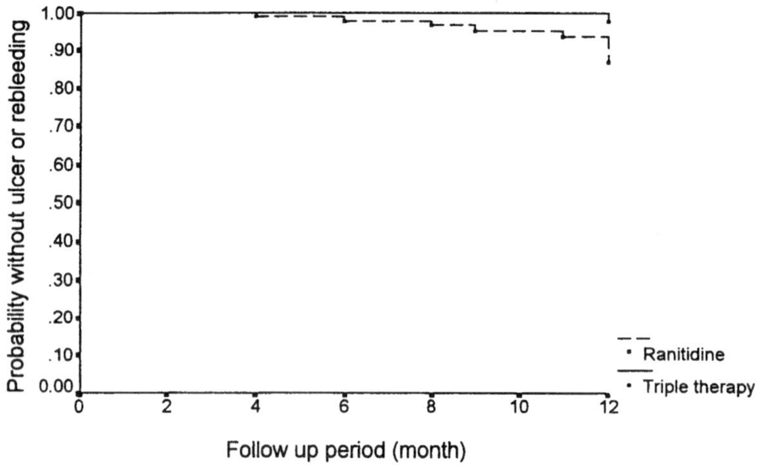

FIGURE 1.—Patients without ulcer recurrence in the ranitidine group and triple therapy group during the 1-year follow-up period ($P = 0.01$). (Courtesy of Sung JJY, Leung WK, Suen R, et al: One-week antibiotics versus maintenance acid suppression: Therapy for *Helicobacter pylori*-associated peptic ulcer bleeding. *Dig Dis Sci* 42:2524-2528, 1997. Plenum Publishing Corporation.)

Methods.—Patients with bleeding gastric ulcer or duodenal ulcer were randomly allocated to receive a 1-week course of triple therapy with bismuth subcitrate (120 mg), metronidazole (400 mg), and tetracycline (500 mg) 4 times daily (n = 126, 22 women) or a 6-week course of ranitidine 300 mg daily (n = 121, 23 women). Endoscopy was performed at baseline and at 6 weeks. Eradication and healing were monitored. Patients treated with anti-*Helicobacter* therapy, nonsteroidal anti-inflammatory drugs, or ulcer surgery and pregnant women were excluded.

Results.—There were 110 antibiotics patients and 115 ranitidine patients in the intent-to-treat group. Patients were studied for a median of 12 months. Ulcers healed in 97 (88.2%) of antibiotics patients and in 99 (86.1%) of ranitidine patients. Recurrent ulcers developed in significantly fewer antibiotics patients than ranitidine patients after 12 months (1 vs. 9) (Fig 1).

Conclusion.—Eradication of *H. pylori* infection is more effective than maintenance treatment with H_2-receptor antagonist therapy for prevention of peptic ulcer bleeding.

▶ Bleeding is a significant complication of peptic ulcer disease. Eradication of *Helicobacter pylori* infection has been demonstrated to heal peptic ulcers and reduce the rate of recurrence. The issue of maintenance therapy after healing of complicated peptic ulcer disease remains unclear. Patients with bleeding duodenal or gastric ulcers and *H. pylori* infection were randomized to receive a 1-week course of bismuth subcitrate, metronidazole, and tetracycline plus ranitidine or a 6-week course of ranitidine alone. After ulcers had healed, 166 patients who received anti-*H. pylori* therapy were given no maintenance therapy, while the group who received ranitidine alone was placed on a maintenance dose of ranitidine, 150 mg per day. *H. pylori* was eradicated in 98.2% of the patients who received the antibiotic therapy vs. 6.1% of the patients who received ranitidine alone. At 6 weeks, ulcer healing was documented to be similar in the 2 groups. Recurrent ulcer developed in 9 of the ranitidine treated patients and one third had recurrent upper gastrointestinal bleeding. One patient in the antibiotic group developed recurrent ulcer without bleeding. This study suggests that, even in peptic ulcer disease complicated with bleeding, anti-*H. pylori* therapy alone vs. maintenance therapy may be sufficient in asymptomatic patients.

G. Aliperti, M.D.

The Clinical and Economic Value of a Short Course of Omeprazole in Patients With Noncardiac Chest Pain

Fass R, Fennerty MB, Ofman JJ, et al (Tucson VA Med Ctr, Ariz; Oregon Health Sciences Univ, Portland; Univ of California Los Angeles; et al)

Gastroenterology 115:42-49, 1998 2–11

Objective.—As many as 60% of patients with noncardiac chest pain (NCCP) may have gastroesophageal reflux disease (GERD). Why acid reflux causes heartburn in some patients and chest pain in others is unknown. The use of high-dose omeprazole as a diagnostic test for GERD in patients with NCCP was evaluated in a double-blind, placebo-controlled, short-term trial, and the cost-savings of this test vs. conventional diagnostic methods were calculated.

Methods.—Baseline symptoms of 39 patients (1 woman), aged 35 to 83 years, with unexplained chest pain were recorded. Patients underwent upper endoscopy and ambulatory 24-hour esophageal pH monitoring and were randomly allocated to receive either placebo or omeprazole (40 mg in the morning and 20 mg in the evening) for 1 week, a washout period for 1 week, a baseline study for 1 week, and a crossover to the other arm for 1 week. Response to the omeprazole test (OT) was the main outcome measure.

Results.—Of the 37 patients who completed the study, 23 (62.2%) received a diagnosis of GERD, and 14 were declared GERD-negative. Chest pain improved significantly with omeprazole treatment in the GERD-positive group, with 18 of 23 (78.3%) having a positive OT. During the treatment period, 12 (52.2%) patients had complete resolution of chest pain and 6 (26.1%) patients had at least 50% improvement. In the placebo group, 11 (50%) patients had no improvement and 5 (22.7%) had at least 50% improvement in chest pain. In the GERD-negative group, chest pain was unchanged in all but 2 (14%) patients after omeprazole treatment. The sensitivity, specificity, and positive and negative predictive values of OT were 78.3%, 85.6%, 90%, and 70.6%, respectively. An economic analysis showed that OT saves $573/patient with NCCP referred for gastrointestinal evaluation, an 81% reduction in endoscopies, a 79% reduction in the utilization of ambulatory 24-hour esophageal pH monitoring, a 28% reduction in total cost per average patient, and a 59% reduction in the total number of diagnostic procedures performed.

Conclusion.—The OT is a safe, reliable, accurate, and simple procedure for diagnosing GERD in patients with NCCP and may reduce costs of unnecessary diagnostic tests for chest pain.

► The most common esophageal cause of noncardiac chest pain is GERD. When patients present with noncardiac chest pain, they often undergo multiple investigations, including upper endoscopy, 24-hour pH monitoring, and/or esophageal manometry. These tests can be invasive and costly. In practice, many physicians have forgone testing and have recommended a short course of high-dose proton pump inhibitor therapy as a diagnostic test for detecting GERD in patients with noncardiac chest pain. The aim of the study was to further evaluate this management strategy. In this double-blind, placebo-controlled study, 39 patients with noncardiac chest pain were randomized to either placebo or omeprazole 40 mg in the morning and 20 mg in the evening for 7 days. Patients were crossed over to the other arm after a washout period. All patients underwent 24-hour pH monitoring and upper endoscopy before randomization. The results showed that, based on investigation, 23 patients were classified as GERD-positive and 14 as GERD-negative. Eighteen, or 78%, of the GERD-positive patients and 2, or 14%, of the GERD-negative patients had a positive response to the omeprazole test. Thus, the authors conclude the sensitivity of the test is 78%, with a specificity of 86%. The study also looks at economic savings and shows that the omeprazole test saves $573.00 per patient evaluated, with a 59% reduction in the number of diagnostic procedures. Overall, this is an excellent study that confirms what many gastroenterologists have often recommended in clinical practice.

G. Aliperti, M.D.

Somatostatin or Octreotide Compared With H2 Antagonists and Placebo in the Management of Acute Nonvariceal Upper Gastrointestinal Hemorrhage: A Meta-analysis

Imperiale TF, Birgisson S (Indiana Univ, Indianapolis; Case Western Reserve Univ, Cleveland, Ohio)

Ann Intern Med 127:1062-1071, 1997 2–12

Background.—Somatostatin, an endogenous peptide, decreases splanchnic blood flow and gastrointestinal (GI) motility, inhibits acid secretion, and may have gastric cytoprotective effects. Octreotide is a long-acting synthetic somatostatin analogue with a similar activity profile. The efficacy of these 2 agents in the treatment of acute nonvariceal upper GI hemorrhages was determined in a meta-analysis of randomized clinical studies.

Methods and Findings.—Fourteen trials published between 1966 and 1996 were included in the analysis. A total of 1,829 patients participated in the studies. All trials compared somatostatin or octreotide with H_2 blockers or placebo in patients with clinical or endoscopic diagnoses of acute nonvariceal upper GI bleeding. The relative risk (RR) for continued bleeding or recurring bleeding was 0.53 in favor of somatostatin, and the number needed to treat (NNT) was 5. In 7 researcher-blinded trials, the RR was 0.73 and the NNT was 11. Somatostatin was effective for peptic ulcer bleeding, and the RR in this instance was 0.48. Also, there was a trend toward efficacy for nonpeptic ulcer bleeding; the RR was 0.62. Overall, findings suggested a reduced need for surgery in the somatostatin group. However, a subgroup analysis of researcher-blinded trials showed a more modest effect that was not significant statistically.

Conclusions.—This meta-analysis of published trials found that somatostatin may decrease the risk for continued bleeding from acute hemorrhages caused by peptic ulcer disease. This agent may be useful as an adjunct before endoscopy or when endoscopy is unsuccessful, contraindicated, or unavailable.

▶ When the emergency room nurse calls us while we are not in the hospital and tells us that our patient has come in with upper GI bleeding, how should we direct the patient's treatment? Initially, our approach is a supportive role with the administration of fluids and blood transfusions. Previously, we did not have a therapeutic agent; however, we now have somatostatin.

Somatostatin or octreotide infusion decreases splanchnic venous blood flow and has been used effectively for patients with bleeding esophageal varices, secondary to portal hypertension. Imperiale and Birgisson have shown in a meta-analysis study that this infusion for at least 48 hours is also effective for treating nonvariceal upper GI hemorrhage originating from peptic ulcer disease.

Thus, in instances when we are called by the emergency room while away from the hospital, our directive should be to resuscitate and monitor the patient, as well as to administer somatostatin.

J.S. Barkin, M.D.

A Comparison of Omeprazole With Ranitidine for Ulcers Associated With Nonsteroidal Antiinflammatory Drugs

Yeomans ND, for the Acid Suppression Trial: Ranitidine Versus Omeprazole for NSAID-associated Ulcer Treatment (ASTRONAUT) Study Group (Univ of Melbourne, Australia; et al)

N Engl J Med 338:719-726, 1998 2–13

Background.—Suppressing acid secretion is believed to decrease the risk of nonsteroidal anti-inflammatory drug (NSAID)–related ulcers. The best way to achieve this, however, is not known.

Methods.—Five hundred forty-one patients needing continuous NSAID treatment because of ulcers or more than 10 erosions in the stomach or duodenum were studied. By random assignment, patients received omeprazole, 20 mg or 40 mg orally per day, or ranitidine, 150 mg orally twice daily, for 4 or 8 weeks depending on the treatment's success. Four hundred thirty-two patients in whom treatment was successful were assigned randomly to maintenance therapy with 20 mg of omeprazole per day or 150 mg of ranitidine twice a day for 6 months.

Findings.—At 8 weeks, treatment was successful in 80% of patients in the 20-mg omeprazole group, in 79% of the patients in the 40-mg omeprazole group, and in 63% of the patients in the ranitidine group. Healing rates for all types of lesions were greater with omeprazole than with ranitidine. During maintenance treatment, the estimated proportions of patients in remission at 6 months in the omeprazole and ranitidine groups were 72% and 59%, respectively. The groups had similar rates of adverse events during both phases. The agents were tolerated well.

Conclusions.—Omeprazole, 20 mg daily, is superior to ranitidine in healing and in preventing gastroduodenal ulcers and erosions in patients taking NSAIDs daily. Omeprazole also proved better at controlling dyspeptic symptoms.

Omeprazole Compared With Misoprostol for Ulcers Associated With Nonsteroidal Antiinflammatory Drugs

Hawkey CJ, for the Omeprazole Versus Misoprostol for NSAID-induced Ulcer Management (OMNIUM) Study Group (Univ Hosp, Nottingham, England; et al)

N Engl J Med 338:727-734, 1998 2–14

Background.—Although misoprostol is effective in the treatment of ulcers associated with regular nonsteroidal anti-inflammatory drug (NSAID) use, it often causes diarrhea and abdominal pain. The efficacy of omeprazole was compared with that of misoprostol in the healing and prevention of NSAID-related ulcers.

Methods.—Nine hundred thirty-five patients were enrolled in the double-blind, randomized trial. All required continuous NSAID treatment and had ulcers or more than 10 erosions in the stomach or duodenum. The patients took 20 mg or 40 mg of omeprazole orally in the morning or 200 µg of misoprostol orally 4 times a day. Treatment was given for 4 or 8 weeks, depending on healing. By random assignment, 732 patients responding to treatment were given maintenance therapy with 20 mg of omeprazole daily, 200 µg of misoprostol twice daily, or placebo for 6 months.

Findings.—At 8 weeks, treatment was successful in 76% of patients receiving 20 mg of omeprazole, in 75% of patients receiving 40 mg of omeprazole, and in 71% of patients receiving misoprostol. Gastric-ulcer healing rates associated with 20 mg of omeprazole were significantly greater than with misoprostol. Healing rates among patients with duodenal ulcers were greater with omeprazole (either dose) than with misoprostol. Healing rates among patients with erosions alone were greater with misoprostol. During maintenance therapy, more patients remained in remission with omeprazole than with misoprostol, and more remained in remission with either active agent than with placebo. Patients receiving misoprostol had more adverse events in the healing phase than did patients given either dose of omeprazole.

Conclusions.—Omeprazole and misoprostol yielded similar overall rates of successful treatment of ulcers, erosions, and symptoms associated with NSAID use. Maintenance therapy with omeprazole was more effective than maintenance therapy with misprostol. However, omeprazole was better tolerated.

▶ Intake of NSAIDs frequently results in gastrointestinal (GI) side effects manifested as dyspepsia and, occasionally, as the occurrence of GI bleeding or perforation. Prevention of these GI problems is a major issue with the extensive use of NSAIDs. These 2 studies (Abstracts 2–13 and 2–14) show that acid suppression is required to prevent NSAID-associated damage.

Omeprazole at a dose of 20 mg per day was found to be superior to 150 mg ranitidine twice a day in the study by Yeomans et al. (Abstract 2–13) In the study by Hawkey et al., omeprazole was found to be equal to misoprostol in preventing mucosal damage. Maintenance therapy with omeprazole was associated with a lower rate of relapse than was maintenance therapy with misoprostol. Hence, until we have selective COX-2 inhibitors, we must continue to prevent the potential side effects of nonselective NSAIDs. The emerging drug of choice seems to be omeprazole at a dose of 20 mg per day.

J.S. Barkin, M.D.

Peptic Ulcer Disease

Clinical and Economic Outcomes of Individuals With Severe Peptic Ulcer Hemorrhage and Nonbleeding Visible Vessel: An Analysis of Two Prospective Clinical Trials

Gralnek IM, Jensen DM, Gornbein J, et al (West Los Angeles VA Med Ctr; Univ of California, Los Angeles; Hennepin County Med Ctr, Minneapolis; et al)

Am J Gastroenterol 93:2047-2056, 1998 2–15

Background.—Peptic ulcer hemorrhage is the most comon cause of acute, severe upper gastrointestinal tract (GI) hemorrhage. The clinical outcomes and the direct medical costs associated with endoscopic hemostasis and with a medical-surgical approach for severe peptic ulcer bleeding and a nonbleeding visible vessel at emergency endoscopy were compared.

Methods.—Data from 2 prospective, randomized, controlled trials were analyzed. One hundred fifty-five patients were assigned to endoscopic hemostasis (group 1) or to medical-surgical treatment (group 2).

Findings.—Compared with group 2, group 1 patients had significantly lower rates of severe ulcer rebleeding, emergency surgery, and blood transfusions. The estimated median direct costs per patient differed in the 2 trials. The first study showed lower costs with endoscopic hemostasis, whereas the second reported lower costs with medical-surgical treatment.

Conclusions.—Endoscopic hemostasis yields significantly better outcomes than medical-surgical therapy in patients with severe ulcer hemorrhage and a nonbleeding visible vessel. The former procedure is also safe. Whether it is less costly than medical-surgical treatment is unclear.

► Endoscopic hemostasis is the universally accepted first line of treatment of bleeding ulcers in modern medicine. Endoscopic and clinical outcomes have demonstrated the efficacy of urgent endoscopy.[1-3] The study adds important information regarding economic outcomes of the accepted algorithm, compared with exclusively medical or surgical treatment. The authors find that endoscopic thermal therapy gives significantly better outcomes in terms of ulcer rebleeding, emergency surgery, and blood transfusion requirements versus exclusively medical or surgical management. The authors assess the results of two consecutive prospective randomized controlled trials with patients assigned to endoscopic hemostasis or medical-surgical treatment. Economic outcomes differed between the two trials, with the first trial resulting in lower cost of endoscopic hemostasis and the second trial yielding lower costs of medical-surgical treatment. However, clinical outcomes were significantly better for endoscopic hemostasis in both trials.

A limitation of this study is that it looks only at direct cost outcomes, which do not estimate indirect costs incurred by the patient and society, such as loss of economic productivity because of loss of life or livelihood. The direct costs in this study were also limited strictly to the hospitalization period and excluded the convalescence period after hospital discharge. In the light of these limitations, one must conclude that the advantage to patient care is inferred by the significantly better clinical outcomes and that management should remain unchanged in the interest of patient care.

G. Aliperti, M.D.

References

1. Kovacs TOG, Jensen DM: Endoscopic control of gastro-duodenal hemorrhage. *Annu Rev Med* 28:267-277, 1987.
2. Longstreth GF, Feitelberg SP: Outpatient care of selected patients with acute non-variceal upper gastrointestinal hemorrhage. *Lancet* 345:108-111, 1995.
3. Longstreth GF, Feitelberg SP: Hospital care of acute nonvariceal upper gastrointestinal bleeding: 1991 versus 1981. *J Clin Gastroenterol* 19:189-193, 1994.

Acute Gastrointestinal Hemorrhage

Influencing the Practice and Outcome in Acute Upper Gastrointestinal Haemorrhage

Rockall TA, for the Steering Committee of the National Audit of Acute Upper Gastrointestinal Haemorrhage (Royal College of Surgeons of England, London)

Gut 41:606-611, 1997 2–16

Introduction.—Many investigations suffer from the inevitable variations in methodology that make comparisons difficult and unreliable, particularly when prospective trials are compared with retrospective ones. Changes in practice and outcome in acute upper gastrointestinal hemorrhage were evaluated in 2 large prospective, multicenter trials using identical methodologies in the same population.

TABLE 1.—Characteristics of Sample Populations in Phase I and II

	Phase I	Phase II
Number of cases	2332	1625
Inpatients/transfers	15.9% (371)	16.4% (266)
Age		
Mean	66	66
Median	71	71
Range	16-103	17-103
% >80 years	27.2% (634)	28.6% (464)
Sex (male)	57.0% (1327)	57.5% (934)
Blood pressure <100 mm Hg on admission	11.2% (256/2293)*	11.8% (191/1613)*
Co-morbidity at presentation		
Any major co-morbidity	59.1% (1378)	59.4% (965)
Malignancy	8.2% (191)	8.9% (145)
Organ failure	15.2% (354)	15.9% (259)
Diagnosis		
None made	23.2% (542)	23.0% (374)
Peptic ulcer	36.1% (842)	36.4% (592)
Upper GI malignancy	4.0% (93)	4.1% (67)
Varices	4.6% (108)	4.9% (80)
Mallory-Weiss tear	5.1% (119)	6.0% (98)
Oesophagitis	10.3% (241)	11.0% (179)
Erosive disease	10.3% (240)	10.9% (177)
Other	6.3% (147)	3.6% (58)
Blood transfusion		
Mean	2.9 units	2.8 units
Median	2.0 units	2.0 units
Rebleeding	15.4% (354/2297)*	16.2 (260/1605)*
Risk score		
0	14.7% (343)	15.7% (255)
1	13.5% (314)	12.6% (205)
2	17.2% (401)	16.2% (263)
3	22.1% (515)	19.5% (317)
4	21.0% (489)	22.6% (368)
5	7.6% (177)	8.7% (141)
6+	4.0% (93)	4.7% (76)

*Denominator is less than total number of cases because of missing values. *Abbreviation: GI*, gastrointestinal.

(Courtesy of Rockal TA, for the Steering Committee of the National Audit of Acute Upper Gastrointestinal Haemorrhage: Influencing the practice and outcome in acute upper gastrointestinal haemorrhage. *Gut* 41:606-611, 1997.)

Methods.—Forty-five hospitals from 3 health regions took part in 2 phases of the audit cycle. Patient management was examined in reference to recommendations in the national (United Kingdom) guidelines for mortality and length of hospital stay. In phase I and phase II, respectively, 2,332 patients over 4 months and 1,625 patients over 3 months who had acute upper gastrointestinal hemorrhage were identified. Phase I was conducted during 1993, and phase II was conducted during 1994 (Table 1).

Results.—After phase I, data from the National Audit were distributed, and specific recommendations for improving practice were made. As a result, the proportion of hospitals with local guidelines or protocols rose from 71% (32 of 45) to 91% (41 of 45). Twelve of the 32 hospitals with existing guidelines at the time of phase I revised their guidelines after the initial survey. There was a small yet significant increase (81% to 86%) in the patients who underwent endoscopy. The proportion of patients who underwent endoscopy within 24 hours of admission rose from 50% to 56%. The use of central venous pressure monitoring in patients with organ failure requiring blood transfusion or those with profound shock increased from 30% to 43%. There were no differences in the use of high-dependency beds or joint medical/surgical management in patients who were at high risk. There were also no significant changes in the crude or risk-standardized mortality rates (13.4% first phase, 14.4% second phase). In the high-risk subgroups, the actual rate of surgical intervention was higher (Table 4), being 21.1% (phase I) and 19.3% (phase II) higher in these high-risk groups than in patients over the age of 60 years who rebled; and 31.1% (phase I) and 22.7% (phase II) higher in those with shock on admission, high transfusion requirements, and rebleeding more than 4 times.

Conclusions.—Many participating hospitals made efforts to improve practice by producing or updating guidelines or protocols, but few hospi-

TABLE 4.—Surgical Practice

	Phase I	Phase II
Operative rate		
For bleeding	134 (5.7%)	82 (5.0%)
For malignancy	18 (0.8%)	12 (0.7%)
For other reason (e.g. peritonitis)	29 (1.2%)	17 (1.0%)
Total	181/2332 (7.8%)	111/1625 (6.8%)
Operator (all patients operated)		
Consultant	91/181 (51.3%)	56/111 (50.5%)
Unsupervised registrar	36/181 (19.9%)	22/111 (19.8%)
Involvement of surgical team in management		
All patients	905/2332 (38.8%)	621/1625 (38.2%)
Over 60 and rebleed	186/270 (68.9%)	125/197 (63.5%)
Shocked, >4 units transfused and rebleed	48/61 (78.3%)	34/44 (77.3%)
Risk >2	543/1274 (42.6%)	377/902 (40.2%)
Consultant informed prior to operation	149/181 (87.6%)	93/111 (85.3%)
Consultant examination prior to operation	102/181 (59.3%)	69/111 (64.5%)

(Courtesy of Rockal TA, for the Steering Committee of the National Audit of Acute Upper Gastrointestinal Haemorrhage: Influencing the practice and outcome in acute upper gastrointestinal haemorrhage. *Gut* 41:606-611, 1997.)

tals had demonstrable changes in any area of practice. Mortality rate may have remained the same because it could not to be improved.

► This large study from the United Kingdom assesses the effects of production and dissemination of guidelines for treating patients with upper gastrointestinal hemorrhage. This study carries out in a prospective, multicenter audit cycle an assessment of outcomes after re-emphasis of national guidelines, in an attempt to assess the effects of the re-emphasis. Unfortunately, this study revealed no changes in the utilization of high-dependency beds of joint medical/surgical management in high-risk cases, and there were no significant changes in crude or risk-standardized mortality. The disappointing findings might be fostered by the multicenter nature of the study, which hinders the uniformity of changes in structure or practice, so that potential benefits at some centers might be obscured by the lack of change at other sites. Secondly, structure and practice varied considerably between the units at the starting point, because of the variation between hospitals with established gastrointestinal bleeding units and district general hospitals with single practitioners. The results might also have been affected by the short time interval between the feedback of data and the second phase of data collection, an interval that might have been sufficient only to increase awareness, but insufficient for costly structural changes leading to significant practice improvements.

G. Aliperti, M.D.

The Effectiveness of Early Endoscopy for Upper Gastrointestinal Hemorrhage: A Community-based Analysis

Cooper GS, Chak A, Connors AF Jr, et al (Case Western Reserve Univ, Cleveland, Ohio)

Med Care 36:462-474, 1998 2–17

Introduction.—Numerous trials have demonstrated the efficacy of upper gastrointestinal (GI) endoscopy in patients with upper GI hemorrhage. Most investigations were performed by expert endoscopists in tertiary care centers. The generalizability of these findings to community practice or to unselected patient populations has not been determined. There also are no available data regarding the relative benefit of early endoscopy in patients with upper GI hemorrhage. A large community-based sample of 3,801 consecutive patients admitted to 30 hospitals in a large metropolitan area was evaluated to determine factors associated with the performance of early endoscopy (within 1 day of hospitalization) and, after adjustment for these factors, to determine correlations between early endoscopy and in-hospital mortality, length of stay, and performance of surgery.

Methods.—Medical records were reviewed for demographic and clinical data (Table 1). Factors that potentially could relate to the decision to

TABLE 1.—Demographic and Clinical Characteristics Associated With the Use of Early Endoscopy in 3,801 Patients With Upper Gastrointestinal Hemorrhage

Characteristic	Number of Patients (%)	Frequency of Early Endoscopy (%)	P
Age (yr)			0.001
<50	750 (19.8)	60.8	
50-60	427 (11.3)	63.9	
61-70	816 (21.5)	62.1	
71-80	1,006 (26.5)	58.2	
≥80	792 (20.9)	52.2	
Race			0.01
Black	753 (19.8)	55.0	
White	2,956 (77.8)	59.7	
Other	88 (2.3)	65.9	
Gender			0.001
Male	2,053 (54.0)	62.0	
Female	1,748 (46.0)	55.4	
Primary health insurance			0.001
Medicare	2,217 (58.6)	55.6	
Commercial*	1.052 (27.8)	67.7	
Medicaid/uninsured	517 (13.7)	55.9	
Admission from nursing home			0.001
No	3,382 (89.0)	60.6	
Yes	419 (11.0)	45.4	
Cancer			0.001
Absent	3,558 (93.6)	60.2	
Present	243 (6.4)	40.7	
End stage renal disease			0.001
Absent	3,721 (97.9)	59.3	
Present	80 (2.1)	40.0	
Chronic obstructive lung disease			0.001
Absent	3,257 (85.7)	60.0	
Present	544 (14.3)	52.4	
Current alcohol use			0.001
Absent	2,109 (55.5)	55.9	
Present	1,692 (44.5)	62.8	
Day of admission			0.001
Sunday	422 (11.1)	61.1	
Monday	642 (16.9)	59.7	
Tuesday	590 (15.5)	63.9	
Wednesday	544 (14.3)	61.8	
Thursday	577 (15.2)	65.3	
Friday	563 (14.8)	57.7	
Saturday	461 (12.1)	39.9	
Abnormal orientation on admission neurological examination			0.001
Absent	3,443 (90.6)	60.1	
Present	358 (9.4)	48.0	
Coma, length, or stupor on admission neurological examination			0.001
Absent	3,681 (96.8)	59.5	
Present	120 (3.2)	42.5	
Abnormal motor examination or pupils on admission			0.001
Absent	3,474 (91.4)	60.2	
Present	327 (8.6)	45.9	

(Continued)

TABLE 1 (cont.)

Characteristic	Number of Patients (%)	Frequency of Early Endoscopy (%)	*P*
Lowest hematocrit in first 2 days (%)			0.001
≤20	508 (13.4)	58.3	
21-25	1,044 (27.4)	63.1	
26-30	1,094 (28.8)	63.4	
31-35	493 (13.0)	55.0	
>35	662 (17.4)	48.3	
Serum albumin (g/dl)			0.03
≤3	1,843 (48.5)	60.8	
>3	1,958 (51.5)	57.2	
Infiltrate on chest x-ray			0.01
Absent	3,588 (94.4)	59.5	
Present	213 (5.6)	50.2	
Number of units of blood in first 2 days			0.001
0	1,818 (47.8)	51.9	
1-2	1,025 (27.0)	64.2	
3-5	800 (21.0)	65.4	
>5	158 (4.2)	72.8	
Admission severity of illness (decile)			0.57
1 (lowest severity)	377 (9.9)	60.7	
2	379 (10.0)	60.7	
3	381 (10.0)	58.8	
4	378 (10.0)	59.3	
5	380 (10.0)	60.3	
6	379 (10.0)	61.2	
7	380 (10.0)	60.8	
8	379 (10.0)	56.7	
9	380 (10.0)	54.7	
10 (highest severity)	381 (10.0)	55.9	

*Includes patients with indemnity or managed care plans.

(Courtesy of Cooper GS, Chak A, Connors AF Jr, et al: The effectiveness of early endoscopy for the upper gastrointestinal hemorrhage: A community-based analysis. *Med Care* 36:462-474, 1998.)

perform endoscopy were used to create a multivariate model. The model was used to determine the propensity (0%-100%) for early endoscopy in each patient (Table 2).

Results.—A total of 2,240 patients (59%) underwent early endoscopy. The procedure was not associated with mortality after adjustment for severity of illness among all patients. It was associated with increased risk of death for patients in the lowest propensity group. Early endoscopy was correlated with diminished likelihood of upper GI surgery in all patients and in the 2 highest propensity groups and with a shorter length of hospital stay for the entire cohort and for all patient subgroups (Table 3).

Conclusion.—When not contraindicated, early endoscopy should be considered in patients with upper GI hemorrhage. It offers reductions in length of hospital stay and in surgical intervention.

► Another larger observational study concludes that early endoscopy reduces length of stay and surgical intervention. This study was carried out in 30 hospitals in a large metropolitan region. Upper endoscopy was the standard of care, utilized in 85% of the patients in this study. Early endoscopy did not affect mortality rates. Early endoscopy was associated with higher in-hospital mortality in the subgroup of patients with higher comorbidities, a

TABLE 2.—Clinical Characteristics of Patients Undergoing and Not Undergoing Early Endoscopy Within Quintiles at Increasing Propensity for Early Endoscopy

	Propensity Quintile									
	1 (Lowest Propensity) Endoscopy		2 Endoscopy		3 Endoscopy		4 Endoscopy		5 (Highest Propensity) Endoscopy	
	Yes	No	Yes	No	Yes	No	Yes	No	Yes	No
Mean age (years)	70.3	70.7	68.1	67.5	64.1	67.0	64.4	62.8	61.0	59.7
Male gender (%)	43	39	41	45	51	53	60	61	76	70
Black gender (%)	29	31	22	21	17	15	14	19	15	13
Commercial Insurance (%)	5	7	14	12	28	24	37	37	57	58
Admission from nursing home (%)	30	31	16	13	6	8	2	5	1	1
Cancer (%)	18	20	5	4	2	4	0.4	0.8	0.7	1
Chronic obstructive lung disease (%)	23	25	19	20	13	13	11	8	5	4
Cirrhosis (%)	4	4	4	3	4	4	6	5	11	12
Chronic renal failure (%)	7	8	1	2	1	1	0.8	0.4	0.2	0.6
Admission to hospital with fellowship (%)	23	22	23	24	19	23	25	28	41	35
Alcohol use (%)	27	27	37	37	45	44	51	52	63	60
Abnormal motor/pupils (%)	27	23	7	11	6	4	2	4	1	2
Coma/lethargy/stupor (%)	10	10	2	4	1	1	0.6	1	1	1
Infiltrate on x-ray (%)	11	10	7	7	4	6	3	3	2	3
Lowest hematocrit (%)	30	30	29	29	27	26	25	24	21	21
Mean predicted risk of death (%)	4	4	3	3	3	3	2	3	3	3
Number units first 2 days	0.8	0.7	1.0	0.8	1.3	1.2	1.7	1.8	3.5	3.4

*$P=0.03$ for differences in age quintile 3; $P=0.07$ for differences in race in quintile four and coma/lethargy/stupor in quintile 2; $P=0.04$ for differences in nursing home admission in quintile 4 and abnormal motor/pupils in quintile 2; $P=0.12$ for differences in alcohol use in quintile 4; $P=0.06$ for differences in hematocrit in quintile 3; $P=0.10$ for differences in hematocrit in quintile 4; $P=0.17$ for differences in number of units transfused in quintile 2; for all other comparisons within strata, $P>0.2$.

(Courtesy of Cooper GS, Chak A, Connors AF Jr, et al: The effectiveness of early endoscopy for the upper gastrointestinal hemorrhage: A community-based analysis. *Med Care* 36:462-474, 1998.)

TABLE 3.—Relationship Between Early Endoscopy and In-Hospital Mortality, Surgery, and Length of Stay Stratified According to the Propensity of Undergoing Early Endoscopy*

Quintile†	Mortality Multivariable Odds Ratio (95% CI)	*P*	Surgery Multivariable Odds Ratio (95% CI)	*P*	Adjusted Length of Stay (95% CI)	*P*
1	2.09 (1.10-4.01)	0.03	0.49 (0.17-1.41)	0.19	-29% (-37%, -21%)	0.0001
2	1.24 (0.55-2.79)	0.60	0.61 (0.21-1.46)	0.27	-28% (-36%, -20%)	0.0001
3	0.76 (0.24-2.42)	0.64	0.66 (0.31-1.43)	0.29	-26% (-34%, -16%)	0.0001
4	1.18 (0.43-3.27)	0.75	0.23 (0.09-0.57)	0.001	-27% (-36%, -15%)	0.0001
5	0.54 (0.22-1.30)	0.17	0.27 (0.17-0.44)	0.0001	-37% (-44%, -30%)	0.0001

Abbreviation: CI, confidence interval.

*Results are shown for multivariable analysis, clustered by hospital and adjusted for admission severity of illness. Multivariable results reflect the odds of death, surgery, or relative length of stay of patients undergoing early endoscopy, compared with patients not undergoing early endoscopy.

†Quintiles are ordered from lowest (1) to highest likelihood (5) of receiving early endoscopy.

(Courtesy of Cooper GS, Chak A, Connors AF Jr, et al: The effectiveness of early endoscopy for the upper gastrointestinal hemorrhage: A community-based analysis. *Med Care* 36:462-474, 1998.)

likely reflection of the associated illnesses. The entire cohort of patients managed with early endoscopy was associated with reduced need for surgical intervention and with a significanly reduced adjusted length of stay. Both of these large observational studies carried out in a community setting show how difficult it is to translate the benefits of early endoscopy demonstrated in carefully randomized trials into the everyday practice.[1,2]

G. Aliperti, M.D.

References

1. Cook DJ, Guyatt GH, Salena BJ, et al: Endoscopic therapy for acute nonvariceal upper gastrointestinal hemorrhage: A meta-analysis. *Gastroenterology* 102:139, 1992.
2. Sacks HS, Chalmers TC, Blum AL, et al: Endoscopic hemostasis: An effective therapy for bleeding peptic ulcers. *JAMA* 264:494, 1990.

Miscellaneous

Randomized Prospective Trial of Early Versus Delayed Feeding After Percutaneous Endoscopic Gastrostomy Placement

McCarter TL, Condon SC, Aguilar RC, et al (Loma Linda Univ Med Ctr, Calif)
Am J Gastroenterol 93:419-421, 1998 2–18

Background.—Percutaneous endoscopic gastrostomy is the preferred method of long-term enteral feeding in patients who cannot take adequate oral nutrition. Most clinicians wait 24 hours after a gastrostomy is placed before using it. It is assumed that this delay allows time for the incision to begin healing and for gastric motility to return to normal, thus reducing the risk of complications. The safety and efficacy of early and delayed feeding after percutaneous endoscopic gastrostomy placement were compared.

Methods.—In a randomized trial, 112 patients with percutaneous endoscopic gastrostomy began tube feedings at 4 hours (group A) or 24 hours (group B) after gastrostomy placement. There were 63 men and 49 women, and the mean patient age was 63. Full-strength Isocal was given as follows: 1,100 mL every 4 hours for 6 feedings on day 1, and 200 mL every 4 hours for 6 feedings on day 2. Gastric residual volume was measured before each feeding, and the next feeding was withheld if there was evidence of gastric retention (residual volume greater than 50%).

Results.—Patients were evaluated on days 1, 2, 7, and 30. The groups were similar in age, sex, nutritional status at baseline, and indications for gastrostomy placement. On day 1, evidence of gastric retention was seen in 25% of the patients in group A and 9% of the patients in group B. On day 2, the percentage of patients with evidence of gastric retention was similar in both groups. On day 2 1 patient from group B died because of aspiration of gastric contents. All other complications were minor and were similar in both groups.

Discussion.—Wound healing follows a well-defined sequence, with the inflammatory phase lasting for 5 to 7 days and the maturation phase beginning around day 20. Thus, 24-hour delayed feeding does not allow sufficient time for any significant wound healing or tract formation. Although a higher incidence of gastric retention was seen in patients who had early feeding, only a small percentage of patients were affected, and only for a day or so. If gastric residual volumes are measured regularly and feedings are temporarily withheld when appropriate, this should not be a significant clinical problem. These results suggest that early feeding after percutaneous endoscopic gastrostomy placement is safe and well tolerated and may reduce costs by shortening the length of parenteral nutritional support and hospital stay.

► This randomized prospective study compares outcomes in patients undergoing endoscopic gastrostomy tube placement. The patients who were randomized received feedings starting 4 hours after insertion of the gastric tube vs 24 hours after. The comparison revealed no significant difference in outcomes. In the current climate of cost containment, the difference might signify a savings of one hospital day or might avoid hospital stay altogether. One caveat is the finding of gastric retention (more than 50% of the prior feeding immediately before the next feeding) in the group of patients fed earlier after gastrostomy placement. This difference may reflect an effect on gastric emptying and motility by the procedure itself, or it may be caused by the sedation required. The authors state that this finding would not constitute a significant clinical problem, provided that gastric residual volumes are routinely measured, and feedings are withheld transiently when appropriate.

G. Aliperti, M.D.

Gastrostomies in Older Patients: The 1990 National Hospital Discharge Survey

Grant MD (West Suburban Hosp Family Practice Residency, Oak Park, Ill)

J Am Board Fam Pract 11:187-192, 1998 2–19

Background.—The use of feeding tubes for older patients generates much discussion about ethical and quality-of-life issues. There is little population-based information concerning the use of gastrostomy in older patients. Numerous published case series describe patient outcome after gastrostomy placement, but generalizing from the results of case studies can present problems. Describing the characteristics and outcomes of older patients fed by gastrostomy may help patients, their families, and clinicians make better informed decisions about gastrostomy placement. Gastrostomy placement in older hospitalized patients was examined in a nationally representative sample.

Methods.—Age, sex, race, primary and secondary diagnoses, and mortality rates were analyzed for hospitalized patients aged 65 years or older who had gastrostomies. Data from the 1990 National Hospital Discharge

TABLE 2.—Percentage of Frequent Primary and Secondary Diagnoses Among Older Patients With Gastrostomies, 1990 National Hospital Discharge Survey

Diagnoses	Percent of Total
Primary diagnoses	
Cerebrovascular disease	19
Pneumonia	12
Neoplasm	11
Fluid or electrolyte disorder	9
Secondary diagnoses	
Fluid or electrolyte disorder	37
Urinary tract infection	25
Nutritional deficiency	21
Dementia	18
Cerebrovascular disease	17
Pneumonia	17
Diabetes	16
Congestive heart failure	13
Chronic obstructive pulmonary disease	12
Ischemic heart disease	12
Neoplasm	11
Decubitus ulcer	11
Swallowing disorders	11
Intestinal disorders*	8
Respiratory failure*	6
Complications	5
Sepsis*	4
Esophageal disorders*	4

From a projected 10,333,000 discharges among patients aged 65 years and older.
*Sample size was between 30 and 59, and estimate might not be reliable.
(Courtesy of Grant MD: Gastrostomies in older patients: The 1990 national discharge survey. *J Am Board Fam Pract* 11:187-192, 1998.)

Survey were used. Mid 1990 Census Bureau population estimates were used to calculate age-specific placement rates.

Results.—An estimated 85,400 patients aged 65 years or older were discharged from hospitals with gastrostomies in 1990. Common primary diagnoses were cerebrovascular disease, pneumonia with or without aspiration, neoplasm, and fluid and electrolyte disorders (Table 2). The in-hospital mortality rate was 16%. Age-specific rates for gastrostomy were 1.2 per 1,000 for patients aged 65 to 74 years and 10.8 for patients aged 85 years or older.

Discussion.—The rate of older hospitalized patients in 1990 who had gastrostomies was higher than expected. The in-hospital mortality rate was considerable. These data indicate that, in 1990, 1% of the U.S. population aged 85 or older was discharged from a hospital with a gastrostomy.

▶ This study reviews utilization of gastrostomy in hospitalized patients age 65 and older. The author concludes that gastrostomies were placed with surprising frequency in hospitalized patients and that the hospital mortality rate was substantial. The conclusions of this study should be taken with due consideration. First, hospitalized patients usually include a select group with an acute health problem superimposed on the usual chronic illness affecting nursing home residents and elderly community patients who require outpatient gastrostomy tube placement. Thus, the association between gastrostomy tube placement and mortality may not be a causal one but might reflect the hope or need to keep the patient hydrated or to attain gastrointestinal decompression during the course of potentially mortal illnesses requiring hospitalization. Of course, encouragement by the author to defer the placement of a permanent feeding tube unless survival seems probable is sound advice for those patients who do not require gastrostomies to resolve immediate needs of decompression or hydration or nutrition.

G. Aliperti, M.D.

Percutaneous Endoscopic Gastrostomy in Children and Adolescents

Behrens R, Lang T, Muschweck H, et al (Univ Children's Hosp Erlangen-Nürnberg, Germany; Gen Hosp Altdorf, Germany; Univ Children's Hosp, Leipzig, Germany)

J Pediatr Gastroenterol Nutr 25:487-491, 1997 2–20

Introduction.—Long-term tube feeding has changed tremendously since introduction of the percutaneous endoscopic gastrostomy (PEG). It is safer, more convenient for the patient, and much less expensive for health maintenance organizations than conventional nasogastric tube feeding. The efficacy, safety, and reliability of PEGs have been established in adults; little information is available on PEGs in children. Reported is experience in the placement and maintenance of PEGs in a large group of children and adolescents.

Methods.—PEGs were placed in 139 patients with an age range of 3 weeks to 36.5 years (mean, 4.4 years) and a weight range of 3.1 to 60 kg (mean, 15 kg). Reason for placement was dysphagia (103); general dystrophy caused by chronic renal failure, congenital heart disease, neoplasm, or cystic fibrosis (26); requirement for a special diet (7); malnutrition related to respiratory insufficiency (2); and gastric volvulus (1). The clinical impact of treatment was evaluated at 6-12 months after PEG placement. Patients and family members or caregivers were asked about changes in the patients' physical status and about handling and care issues.

Results.—The PEGs were placed in the stomach or duodenum in 122 and 15 patients, respectively. Two patients underwent a direct percutaneous endoscopic jejunostomy when duodenal placement proved impossible. Intravenous sedation with midazolam, etomidate, or diazepam was used for placement of PEGs. No patients required general anesthesia. There were 19 complications: dislocation of the duodenal part into the stomach (5), inflammation of the insertion site (3), perforation of the stomach (which healed with conservative treatment) (2), disconnection of the retention disk (4), occlusion of the tube (4), and chronic vomiting (1). Mean PEG lifetime was longer than 1 year.

Conclusion.—For children who require long-term tube feeding, PEG is superior to nasogastric tube feeding. The high efficacy and low rates of complications observed with PEG suggest that it should be considered more frequently, even in infants.

▶ This study summarizes the authors' positive experience with the utilization of fitting feeding gastrostomies in infants. The follow-up of 10 to 12 months is adequate to monitor potential complications and the impact on nutrition and quality of life and to detect technical complications. The absence of mortality in these series may reflect the relatively small number of patients. The mortality rate with percutaneous endoscopic gastrostomy placement in the adult population has been reported in the neighborhood of 1%, and this series lacks the power to clearly state that the mortality rate of this procedure in the pediatric population is lower than in adults. However, the higher mortality rate in the elderly adult population certainly is inflated by the concomitant illnesses of older patients.

G. Aliperti, M.D.

Gastrointestinal Bleeding in the Hospitalized Patient: A Case-Control Study to Assess Risk Factors, Causes, and Outcome

Terdiman JP, Ostroff JW (Univ of California, San Francisco)

Am J Med 104:349-354, 1998 2–21

Introduction.—The usual source of gastrointestinal (GI) bleeding in hospitalized patients is gastroduodenal ulcers, frequently coupled with an erosive gastropathy. These ulcers are believed to form in response to the stress of critical illness and to be distinct in etiology from routine peptic

TABLE 2.—Sources of Clinically Important Nosocomial Gastrointestinal Bleeding in 67 Patients

Source	Percent
Upper Gastrointestinal Tract	
Duodenal ulcer	36
Gastric ulcer	10
Esophagitis	10
Mallory-Weiss tear	6
Gastropathy/duodenopathy	5
Varices	3
Mass lesion	3
No endoscopic evaluation*	13
Lower Gastrointestinal Tract	
Colitis	6
Colonic vascular ectasia	1
No lesion found†	6

*No endoscopic evaluation performed, but upper gastrointestinal bleed based on clinical impression.
†Negative endoscopic evaluation (esophagogastroduodenoscopy and colonoscopy performed in 2 cases, esophagogastroduodenoscopy alone in 1 case and colonoscopy alone in 1 case). No definite bleeding lesion found, but lower gastrointestinal bleed based on clinical impression.
(Courtesy of Terdiman JP, Ostroff JW: Gastrointestinal bleeding in the hospitalized patients: A case-control study to assess risk factors, causes and outcome. *Am J Med* 104:349-354. Copyright 1998, with permission from Excepta Medica Inc.)

ulcers. The risk factors, cause, and outcome of nosocomial GI bleeding was assessed in a heterogeneous group of both ICU and non-ICU patients; these patients were evaluated to determine whether their nosocomial ulcer disease was distinct in etiology from that observed in outpatients.

Methods.—Consecutive patients in whom GI bleeding developed more than 24 hours after admission were compared with 2 control populations: (1) hospitalized patients without GI bleeding, matched for age, gender, and length of stay, and (2) patients admitted to the hospital with clinically important gastroduodenal ulcer bleeding. Medical records were reviewed

TABLE 4.—Comparison of Patients With Nosocomial Gastroduodenal Ulcer Bleeding and Patients Admitted With Gastroduodenal Ulcer Bleeding

	Nosocomial Ulcer Bleeders (n = 31)	Admitted with Ulcer Bleeding (n = 66)	*P* Value
Risk factor			
History of peptic ulcer	13%	50%	<0.01
Nonsteroidal anti-inflammatory drug use	48%	68%	<0.08
Helicobacter pylori infection*	14%	62%	<0.0001
Chronic active gastritis*	29%	91%	<0.0001
Outcome			
Persistent or recurrent bleeding	39%	9%	0.001
Total red cell transfusions, units†	7 ± 6	5 ± 5	<0.05
Subsequent length of stay, days†	12 ± 8	5 ± 5	0.0001
Subsequent intensive care unit length of stay, days†	6 ± 7	2 ± 3	0.0004
Mortality	29%	3%	0.0005

*Based on histologic examination of gastric biopsies in 67% of the cases and 68% of the controls respectively.
†Plus-minus vales are mean ± SD.
(Courtesy of Terdiman JP, Ostroff JW: Gastrointestinal bleeding in the hospitalized patients: A case-control study to assess risk factors, causes and outcome. *Am J Med* 104:349-354. Copyright 1998, with permission from Excerpta Medica Inc.)

to determine length of hospital stay and length of ICU stay subsequent to onset of bleeding, persistent or recurrent bleeding, surgical or angiographic intervention to arrest bleeding, total number of units of red blood cells transfused, death, and death from uncontrolled bleeding. The presence of *Helicobacter pylori* infection and chronic active gastritis was determined histologically.

Results.—Sixty-seven inpatients had clinically important nosocomial GI bleeding after a mean of 14 days in the hospital (Table 2). Sixty-four percent of the patients were not hospitalized in the ICU when bleeding started. Of these, 72% had received some form of bleeding prophylaxis. Multivariate analysis revealed that prior ICU stay and mechanical ventilation were independent risk factors for onset of bleeding. Nosocomial GI bleeding was correlated with poor outcome and an associated mortality rate of 34%. Duodenal ulcer disease was the most frequent cause of GI bleeding (36% overall). Patients with nosocomial bleeding were less likely to have a previous history of ulcer disease (13% vs. 50%; $P < 0.05$), *H. pylori* infection (14% vs. 62%; $P < 0.0001$), chronic acute gastritis (29% vs. 91%; $P < 0.0001$), or to be taking nonsteroidal anti-inflammatory drugs (NSAIDs) (48% vs. 68%; $P < 0.08$), than patients admitted to the hospital with bleeding ulcer (Table 4).

Conclusion.—Gastrointestinal bleeding is an important complication of hospitalization and is highly correlated with mortality. Bleeding is most likely to occur after a prolonged hospital stay and in patients with more severe underlying illnesses. The most common cause of this type of GI bleeding is duodenal ulcer. Nosocomial gastroduodenal ulcer disease is distinct in etiology from ulcer disease observed in outpatients.

▶ Clinically significant GI bleeding is known to occur in the subset of hospitalized patients with more severe underlying disease. This retrospective study reminds us that the risk factors include prior ICU stay and mechanical ventilation. Bleeding in these patients was associated with a high mortality rate. The authors found that duodenal ulcer disease was the most common source of bleeding in these patients, despite the low incidence of prior peptic ulcer disease and *H. pylori* infection in this subgroup. The authors stress that bleeding nosocomial "ulcer disease" appears to have an etiology that is distinct from the ulcer disease seen in patients admitted with GI bleeding as the primary indication.

G. Aliperti, M.D.

Demography, Clinical Characteristics, Psychological and Abuse Profiles, Treatment, and Long-term Follow-up of Patients With Gastroparesis

Soykan I, Sivri B, Sarosiek I, et al (Univ of Kansas, Kansas City; Univ of Virginia, Charlottesville)

Dig Dis Sci 43:2398-2404, 1998 2–22

Background.—Little is known about the natural history of gastroparesis or the characteristics of the patients who have this gastric motility disorder. These authors describe patient and treatment factors associated with outcomes in patients with gastroparesis.

Methods.—Data from 146 patients (26 men and 120 women; mean age, 45.5 years) with gastroparesis of more than 3 months' duration were reviewed (average age at onset, 33.7). Each patient underwent a gastric emptying study and was interviewed to determine gastrointestinal symptoms, psychological status, sexual and physical abuse status (women only), somatization, depression, and personality functioning.

Findings.—Causes of the gastroparesis were diabetes in 42 patients (29%), gastric surgery in 19 patients (13%), Parkinson's disease in 11 patients (7.5%), collagen vascular disorders in 7 patients (4.8%), intestinal pseudo-obstruction in 6 patients (4.1%), miscellaneous causes in 9 patients (6%), and idiopathic in 52 patients (35.6%). Within the patients with idiopathic gastroparesis, 25 (48%) had severe abdominal pain, 12 (23%) likely had a viral etiology, 12 (23%) were believed to be depressed, and 10 (19%) had gastroesophageal reflux disease and nonulcer dyspepsia. Almost two thirds of the women with idiopathic gastroparesis (29, or 62%) had a history of physical or sexual abuse; physical abuse was significantly associated with greater abdominal pain, somatization, depression, gastrointestinal symptoms, and more previous abdominal surgical procedures. Patients were treated with oral cisapride (n = 47), oral domperidone (n = 42), subcutaneous metoclopramide (n = 25), intravenous or oral erythromycin (n = 25), or lueprolide acetate (n = 1), or received no prokinetic therapy (n = 6). The overall response rate to these drugs was 74%; response rates for cisapride, domperidone, metoclopramide, and erythromycin were 65%, 80%, 75%, and 64%, respectively. Eight patients (5%) had undergone gastrectomy, and 9 (6.2%) had undergone gastric electrical stimulation for gastric pacing. In addition, 21% of the patients had at some point required parenteral nutrition or enteral feeding with a jejunostomy tube. Patients with virus-associated idiopathic gastroparesis rated their quality of life as significantly better than did the other patients in the idiopathic group. Overall, in the idiopathic group, 55% of the patients were employed, 35% reported a good quality of life, and 70% required continuous prokinetic therapy. Ten patients died (7%) of metabolic disarray and cardiac complications, suicide, or bowel ischemia.

Conclusions.—Different etiologic and psychological factors associated with gastroparesis were associated with different responses to prokinetic therapy. In general, good responses can be expected from patients with idiopathic virus- or dyspepsia-associated disease, Parkinson's disease, or diabetes. Poorer responses can be expected in patients with gastroparesis caused by gastrectomy, connective tissue disease, or idiopathic disease associated with abdominal pain and physical or sexual abuse.

3 The Spleen

Laparoscopic Splenectomy

Laparoscopic Versus Open Splenectomy in the Management of Splenomegaly: Our Preliminary Experience

Terrosu G, Donini A, Baccarani U, et al (Univ Hosp, Udine, Italy)

Surgery 124:839-843, 1998 3–1

Objective.—Laparoscopic splenectomy is usually contraindicated when the volume of the spleen is large. Experience with 8 consecutive cases of laparoscopic splenectomy in the management of splenomegaly was reviewed retrospectively.

Methods.—Between 1989 and 1997, 23 patients with splenomegaly (spleens weighing > 500 g) were operated on using the laparoscopic approach (n = 8, group 1) or using the traditional open approach (n = 15, group 2). Data were compared with those from 27 patients having laparoscopic splenectomy for normal-sized spleens (group 3). Outcome measures were operative time, intraoperative blood loss, blood transfusion requirement, postoperative ileus, postoperative stay, mortality rates, and morbidity rates.

Results.—There were significant differences between groups 1 and 2 with respect to operating time, blood transfusion requirement, and postoperative course (Table 2). Only operative time differed when groups 1 and 3 were compared (Table 3).

TABLE 2.—Laparoscopic Splenomegaly Versus Open Splenomegaly

Results	Laparoscopic Splenomegaly	Open Splenomegaly	*P* Value*
Mean ± SD operating room time (min) (range)	197 ± 65 (110-300)	110 ± 21 (85-150)	<.01
No. of patients transfused (mean units blood/patient)	1 (2)	10 (1.3)	<.01
Mean ± SD days to liquid diet (range)	2 ± 1 (1-5)	4 ± 0.6 (3-5)	<.005
Mean ± SD postoperative stay (days) (range)	6 ± 3 (4-12)	9 ± 3 (6-14)	<.02
Postoperative complications (n) (%)	1 (12.5)	5 (33)	.27

*Student *t* test or chi-squared test.

(Courtesy of Terrosu G, Donini A, Baccarani U, et al: Laparoscopic versus open splenectomy in the management of splenomegaly: Our preliminary experience. *Surgery* 124:839-843, 1998.)

TABLE 3.—Laparoscopic Splenomegaly Versus Laparoscopic Normal-sized Spleen

Results	Laparoscopic Splenomegaly	Laparoscopic Normal Spleen	*P* Value*
Mean ± SD operating room time (min) (range)	197 ± 65 (110-300)	117 ± 51 (42-200)	<.01
Conversion rate (n) (%)	0	1 (4)	.58
Mean ± SD estimated blood loss (mL) (range)	393 ± 239 (100-800)	228 ± 226 (0-1100)	.13
No. of patients transfused (mean units blood/patient)	1 (2)	0	.06
Mean ± SD days to liquid diet (range)	2 ± 1 (1-5)	1.6 ± 0.6 (1-3)	.19
Mean ± SD postoperative stay (days) (range)	6 ± 3 (4-12)	5 ± 3 (2-18)	.32
Postoperative complications (n) (%)	1 (12.5)	2 (8)	.65

(Courtesy of Terrosu G, Donini A, Baccarani U, et al: Laparoscopic versus open splenectomy in the management of splenomegaly: Our preliminary experience. *Surgery* 124:839-843, 1998.)

Conclusion.—Laparoscopy for splenomegaly is safe and effective, resulting in a lower intraoperative blood requirement and a less complicated operative course.

▶ This article reports a single-institution case series with comparison of 3 groups of patients: patients with splenomegaly undergoing open splenectomy, patients with splenomegaly undergoing laparoscopic splenectomy, and patients undergoing laparoscopic splenectomy in the setting of small, normal spleen size. The authors suggest that patients undergoing laparoscopic surgery regardless of spleen size gain the usual benefits of laparoscopic procedures, namely, a shorter hospital stay, decreased postoperative discomfort with earlier resumption of diet, and return to normal activities. They do demonstrate that management of larger spleens via laparoscopic approach requires more time than either management of smaller spleens via the laparoscope or management of large spleens via an open technique, although the increase in time was not prohibitive. One criticism of this study is that the authors identify any spleen of greater than 500 g as meeting the criteria for splenomegaly. Although the average spleen weight in the splenomegaly group was 1.7 kg, several spleens were clearly much smaller than this and may have helped minimize the difference in data between laparoscopic splenectomy for normal and enlarged spleens. An additional concern not dealt with by the authors is the question of tumor cell dissemination. In some cases, lymphoma of the spleen is an isolated finding, although often it is simply a sequela of systemic disease. Certainly the risk of splenic injury or rupture in this setting should give one pause when pursuing a laparoscopic approach. Laparoscopic splenectomy does appear to be a procedure like laparoscopic cholecystectomy and Nissen fundoplication that, overall, has significant patient benefits when compared with an open technique and will no doubt become the standard approach to splenectomy in many circumstances. It is hoped that randomized, prospective trials in the setting of specific problems, such as the very large spleen and/or patients with neoplasia of the spleen, will assist in determining which patients are appropriately managed by this strategy.

J.A. Drebin, M.D., Ph.D.

Laparoscopic Versus Open Splenectomy for Immune Thrombocytopenic Purpura

Lozano-Salazar RR, Herrera MF, Vargas-Voráckova F, et al (Instituto Nacional de la Nutrición Salvador Zubirán, México City)

Am J Surg 176:366-369, 1998 3–2

Background.—For patients with immune thrombocytopenic purpura (ITP) in whom medical therapy is unsuccessful, splenectomy can usually achieve an adequate response. Open splenectomy (OS) is more commonly performed, but several studies have advocated laparoscopic splenectomy (LS). The therapeutic responses between OS and LS in patients with ITP were compared.

Methods.—The subjects were 49 patients with ITP who underwent splenectomy. OS was performed in the first 27 patients (8 men and 19 women; mean age, 38 years) and LS was performed in the last 22 patients (7 men and 15 women; mean age, 39 years). Average spleen sizes were similar in the OS and LS groups (11 vs. 10 cm). Preoperatively, platelet counts were significantly higher in the LS group (50 vs. 16 $\times$ 10^9/L). A complete response was defined as a sustained increase in a platelet count of more than 150 $\times$ 10^9/L for 2 months or more without medication. A partial response was defined as either a platelet count greater than 50 $\times$ 10^9/L without treatment, a normal platelet count with maintenance treatment, or a response followed by a recurrence.

Findings.—Mean operative time was significantly longer in the LS group (4.5 ± 1 vs. 2.7 ± 0.7 hours), and 2 patients in the LS group required conversion to laparotomy. Only 3 patients in the OS group and 2 patients in the LS group required blood transfusion, despite significantly lower preoperative platelet counts in the OS group. Ten patients in the OS group experienced a total of 14 complications, including 2 cases each of pulmonary atelectasis, subphrenic abscess, upper gastrointestinal (GI) bleeding, and wound infection. Six patients in the LS group experienced a total of 8 complications, including 2 cases each of wound infection and pneumonia. Two patients in the OS group died (of GI and intracranial bleeding or GI bleeding and bronchoaspiration) and 1 patient in the LS group died (of intra-abdominal bleeding and stroke); all 3 of these patients had preoperative platelet counts less than 16 $\times$ 10^9/L. Mean postoperative hospital stay was significantly shorter in the LS group (4 vs. 6 days). Median follow-up times in the OS and LS groups were 35 and 14.5 months, respectively. At follow-up, 59% of the patients in each group had achieved a complete response, and 29% of the OS group and 27% of the LS group had achieved a partial response.

Conclusions.—Outcomes after LS are similar to those after OS, and hospital stays are shorter with LS. Despite the longer operative time with LS, the incidence of pulmonary atelectasis, deep venous thrombosis, surgical infection, or elevated metabolic trauma response was not significantly different from that after OS. Additional experience with the LS approach is expected to reduce operative times in the future.

▶ This article addresses the appropriate operative strategy of performing splenectomy in the setting of ITP. ITP represents a relatively ideal setting in which to carry out LS inasmuch as the spleens in such patients are often normal or even small in size. The authors compare a group of patients who underwent OS with a group undergoing LS with regard to outcomes and complications. The overall complication rate in this study was rather high in both groups, with mortality rates that would be considered unacceptable in this country. However, it is apparent that the laparoscopic group had results that were comparable or even superior to those who had open surgery. Moreover, the therapeutic response from the point of view of the patients' ITP was equivalent in the 2 groups, with about 90% of the patients showing at least a partial response. This manuscript adds to the evidence that LS is appropriate in the approach to managing ITP.

J.A. Drebin, M.D., Ph.D.

A New Technique for Laparoscopic Splenectomy With Massively Enlarged Spleens

Hebra A, Walker JD, Tagge EP, et al (Med Univ of South Carolina, Charleston)
Am Surg 64:1161-1164, 1998 3–3

Background.—Current methods of removing the spleen in children with sickle-cell disease (SCD), splenomegaly, and recurrent splenic sequestration place the patient at high risk of postoperative complications. These authors described a method of laparoscopic splenectomy (LS) based on intracorporeal splenic fragmentation.

Methods.—The patients were 5 children who had SCD, splenomegaly, and splenic sequestration. Age ranged from 22 months to 11 years and weight ranged from 13.2 to 30.1 kg. Patients were examined preoperatively by ultrasound, which revealed a spleen size index of 0.42 to 0.76. To perform the procedure, general anesthesia is induced, and the patient is placed in the lateral decubitus position, and 4 trocars are placed. (Note that in 1 patient who also required laparoscopic cholecystectomy, 6 trocars were placed and 2 were used for both procedures.) Then the spleen is devascularized and pushed against the diaphragm to keep it stable. An electromechanical morcellator is introduced, and the spleen is systematically cored until it is completely removed. Afterward, the left upper quadrant is irrigated and the entire peritoneal cavity is examined for residual fragments, which, if present, are easily removed via the ports. For 24 hours postoperatively, patients receive supplemental oxygen and IV fluids.

Findings.—None of the procedures required conversion to open surgery or required larger incisions to remove the spleen. Operative time averaged 190 minutes (245 minutes in the patient who underwent cholecystectomy and LS). No patient required intraoperative or postoperative blood transfusion, and average blood loss was less than 50 mL. Patients were discharged within 2 days after surgery, and there were no postoperative sickle-cell crises. At follow-up, a nuclear scan was performed to search for remnant splenic tissue; none was found, nor was there any evidence of splenosis.

Conclusions.—Even in the youngest child in this series, LS with intracorporeal splenic fragmentation completely removed the massively enlarged spleens in these children with SCD. Patients quickly recovered postoperatively and experienced minimal pain and scarring. This laparoscopic approach avoids the need for intracorporeal bags and additional large incisions for removing the spleen. This method should extend the benefits of laparoscopic surgery to children with hematologic disorders and splenomegaly who have significant co-morbidities that make open surgery or other approaches risky.

▶ This article addresses the problem of performing splenectomy in the setting of splenomegaly. The authors have used an electromechanical morcellator to break up and aspirate the spleen intracorporeally after ligation of the vascular pedicle of the spleen. This approach obviates the need for placing the spleen in a bag and facilitates the removal of such large spleens. The authors have performed this approach on children with splenomegaly secondary to SCD with good success. However, I think there are some major limitations to this approach, namely, that the spleen and splenic capsule are violated intracorporeally by this approach. Thus, in patients with idiopathic thrombocytopenic purpura, this would not be a satisfactory approach because secondary splenosis would likely result. Similarly, in patients who may have a diagnosis of lymphoma or other neoplasm involving the spleen, violating the splenic capsule into the abdomen would clearly be contraindicated. A selective group of patients in whom the fragmentation of the spleen and dispersal of splenic tissue into the abdomen is not contraindicated and may, in fact, be desirable—such as patients with SCD—could potentially benefit from this approach.

J.A. Drebin, M.D., Ph.D.

Laparoscopic Splenectomy: Outcome and Efficacy in 103 Consecutive Patients

Katkhouda N, Hurwitz MB, Rivera RT, et al (Univ of Southern California, Los Angeles; Univ of Nice, France)

Ann Surg 228:568-578, 1998 3–4

Objective.—A number of small studies have demonstrated that laparoscopic splenectomy (LS) can be performed with low morbidity and mortality rates, but the efficacy of the procedure in patients with hematologic disorders has not been demonstrated. Clinical outcome data from 103 consecutive patients undergoing LS were evaluated, and the efficacy of the procedure was analyzed.

Methods.—Between June 1992 and October 1997, 103 patients underwent LS for idiopathic thrombocytopenic purpura (ITP), hereditary spherocytosis, autoimmune hemolytic anemia, thrombotic thrombocytopenic purpura, and reasons other than trauma or carcinoma. Perioperative adverse events, blood transfusion requirement, death, and surgical time were recorded.

Results.—Four (3.9%) patients were converted to the open procedure. Spleen dimensions and weight averaged 14 cm in the longest dimension and 263 g, respectively. Accessory spleens were found in 20 patients, including 15 in 12 patients with ITP and 5 in patients without ITP. Surgical time averaged 161 minutes. Bowel sounds returned in 29 hours on average. Six patients required an average of 2.9 U of packed cells, and 2 required transfusions. Six patients had complications, and 1 required a second surgery for bowel obstruction. The average hospital stay was 2.5 days. ITP patients were examined for an average of 38 months during which 4 (6%) patients experienced relapse. The global failure rate was 22.4%. Eleven of 12 hereditary spherocytosis patients had a positive response during an average follow-up period of 27 months. Hematocrit levels increased significantly in 7 (70%) patients with warm antibody autoimmune hemolytic anemia. Four (67%) of 6 patients with thrombotic thrombocytopenic purpura responded. All patients with HIV and systemic lupus erythematosus had a positive response, and AIDS did not develop in the HIV patients during the follow-up period. The single patient with hairy-cell leukemia is alive without recurrence 19 months after splenectomy.

Conclusion.—LS is safe and effective for treatment of benign hematologic disorders. Morbidity rates are lower than for the open procedure, and mortality and efficacy rates are comparable.

▶ This article provides a single-institutional summary of more than 100 patients undergoing LS in a 5-year period. The majority of patients underwent splenectomy for ITP, and the majority of spleens removed were small. The authors demonstrate good long-term outcomes with rates of resolution of ITP or consumptive red blood cell disorders comparable to those achieved using open techniques. In addition, the authors specifically address the question of accessory splenosis and point out that these can often be easily identified through the laparoscope. In fact, such accessory spleens were identified in 20% of patients. Only 4% of patients required conversion to open splenectomy, and transfusions were only required in a total of 6% of the patients, including the 4% who underwent conversion and 2% of patients successfully undergoing LS. This study shows the quality of results that can be achieved using a laparoscopic technique and demonstrates that the most likely complication of LS is bleeding, which requires conversion to an open procedure. The usual benefits of laparoscopic surgery, including diminished hospital stay and discomfort, were noted in patients undergoing LS. Furthermore, the authors suggest there is a specific learning curve for this procedure with decreased operating time coming with increased surgical experience. LS clearly is the preferred method of management for patients requiring splenectomy for a variety of disorders, particularly those in which the spleen is not massively enlarged. An aggressive search for accessory splenosis is important in patients undergoing splenectomy for ITP because failure to recognize this relatively common problem may result in treatment failure.

J.A. Drebin, M.D., Ph.D.

4 The Small Intestine

General

Palliation of Malignant Gastric and Small Intestinal Strictures With Self-expandable Metal Stents

Yates MR III, Morgan DE, Baron TH (Univ of Alabama at Birmingham)

Endoscopy 30:266-272, 1998 4–1

Objective.—The feasibility, effectiveness, safety, and outcome of using expandable metal stents to provide palliation was evaluated in patients with inoperable malignant stricture of the stomach and small intestine.

Methods.—Between July 1994 and May 1996, 11 consecutive patients, aged 49 to 90 years, with unresectable malignant gastric or small intestinal obstruction were treated with 19 uncovered expandable metal stents,

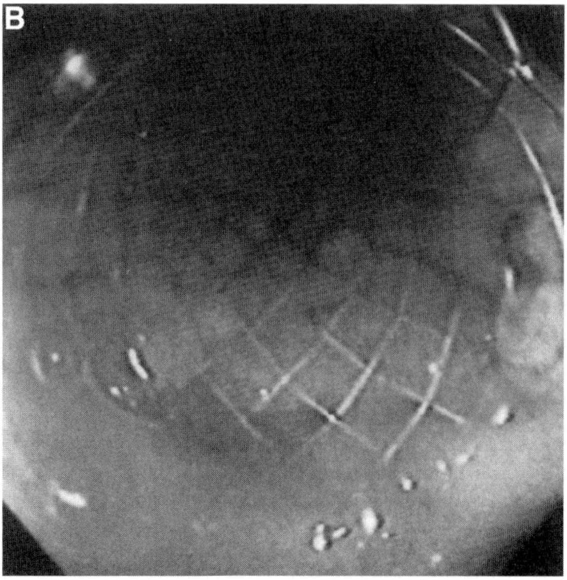

FIGURE 3.—Recurrent gastric adenocarcinoma at the gastrojejunal anastomosis. **B**, endoscopic view of a 10-mm biliary Wallstent placed within the jejunum. (Courtesy of Yates MR III, Morgan DE, Baron TH: Palliation of malignant gastric and small intestinal strictures with self-expandable metal stents. *Endoscopy* 30:266-272, 1998. Georg Thieme Verlag.)

under endoscopic and fluoroscopic guidance, for palliation of symptomatic obstruction (Fig 3). Stent patency was confirmed by contrast radiograph. Success was defined as improvement in the patient's peroral intake.

Results.—The procedure was successful in 9 (82%) patients. In 1 patient whose stent did not completely traverse the entire duodenal stricture, another stent was inserted that successfully relieved the stricture. The final success rate was 10 of 11 (91%). There were no major complications, but 5 stents were occluded by tumor ingrowth or overgrowth at 3.5 to 11 weeks after the procedure. The duration of success ranged from 5 to 294 days. Nine patients died of their disease, and 2 died of pneumonia.

Conclusion.—Expandable metal stents provide effective and safe palliation and an alternative to surgery for patients with malignant gastric and small intestinal strictures.

▶ Expandable metal stents have, more recently, also been used in gastric outlet obstruction and small intestinal strictures. This article and one by Bethge et al.[1] describe 17 patients with such malignancies in whom metal stents were placed. Success was achieved in 16 of the patients and placement was impossible in 1 patient because of severe anastomotic angulation and distal luminal obstruction. The follow-up of these patients goes through 294 days, with a mean of approximately 2 months. The improvement in quality of life in patients with inoperable malignancies and short survival makes the rate of complications acceptable in this group of patients.

G. Aliperti, M.D.

Reference

1. Bethge N, Breitkreutz C, Vakil N: Metal stents for the palliation of inoperable upper gastrointestinal stenoses. *Am J Gastroenterol* 93:643-645, 1998.

Intestinal Ischemia

Percutaneous Transluminal Angioplasty in the Treatment of Chronic Mesenteric Ischemia: Results and 3 Years of Follow-up in 23 Patients

Maspes F, Mazzetti di Pietralata G, Gandini R, et al (Università degli Studi di Roma "Tor Vergata," Rome; Univ of Perugia, Italy)

Abdom Imaging 23:358-363, 1998 4–2

Objective.—Surgical revascularization, the treatment of choice for chronic mesenteric ischemia (CMA), carries high mortality and morbidity rates. The clinical efficacy of percutaneous transluminal angioplasty (PTA) in the treatment of CMA was retrospectively evaluated in patients with CMA.

Methods.—Charts of 23 patients, aged 49 to 76 years, who underwent 41 PTAs of visceral arteries between 1982 and 1995 were reviewed. Angiography revealed 42 lesions. All were atherosclerotic except for 1 superior mesenteric artery fibrodysplastic stenosis, and 13 were located in the ostial tract. Patients were examined at 2, 6, 12, 24, and 36 months.

Measures of outcome were remission of symptoms and recovery of body weight.

Results.—PTA was technically successful in 37 lesions (90%). Symptoms improved in 17 of 22 patients by 2 months. Two patients with restenosis underwent a second PTA, which was successful. Their symptoms resolved at 24 and 36 months, but 1 underwent an aortomesenteric bypass. At follow-up, 13 (68%) of 19 patients had gained 40% to 100% of their weight, and 3 patients had unchanged body weight. Two patients (12%) had relapse of symptoms. Clinical success at 3 years was 88%. Two patients underwent successful repeat angioplasty at 2 and 3 years. There were 2 complications—1 hematoma at the approach site and a balloon rupture that did not require additional hospitalization or treatment.

Conclusion.—In contrast to the high mortality and morbidity rates after surgical treatment of CMA, PTA carries a low complication rate.

▶ The use of PTA for treatment of vascular lesions has been standardized for the heart and seems to be uniquely amenable to the treatment of lesions at vessel origins arising from the abdominal aortic and mesenteric vessels. Not only are these lesions acceptable for treatment by angioplasty, but they are potentially treatable by the intraluminal grafting procedures that have been developed for treatment of abdominal aortic aneurysms and other problems. Certainly, for high-risk patients, percutaneous angioplasty is much safer and less morbid than an operation. The authors admit that surgical bypass remains the treatment of choice for mesenteric vascular disease and chronic intestinal ischemia. One should still keep in mind the possibility of angioplasty in these patients.

J.W. Fleshman, Jr., M.D.

Intestinal Infarctions: A Reappraisal of the Factors Predictive of Operative Mortality

Goudet P, Michelin T, Rousseau P, et al (Univ Hosp of Burgundy, Dijon, France)

Eur J Surg 164:593-598, 1998 4–3

Objective.—Mortality rates after acute intestinal infarction vary from 40% to 93%. Predictive factors of operative mortality, including referral, in a series of 144 intestinal infarctions were evaluated retrospectively by means of univariate and multivariate analysis.

Methods.—A total of 144 patients (71 women), aged 27 to 93 years, were operated on between January 1980 and August 1995 for infarction of the gastrointestinal tract between the duodenojejunal junction and the rectum. Cases of chronic ischemia and strangulation were excluded.

Results.—The operative mortality rate, which remained relatively constant over the study period, was 67%. Most deaths occurred within 45 days after surgery. Women were significantly older than men (78 vs. 68

years). Univariate analysis revealed that age over 75 years, female sex, the existence of shock, the extent of infarction, and cardiovascular referral were predictive of operative mortality. However, multivariate analysis reduced these predictors of operative mortality to the extent of infarction, age older than 75 years, the existence of shock, and recent cardiac or vascular surgery.

Conclusion.—Age older than 75 years, the existence of shock, the extent of infarction, and recent cardiac or vascular surgery were predictive of operative mortality in patients with intestinal infarction. The wide range of mortality rates is probably the result of the type of referral.

▶ Once again we see that the high-risk factors for intestinal ischemia include cardiovascular diseases and previous cardiovascular operations. Independent prognostic factors after operation for intestinal ischemia included the extent of infarction, age over 75, the presence of shock, and recent cardiac or vascular surgery. Interestingly, these seem to correlate with the referral pattern within the hospital. Patients referred from cardiac and medical or surgical ICUs were more likely to succumb to their disease than those from the general surgery floor or the medical floor. Early diagnosis and management remain the treatment of choice in these individuals; however, this information can certainly help us determine those who are more likely to survive an operation.

J.W. Fleshman, Jr., M.D.

Small Bowel

General and Cancer Specific Mortality of a Population Based Cohort of Patients With Inflammatory Bowel Disease: The Florence Study

Palli D, Trallori G, Saieva C, et al (Ospedaliera CAREGGI, Firenze, Italy)
Gut 42:175-179, 1998 4–4

Background.—Recently the incidence and prevalence of inflammatory bowel disease have been increasing in the area surrounding Florence, Italy. These authors analyzed differences in the causes of death for all patients in whom ulcerative colitis (UC) or Crohn's disease (CD) developed during a 15-year period.

Methods.—Between 1978 and 1992, 920 patients were given diagnoses of either UC (n = 689; 410 men and 279 women) or CD (n = 231; 115 men and 116 women). All patients were followed up until death or until Dec. 31, 1996. Only 8 patients could not be traced for the full follow-up period; their data are included up to the date when they were lost to follow-up. Overall, patients with UC provided 7,380 person-years of follow-up, and patients with CD provided 2,560 person-years of follow-up. During follow-up, 70 deaths (36 men, 34 women) occurred, and cause of death was determined. The number of expected deaths was estimated on the basis of age, gender, and national mortality rates, and standardized mortality ratios (SMRs) were calculated.

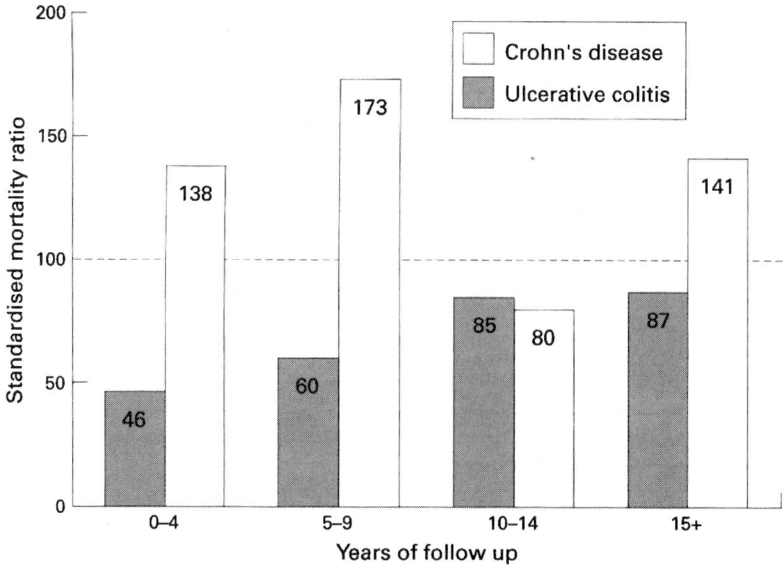

FIGURE 1.—Total mortality SMRs for each 5-year follow-up period by type of inflammatory bowel disease. (Courtesy of Palli D, Trallori G, Saieva C, et al: General and cancer specific mortality of a population based cohort of patients with inflammatory bowel disease: The Florence study. *Gut* 42: 175-179, 1998.)

Findings.—Of the 70 patients who died, 47 had UC and 23 had CD. The number of deaths expected in this group overall was 92; thus, the SMR of 0.76 was significantly lower than expected. Mortality in the patients with UC was significantly lower than expected (SMR, 0.62), mainly because the number of deaths due to cardiovascular diseases was almost half the number expected (SMR, 0.58). In fact, the only cause of death responsible for a higher-than-expected death rate was gastrointestinal disease, and this was associated with only a moderate increase in deaths (SMR, 1.57). Mortality in the patients with CD was slightly (but not significantly) higher (SMR, 1.36), mainly because of a significant increase in deaths caused by gastrointestinal diseases (SMR, 4.31) and a slight increase in deaths caused by neoplasms (SMR, 1.90). Deaths caused by colorectal cancer were not significantly increased in either patient group. However, there were fewer cancers of the respiratory tract in patients with UC (SMR, 0.16; $P < 0.05$) and more of these neoplasms in patients with CD (SMR, 2.63). When SMRs were analyzed according to the time since the start of follow-up, 2 distinct patterns emerged (Fig 1). Patients with UC had a lower mortality rate early in the follow-up period, but rates increased as time progressed. Alternatively, patients with CD had high SMRs at the beginning of follow-up that stayed high through 15 years of follow-up. The median ages at death for patients with UC or CD were 60 and 73 years, respectively.

Conclusions.—In this Mediterranean study, patients with UC had a different mortality pattern than patients with CD. Mortality rates for the patients with UC were significantly lower than expected, mainly because of fewer cardiovascular-related deaths. Mortality rates for the patients with CD were slightly higher than expected, probably because more of these patients smoked and the severity of the CD was greater.

▶ The morbidity of inflammatory bowel diseases is extensive and their burden is well described. Less certain is the impact of these diseases on overall mortality, not just those deaths due to gastrointestinal (GI) complications. This population-based study of Italian patients identified a divergence in mortality between patients with UC, having an SMR lower than expected, and patients with CD, having a slightly higher than expected SMR. The critical factor in this difference may be attributable in large part to cigarette use, which was less in patients with UC and greater in patients with CD. However, other factors may be important as well. The maintenance use of mesalazine products, more standard in UC than in CD may also have an anticarcinogenic effect and has been suggested to reduce cardiovascular mortality. Genetic predispositions or socioeconomic factors may also influence these findings. Significantly, these influences are not only in relation to GI-related mortality. Increased vigilance for colon cancers, increased attentiveness to maintenance medication, and early surgery for patients with UC may have an impact not only on GI-related mortality but on other areas as well. In general agreement with similar studies, these possible lessons are important for patient education as well to provide them a fuller sense of the picture and to show them that, although concern for colon cancer persists, the broader outlook is not universally grim.

G. Aliperti, M.D.

Clinical Course and Management of Inflammatory Bowel Disease After Liver Transplantation

Befeler AS, Lissoos TW, Schiano TD, et al (Univ of Chicago)

Transplantation 65:393-396, 1998 4–5

Background.—Some studies have reported that up to two thirds of all patients who have a history of inflammatory bowel disease (IBD) will experience symptomatic IBD after orthotopic liver transplantation (OLT). As many as one third of these high-risk patients will require colectomy. The experience of these authors, however, is that IBD and the need for colectomy after OLT occur less frequently. To explain the differences between their results and reports in the literature, they reviewed their experience with management of IBD after OLT.

Methods.—The subjects were 35 patients (21 men and 14 women; median age, 47 years) who underwent OLT and who had a preoperative diagnosis of IBD (n = 29) or primary sclerosing cholangitis (PSC) without IBD (n = 6). Ulcerative colitis (UC) was present in 25 of the 29 patients with IBD, and 8 of them underwent total or partial colectomy before OLT. Crohn's disease was present in 4 of the 29 patients with IBD, and 2 of them underwent partial colectomy before OLT. Patients were categorized as

TABLE 1.—Summary of Previously Reported Inflammatory Bowel Disease Activity After Orthotopic Liver Transplantation of At-Risk and High-Risk Patients

Reference	No. "High Risk"	Symptomatic (%)	Surgery (%)	No. "At Risk"	Symptomatic (%)	Surgery (%)
Knechtle et al. (2)	21	33	29	33	21	18
Stephens et al. (3)	27	33	15	—[a]	—[a]	—[a]
Miki et al. (6)	26	35	—[a]	—[a]	—[a]	—[a]
Shaked et al. (7)	24	45	13	31	35	10
Fabry et al. (4)	13	23	0	34	12	0
Kitis et al. (5)	33	67	9	—[a]	—[a]	—[a]
Current report	*23*	*26*	*0*	*29*	*24*	*0*

*Not reported.

(Courtesy of Befeler AS, Lissoos TW, Schiano TD, et al: Clinical course and management of inflammatory bowel disease after liver transplantation. *Transplantation* 65:393-396, 1998.)

high risk if they had a history of IBD but no colectomy (n = 23). Patients in the at-risk category (n = 29) included the high-risk patients plus those with a history of PSC but not IBD or colectomy. After OLT, patients received immunosuppression with cyclosporine, prednisone, and azathioprine (n = 34) or tacrolimus and prednisone (n = 1) and were followed up for a mean of 37 ± 6.4 months.

Findings.—After OLT, only 1 patient (17%) who had PSC but not IBD preoperatively had IBD postoperatively. None of the patients required surgery for active IBD; nor did any patient require IV steroids. Five of the at-risk patients (17%) had no IBD at all after OLT. Seventeen of the high-risk patients (74% of the high-risk group and 59% of the at-risk group) had quiescent disease and required only immunosuppressive drugs. Mild IBD flares developed in 6 high-risk patients (26%) and in 7 at-risk patients (24%), but these were controlled with increases in oral steroid dosages in 2 patients and the addition of 5'-aminosalicylates in 5 patients.

Conclusions.—Many of the immunosuppressive drugs used to treat IBD are the same as those used with OLT, including steroids, azathioprine, and cyclosporine. In most of these patients, post-OLT immunosuppressive regimens were able to control symptoms of IBD. In approximately one fourth of the patients, mild IBD flares developed and were treated with oral steroids or 5'-aminosalicylates. In fact, 5'-aminosalicylates were helpful, even when patients were already taking steroids, azathioprine, or cyclosporine. These findings are at odds with reports in the literature documenting the need for aggressive medical therapy or surgery in these patients after OLT (Table 1). These differences might be explained by the fact that IBD symptoms in these patients were controlled before OLT and that all but 1 patient received azathioprine (which has documented effectiveness against IBD) postoperatively.

► The clinical course of patients with IBD undergoing liver transplantation has been reported as being frequently difficult to control despite the presence of potent immunosuppression. Curiously, a number of patients with new-onset IBD after their transplants have been described. This report suggests a more sanguine course of IBD in the posttransplant individual. Most patients in this report had UC, skewed by the many patients undergoing transplantation because of PSC. Flares were often easily controlled with 5'-aminosalicylates or steroids. The authors suggest that there may be 2 possible reasons for the discrepancy between this report and others: (1) their patients were generally under good control at the time of transplant and (2) azathioprine was more frequently used in their population. In addition to the potential practical lessons in this subgroup of patients, this report reinforces the concept that azathioprine modulates the immune system in a particular way, quite different from other immunosuppressants, which has been poorly defined but offers important insights into the pathogenesis of IBD.

G. Aliperti, M.D.

Small Bowel Obstruction in Patients Previously Operated on for Colorectal Cancer

Edna T-H, Bjerkeset T (Innherred Hosp, Levanger, Norway)

Eur J Surg 164:587-592, 1998 4–6

Background.—Colorectal cancer is the most common primary tumor causing metastatic small-bowel obstruction. The incidence, etiology, and outcomes of patients undergoing surgery for small-bowel obstruction after previous surgery for colorectal cancer were reported.

Methods.—Four hundred seventy-two consecutive patients undergoing surgery for colorectal cancer were studied. Resection was done with curative intent in 351 patients and with palliative intent in 121. The median follow-up was 5.5 years.

Findings.—Surgery was performed for small-bowel obstruction after curative resection in 36 patients (10%) and after palliative surgery in 5 patients (4%). Obstructions were caused by benign adhesions in 21 patients, local recurrence in 17, and peritoneal carcinomatosis in 3. One patient died of myocardial infarction and 6 died of cancer within 30 days of surgery for obstruction. The estimated median survival was 1.9 years after surgery for benign obstruction and 0.36 years after surgery for malignant obstruction. Adhesions were associated with greater blood loss during primary surgery. Obstructive adhesions did not develop in any of the 62 patients who took thiazide diuretics at the time of the primary surgery.

Conclusions.—Small-bowel obstruction developed after primary surgery for colorectal cancer in 9% of these patients. The etiology of obstruction was benign in about half and malignant in the other half. Patients with benign obstruction had a much better survival after surgery than those with malignant obstruction.

▶ This paper emphasizes the need to approach most individuals with late small-bowel obstruction after curative operations for colorectal cancer in an aggressive surgical manner. Approximately 50% of these patients were found to have benign causes of small-bowel obstructions that resolved with operative therapy. However, for patients with known carcinomatosis and extensive disease, it is more appropriate to pursue nonoperative therapy, if at all possible, because the outcome after operation in these patients is dismal.

This article re-emphasizes the high incidence of adhesive disease after colorectal procedures and the need for some form of anti-adhesive therapy. The authors suggest that thiazide diuretics may be such an agent. They found this serendipitously in their review of the relationship between antihypertensives and colorectal cancer. More realistic, however, is the use of anti-adhesive barriers such as carboxymethylcellulose and sodium hyaluronate uronate acid sheets. This may prevent the need for reoperation for small-bowel obstruction in approximately 14% of patients who have undergone operation for colorectal cancer.

J.W. Fleshman, Jr., M.D.

Small Bowel Obstruction After Total or Subtotal Colectomy: A 10-Year Retrospective Review

Nieuwenhuijzen M, Reijnen MMPJ, Kuijpers JHC, et al (Univ Hosp Nijmegen, The Netherlands)

Br J Surg 85:1242-1245, 1998 4–7

Background.—Adhesions are the leading cause of small-bowel obstruction (SBO) and secondary female infertility. Such adhesions may be related to chronic abdominal pain. The cumulative incidence of adhesive SBO

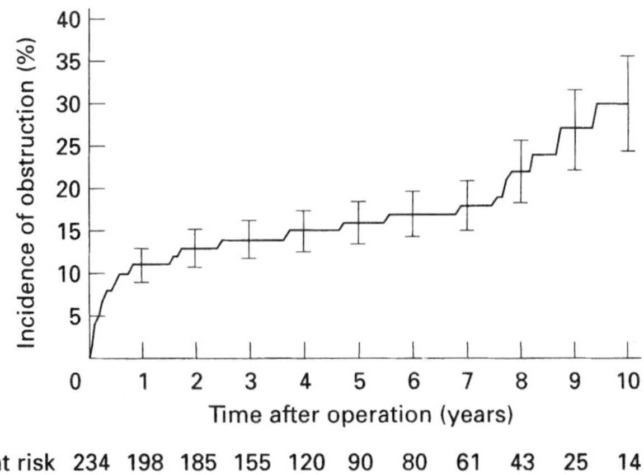

FIGURE 1.—Cumulative incidence of adhesive small-bowel obstruction using the Kaplan-Meier method for time-related incidence. This method adjusts the incidence ratio to account for various lengths of follow-up and losses to follow-up. *Standard error bars* are shown. (Courtesy of Nieuwenhuijzen M, Reijnen MMPJ, Kuijpers JHC, et al: Small bowel obstruction after total or subtotal colectomy: A 10-year retrospective review. *Br J Surg* 85:1242-1245, 1998. Published by Blackwell Science Ltd.)

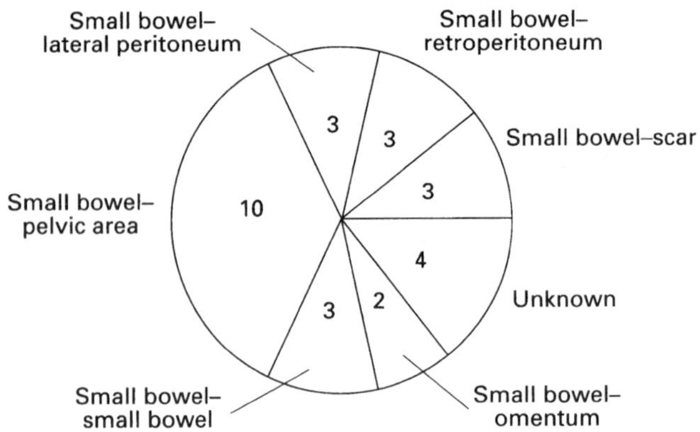

FIGURE 2.—Distribution of adhesions that caused small-bowel obstruction in 28 patients, as identified at laparotomy. (Courtesy of Nieuwenhuijzen M, Reijnen MMPJ, Kuijpers JHC, et al: Small bowel obstruction after total or subtotal colectomy: A 10-year retrospective review. *Br J Surg* 85:1242-1245, 1998. Published by Blackwell Science Ltd.)

after total or subtotal colectomy was determined, and the site of the obstructive adhesions in the abdominal cavity was investigated.

Methods.—The records of 234 patients undergoing colectomy between 1985 and 1994 were reviewed. The mean follow-up was 63 months.

Findings.—Twenty-four percent of the patients were found to have SBO. Eighteen percent had adhesive obstruction. The risk of SBO resulting from adhesions within 1 year was 11%, increasing to 30% 10 years after colectomy. No risk factors were identified for adhesive SBO in a univariate analysis that included previous laparotomy, septic complications, and omental resection. The pelvis was the most common site of obstructing lesions (Figs 1 and 2).

Conclusion.—The incidence of SBO is high after colectomy. This procedure may be a suitable model for studying ways to prevent adhesion.

▶ This retrospective review of a fairly large number of patients undergoing subtotal colectomy reveals that SBO develops in 30% of patients by 10 years after operation. This is a significant finding and suggests that the removal of the abdominal colon is a procedure which is adhesiogenic. Therefore, measures should be taken to avoid the development of adhesions and SBO in the future. In three fourths of all patients, SBO developed because of adhesions and required laparotomy. This is a costly complication of an operation and preventative measures are indicated. I agree with the authors that some form of anti-adhesive therapy should be applied.

J.W. Fleshman, Jr., M.D.

5 The Colon

Introduction

A major portion of this chapter covers several aspects of neoplastic disease seen by the colon and rectal surgeon—screening, postoperative surveillance, and genetic predisposition along with comparative studies of surgical choices and diverse populations. The largest of these studies on invasive colon cancer involves more than 34,000 patients in the United States; other studies included are from Great Britain, The Netherlands, France, and Australia.

The section on inflammatory bowel disease presents surgical, laparoscopic, and medical decisions involved in treating ulcerative colitis and Crohn's disease, including genetic and autoimmune aspects of these related but distinct diseases. The next section addresses some problems encountered when the anorectum fails to function normally, from incontinence and obstruction to hemorrhoids and fissures. Another section concerning dysfunction covers diverticular disease. Two articles address the Hartmann procedure, and a study from Finland discusses when to operate for diverticulosis of the colon to obtain optimal treatment for patients of all ages.

This chapter also presents an assortment of articles on situations or decisions that confront the surgeon, including rectal trauma, colitis, and surgical techniques. A large portion of this section offers various viewpoints and studies on laparoscopic colorectal surgery.

Giuseppe Aliperti, M.D.

Gastrointestinal Infection

Prevalence of Infection With *Cryptosporidium parvum* and *Cyclospora cayetanensis* Among International Travellers

Jelinek T, Lotze M, Eichenlaub S, et al (Univ of Munich)
Gut 41:801-804, 1997 5–1

Background.—Two possible causes of traveler's diarrhea have been recently identified. *Cyclospora cayetanensis* is common in developing countries; for example, in Lima, Peru, almost 1 of every 5 children was found to be infected. *Cryptosporidium parvum* commonly causes diarrhea in immunocompromised patients. It, too, is common in developing countries, accounting for 6.1% of diarrheal illnesses in immunocompetent patients. These authors examined the prevalence of *Cyc. cayetanensis* and *C. parvum* in travelers returning from international vacations.

Methods.—Upon their return home, 975 German citizens who had traveled abroad visited an outpatient clinic because of diarrhea (459 patients, or 59%), fever (167, or 21%), skin problems (83, or 10.4%), or for a medical check-up although they were not experiencing any symptoms (76, or 9.6%). The patients provided 978 stool samples that were examined by microscopy and antigen capture enzyme-linked immunosorbent assay to detect *Cryptosporidium* oocysts.

Findings.—Thirteen patients provided 15 specimens that were positive for *C. parvum* (1.6% of total patients, 2.8% of patients with diarrhea). Five patients provided 5 specimens that were positive for *Cyc. cayetanensis* (0.6% of total patients, 1.1% of patients with diarrhea). All patients with these infections experienced watery diarrhea with or without nausea, anorexia, and itching of the skin. The mean duration of symptoms was 19.8 days in the patients with *C. parvum* infection and 36.2 days in the patients with *Cyc. cayetanensis* infection. Microscopy was markedly more sensitive than antigen capture enzyme-linked immunosorbent assay in detecting *C. parvum* in stool (93% vs. 67%). Stool examination revealed the presence of other parasites in 201 patients (25.3%), most commonly *Giardia duodenalis* (74 patients), *Entamoeba dispar/histolytica* (74 patients), and *Blastocystis hominis* (73 patients).

Conclusions.—Given their low prevalences in these patients, neither *C. parvum* nor *Cyc. cayetanensis* seems to be a major cause of traveler's diarrhea. Nonetheless, for patients who experience prolonged, unexplained watery diarrhea after traveling abroad, the differential diagnosis should include these 2 pathogens.

Risk Factors for and Prevention of Sporadic Infections With Vero Cytotoxin (Shiga Toxin) Producing *Escherichia coli* 0157

Parry SM, Salmon RL, Willshaw GA, et al (Welsh Combined Centres for Public Health, Cardiff, Wales; Abton House, Cardiff, Wales; Central Public Health Lab, London)

Lancet 351:1019-1022, 1998 5–2

Background.—Worldwide, vero cytotoxins (shiga toxins) producing *Escherichia coli* O157 (VTEC O157) are becoming a recognized foodborne pathogen. Most of the current information about VTEC O157 comes from studies during outbreaks. These authors examined foodborne, person-to-person, and zoonotic transmission of VTEC O157 in sporadic cases in Wales.

Methods.—Eighty-five people who had experienced sporadic infection with VTEC O157 over 2 years were identified. One or 2 age- and sex-matched controls were selected for each patient from the patient's physician's practice list, for a total of 142 controls. All participants were questioned about exposures to food, animals, farms, and other factors (e.g., day care, bathing in recreational waters, etc.) for 7 days before the onset of symptoms (for patients) or during the same period (for controls). When patients reported eating beef burgers or cooked sliced meats from a catering establishment or having contact with a farm, the authors visited the site to examine its cooking and animal-handling policies.

Findings.—One of the catering establishments visited by patients was a national fast-food chain with a policy ensuring that beef burgers were cooked thoroughly. When this restaurant was removed from the analysis, VTEC O157 infection was significantly associated with eating a beef burger prepared in a commercial (relative risk [RR], 4.63) or mobile (RR, 2.33) site. Eating any cold, loose, cooked, sliced meat from a catering site (not from a butcher, supermarket deli counter, or general store) was significantly associated with VTEC O157 infection (RR, 3.36). Furthermore, patients were significantly more likely than controls to have farm exposure (e.g., a household member who worked with farm animals or had contact with farm animal manure; RR, 2.71). Other environmental exposures that were significantly associated with VTEC O157 infection included travel for 1 night or more within the United Kingdom (RR, 8.50) or abroad (RR, 3.40), contact with a household member who had had diarrheal illness 5 days or less before the patient's symptom onset (RR, 6.83), and bathing in an outdoor swimming pool (RR, 6.50).

Conclusions.—Foodborne, person-to-person, and zoonotic transmission of VTEC O157 can occur. The national chain restaurant with policies to ensure thorough cooking of beef burgers required cooking the burger from the top and bottom simultaneously for 44 or 122 seconds (depending on thickness) determined by a timer. Ensuring that catering establishments thoroughly cook their beef burgers is critical to reducing the risk of VTEC O157 transmission. Educating the public to send back undercooked, pink beef burgers, and to be aware of situations in which person-to-person and zoonotic spreads are more likely, is also helpful.

A Foodborne Outbreak of Cyclosporiasis Caused by Imported Raspberries

Cáceres VM, Ball RT, Somerfeldt SA, et al (Ctrs for Disease Control and Prevention, Atlanta, Ga; South Carolina Dept of Health & Enviromental Control, Columbia)

J Fam Pract 47:231-234, 1998 5–3

Background.—Cyclosporiasis is characterized by prolonged diarrhea, fatigue, and weight loss. Previous studies have implicated waterborne transmission of *Cyclospora cayetanensis* as the cause of the illness. This article implicates the foodborne transmission of this parasite in contaminated raspberries.

Methods.—Several attendees at a luncheon near Charleston, SC, on May 23, 1996, reported a prolonged diarrheal illness for which no cause could be identified by routine stool examinations. The South Carolina

Department of Health and Environmental Control questioned all 64 attendees and the chef about exposure to food and beverages. A case was defined as the onset of diarrhea (3 or more loose stools per day, or 2 or more loose stools per day if the attendee was using antimotility agents) after attending the luncheon. The Department of Health and Environmental Control also identified 6 other sporadic cases of cyclosporiasis between late May and early June.

Findings.—More than half (38 of 64, or 59%) the luncheon attendees met the case definition. The illness had a median incubation of 7 days and lasted 2 or more weeks. It caused symptoms of diarrhea in 100% of the patients, fatigue in 79%, weight loss in 61%, and abdominal pain in 55%. Attendees who ate raspberries (relative risk [RR], 5.4), strawberries (RR, 2.3), or potato salad (RR, 1.8) were at significantly increased risk of illness. Statistical analysis controlling for exposure to raspberries indicated that exposure to strawberries was no longer a significant risk factor, but exposure to potato salad still was (although the RR was decreased to 1.5). Some of the attendees provided stool samples; none of the samples from 6 healthy attendees was positive for *Cyclospora*, but oocysts were found in 11 samples from 13 patients (85%). Community surveillance of this cluster of outbreaks and the 6 sporadic cases revealed that the contaminated raspberries had originated in Guatemala.

Conclusions.—The transmission of *Cyclospora* via raspberries was strongly implicated in this outbreak of cyclosporiasis. In recent years the incidence of cyclosporiasis in the United States has been increasing. The more frequent importation of foods may play a role in this increased rate. Cyclosporiasis should be part of the differential diagnosis for patients who experience prolonged, unexplained diarrhea.

First Reported Outbreak in the United States of Cryptosporidiosis Associated With a Recreational Lake

Kramer MH, Sorhage FE, Goldstein ST, et al (Ctrs for Disease Control and Prevention, Atlanta, Ga; New Jersey Dept of Health, Trenton)
Clin Infect Dis 26:27-33, 1998 5–4

Background.—Outbreaks of *Cryptosporidium parvum* have been associated with exposure to contaminated drinking water and water from swimming pools and parks. These authors describe an outbreak of *C. parvum* associated with exposure to contaminated lake water.

Methods.—In the summer of 1994, the New Jersey State Department of Health identified an outbreak of cryptosporidiosis among people who had swum in a state park lake. A press release prompted 426 people who had suffered gastrointestinal illness after visiting the park to contact a health department. From this list, 185 persons who reported a single park visit were enrolled in a cohort study (median age, 33.5; 34.1% were children; 53.5% were female). These participants or their proxies answered questions about whether they had had contact with lake water, whether they had consumed food or water while at the park, whether they had experienced any gastrointestinal illness after their visit, and whether they had had other exposures that could have caused the gastrointestinal illness. A confirmed case was noted when the patient developed gastrointestinal symptoms within 2 to 14 days after visiting the park and had a positive stool specimen for *Cryptosporidium*. A probable case was noted when the patient developed diarrhea within 2 to 14 days after visiting the park and when the diarrhea lasted 2 days or more.

Findings.—Among the cohort, 4 people had confirmed cryptosporidiosis and 34 had probable cryptosporidiosis, for a total of 38 cases (20.5%). Compared with people who had had no exposure to lake water, people who had had any exposure had a significantly elevated risk of cryptosporidiosis (relative risk [RR], 11.05). The risks were particularly elevated for facial contact with lake water (RR, 9.23), oral contact (RR, 16.30), and a duration of contact > 30 minutes (RR, 19.23). Water samples taken at various times and sites from the lake indicated that the outbreak lasted 4 weeks and was most likely caused by contaminated runoff of rainwater from an area where the septic tank had backed up. Also, anecdotal evidence suggested that the sources of contamination were infected people (especially children wearing diapers) going into the water and people rinsing soiled diapers in the water.

Conclusions.—This is the first documented outbreak of cryptosporidiosis associated with recreational lake water in the United States. Thus, people at high risk for severe cryptosporidiosis, such as people with acquired immunodeficiency syndrome, must be made aware that exposure to recreational lake water can be a source of *Cryptosporidium* infection. Public education efforts should include posting signs that warn against drinking lake water and against defecating or rinsing diapers in lake water. Furthermore, lake recreational areas must provide adequate toilet, handwashing, and diaper-changing facilities to avoid contamination of the lake water.

► The safety of our food supply has become a national issue. Outbreaks of *Escherichia coli* 0157, resulting in deaths when undercooked beef burgers or unpasteurized apple juice were ingested, may have changed our eating habits. The risk of contracting *E. coli* 0157 infection was re-examined in a case-controlled study of sporadic *E. coli* 0157 infection in the United Kingdom. Parry et al. (Abstract 5–2) found that *E. coli* resulting from consumption of cooked, sliced meat from caterers was related to food handling but not to the butchers. *E. coli* was not found to result from ingesting hamburgers from fast food chains, because the chains ensured adequate cooking. Therefore, along with ingestion of undercooked ground beef, food handling is now considered a source of contamination with *E. coli* 0157.

Cyclospora ingestion may cause prolonged diarrhea, fatigue, and weight loss, for which there is effective treatment (trimethoprim sulfamethoxazole). Cyclospora may be acquired from ingestion of fruits such as raspberries (Abstract 5–3). Unfortunately it can also be contracted from a contaminated drinking water supply, as well as water in recreational lakes, swimming pools, and water parks (Abstract 5–4). This, like *Cryptosporidium parvum* should be sought as an offending agent in travelers' diarrhea (Abstract 5–1).

J.S. Barkin, M.D.

Crohn's Disease

Conflicting Results of Ileoscopy and Small Bowel Double-Contrast Barium Examination in Patients With Crohn's Disease

Tribl B, Turetschek K, Mostbeck G, et al (Univ of Vienna, Austria)
Endoscopy 30:339-344, 1998 5–5

Introduction.—Ileoscopy is widely used to inspect the terminal ileum in patients with suspected Crohn's disease (CD). Although barium studies are regarded as highly accurate in the diagnosis of terminal ileitis, endoscopic and/or histologic verification are lacking. Small bowel barium studies and ileoscopy were compared for diagnostic performance in patients with CD of the terminal ileum.

Methods.—The retrospective study included 55 patients with confirmed CD who underwent successful ileocolonoscopic and barium examinations within 1 month. There were 34 women and 21 men (median age, 26 years) in the study. First, the routine radiologic reports were compared with the ileoscopy findings. The barium films were then interpreted in blinded fashion on 2 occasions by 2 expert gastrointestinal radiologists, who scored the quality of the examination. This permitted assessment of the effects of image quality on diagnostic information, as well as interobserver and intraobserver variation.

Results.—Based on the routine radiology reports, barium studies had a sensitivity of 66% and specificity of 82% for inflammatory changes of the terminal ileum. In the expert radiologist study, sensitivity improved to 68% and specificity to 91%. Disagreement between the endoscopic and radiologic findings decreased from 31% in the first part of the analysis to 27% in the second, mainly reflecting the influence of false-negative barium studies. High-quality barium studies were associated with a sensitivity of 91% and specificity of 100%.

Conclusions.—In patients with CD of the terminal ileum, ileoscopy offers superior diagnostic performance to barium examination. However, barium studies still have an important role, and their sensitivity and specificity are high if the studies are of good quality. The radiologic report should include information about the quality of the barium study.

Adult Crohn Disease: Can Ileoscopy Replace Small Bowel Radiology?

Halligan S, Saunders B, Williams C, et al (St Mark's Hosp, Middlesex, England)
Abdom Imaging 23:117-121, 1998 5–6

Objective.—In the diagnosis of Crohn's disease (CD), ileoscopy may help to avoid the need for radiologic examination, or selective studies that

TABLE 2.—Severity of Small Bowel CD Related to Disease Site

Disease Site	Disease Stage Early	Advanced	Early + Advanced
Proximal (n = 18)	12	3	3
Ileum (n = 38)	6	12	20
Terminal ileum (n = 62)	12	29	21

(Courtesy of Halligan S, Saunders B, Williams C, et al: Adult Crohn disease: Can ileoscopy replace small bowel radiology? *Abdom Imaging* 23:117-121, 1998.)

use visualization of the distal ileum may replace total small bowel radiology. Various techniques of small bowel radiology have been proposed, including infusion methods and conventional barium follow-through (BaFT). Using the BaFT technique, the radiologic features and distribution of small bowel CD were analyzed.

Methods.—The retrospective study included the BaFT studies of 121 adult patients with confirmed CD (median age, 33 years). The reviewers reached a consensus regarding the presence and staging of small bowel CD in the proximal, mid ileal, and terminal ileal areas. Thirty-seven patients underwent colonoscopy with attempted ileoscopy. In this group, the BaFT and ileoscopic results were compared (Table 2 and Table 3).

Results.—Seventy-four percent of BaFT studies showed a normal villous pattern. In 59% of patients, BaFT led to the diagnosis of small bowel CD. In 87% of patients with small bowel CD, the terminal ileum was involved. However, almost two thirds of patients had more proximal small bowel involvement, including 13% with normal findings in the terminal ileum. Seventy-three percent of patients had early mucosal changes consistent with CD; in 21%, these changes were the only sign of CD.

Ileal intubation was not achieved in 38% of patients undergoing colonoscopy. Of these 14 patients, 9 had CD on BaFT. When ileoscopy was successfully carried out, the results agreed with those of BaFT in 96% of cases. The BaFT studies played an important role in the decision to perform surgery.

Conclusions.—In adult patients with small bowel CD, BaFT studies provide important information on the stage and extent of disease. Because most patients have disease proximal to the terminal ileum, reliance on

TABLE 3.—Findings at Attempted Ileoscopy in 37 Patients With CD

Small Bowel Disease on Follow Through	Ileoscopy During Colonoscopy, n (%) Possible	Not Possible
Present	14 (38)	9 (24)
Absent	9 (24)	5 (14)
Total	23 (62)	14 (38)

(Courtesy of Halligan S, Saunders B, Williams C, et al: Adult Crohn disease: Can ileoscopy replace small bowel radiology? *Abdom Imaging* 23:117-121, 1998.)

ileoscopy without small bowel radiologic studies would underestimate the extent of CD or miss the diagnosis in many patients. Among patients undergoing colonoscopy, ileoscopy is not always possible.

▶ Diagnosing small bowel involvement in inflammatory bowel disease is a critical element in distinguishing Crohn's disease from ulcerative colitis and in the care of patients with Crohn's disease. These conflicting studies (Abstracts 5–5 and 5–6) address the reliability of ileoscopy compared to dedicated small bowel follow through in diagnosing small bowel Crohn's disease. These studies, each supportive of a differing approach, may be somewhat reconciled. The study supportive of ileoscopy (Tribl et al.) subgroups small bowel follow-throughs (SBFTs) by quality of exam. In those studies that were technically good and reevaluated by 2 gastrointestinal radiologists, the specificity and sensitivity was extremely high, appearing at least as reliable as the other study suggested. In addition, in the study by Halligan et al., a sizable proportion of patients (13%) had normal terminal ileums by both modalities, but had more proximal small bowel disease identified only by SBFT. False negatives were also noted in SBFT compared with active disease found on ileoscopy, even in some patients with severe disease. Both modalities may provide complementary information although with much overlap. This does not imply that all patients need both studies. Either, if done adequately, may be sufficient. But both tests should be interpreted with skepticism to determine if further evaluation is needed.

G. Aliperti, M.D.

Budesonide Versus Prednisone in the Treatment of Active Crohn's Disease

Bar-Meir S, and the Israeli Budesonide Study Group (Chaim Sheba Med Ctr, Tel Hashomer, Israel; et al)

Gastroenterology 115:835-840, 1998 5–7

Purpose.—Because of its extensive first-pass metabolism, budesonide is a promising treatment for Crohn's disease (CD). Studies using a pH-dependent budesonide preparation that releases the drug into the terminal ileum and ascending colon have shown budesonide effectively treats active CD. This study compared budesonide and prednisone for the treatment of active CD involving the terminal ileum, colon, or both.

Methods.—The randomized, double-blind trial included 201 adult patients with mild to moderate active CD involving the terminal ileum, colon, or both. One group received budesonide, 9 mg once daily for 8 weeks; the other received prednisone once daily for 2 weeks, tapering thereafter to 5 mg/day. In a double-dummy design, patients in the budesonide group received prednisone placebo, and vice-versa. The 2 treatments were compared for their effects on disease activity, quality of life, and laboratory parameters, including osteocalcin as an indicator of bone metabolism. The study definition of treatment efficacy was a Crohn's Disease Activity Index of less than 150.

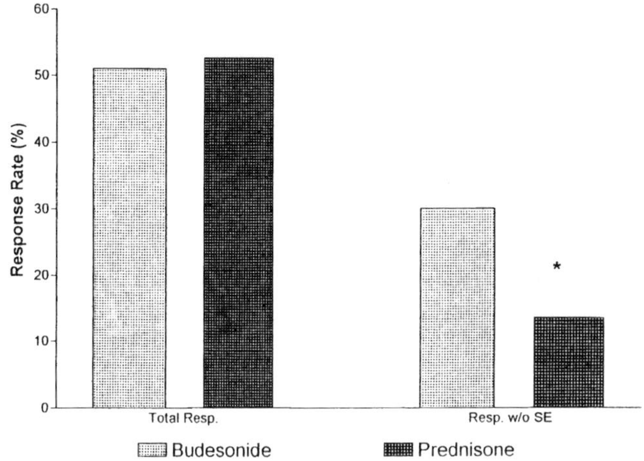

FIGURE 1.—Efficacy results and steroid side effects with PRED and BUD therapy. *$P = 0.006$, 90% confidence interval (two-sided). Difference in response rate, 1.48%; lower limit, −13.07; upper limit, 10.12; $P = 0.8881$. (Courtesy of Bar-Meir S, and the Israeli Budesonide Study Group: Budesonide versus prednisone in the treatment of active Crohn's disease. *Gastroenterology* 115:835-840, 1998.)

Results.—Treatment efficacy was reached in 51% of the budesonide group and 52.5% of the prednisone group. On analysis of patients who completed 8 weeks of treatment, the treatment efficacy rate was 64.9% and 61.5%, respectively. Side effects were significantly more common with prednisone: the percentage of treatment responders without side effects was 30% with budesonide vs. 14% with prednisone (Fig 1). More than 80% of the reduction in Crohn's disease activity scores took place in the first 2 weeks of treatment. The 2 groups had similar results on quality-of-life and laboratory examinations.

Conclusions.—For patients with active CD involving the terminal ileum and right colon, budesonide is as effective as prednisone, but with fewer steroid side effects. Among treatment responders, side effects are about half as frequent with budesonide as with prednisone. The observed lack of difference in quality of life may result from the short duration of the study.

Budesonide Enema for the Treatment of Active, Distal Ulcerative Colitis and Proctitis: A Dose-Ranging Study

Hanauer SB, for the Budesonide Enema Study Group (Univ of Chicago; Univ of Oklahoma, Oklahoma City; Nashville Med Research Inst, Tenn; et al)
Gastroenterology 115:525-532, 1998 5–8

Background.—Because of its high first-pass hepatic metabolism, budesonide treatment for various conditions offers good efficacy with a low rate of side effects. Budesonide suspension enema formulation, which can deliver drug to the distal colon, has been as effective as other steroid and mesalamine enemas. This randomized, placebo-controlled trial compared

3 different doses of budesonide enema preparation for patients with active distal ulcerative colitis or proctitis.

Methods.—The study included 233 adult patients with active, distal ulcerative colitis with a sigmoidoscopic inflammation grade score of 2 or greater. They were assigned to receive either a placebo enema or 1 of 3 doses of budesonide enema: 0.5, 2.0, or 8.0 mg/100 mL. All enemas were given once daily at bedtime for 6 weeks. The treatments were compared for their effect on sigmoidoscopic inflammation grade, total histopathology score, and remission rates.

Results.—The 2.0 and 8.0 mg doses of budesonide offered significantly greater improvement in sigmoidoscopy and histopathology scores than placebo. The remission rate was 19% for patients receiving the 2.0 mg dose and 27% for those receiving the 8.0 mg dose, compared with 7% for those receiving the 0.5 mg dose and 4% for those receiving placebo. At last follow-up, the adrenocorticotropin-stimulated cortisol response was normal in 90% of patients receiving budesonide. There were no significant differences in adverse events between groups.

Conclusions.—This trial demonstrates the safety and efficacy of budesonide enema for patients with active distal ulcerative colitis or proctitis. Budesonide enemas are safe and well tolerated, with little effect on the hypothalamic-pituitary-adrenal axis. The lowest effective dose appears to be 2.0 mg/100 mL budesonide.

▶ Glucocorticosteroids remain a pillar of therapy in inflammatory bowel disease despite their association with a high burden of adverse effects that make them unpopular among many patients and physicians despite their efficacy. The search for a more user-friendly steroid has promoted budesonide in a number of promising trials. Budesonide has a high first-pass metabolism with low oral availability (11% for budesonide vs. 80% for prednisone) producing a largely topical benefit with presumably lower systemic toxicity. These recent studies (Abstracts 5–7 and 5–8) have further defined the benefits and risks of budesonide in inflammatory bowel disease. In the study by Bar-Meir et al. (Abstract 5–7), budesonide, delivered principally to the terminal ileum and ascending colon by a pH-sensitive preparation, demonstrated equivalent efficacy to prednisone for disease in the ascending colon or terminal ileum. A significant few with left-sided disease responded in the budesonide group. Fewer side effects were noted, although principally a decrease in moon faces, buffalo hump, and acne, while other side effects were noted in this 8-week study. Budesonide enemas tested in 3 doses against placebo demonstrated a statistically significant response, although not dramatically robust remission rates of 27% in the highest dose studied. Little effect was noted on the hypothalamic-pituitary-adrenal axis. Budesonide represents an advance, but is only a small step forward. With many patients either not responding or becoming dependent on steroids, alternatives to steroids, of any kind, offer a more promising long-term path.

G. Aliperti, M.D.

A Short-term Study of Chimeric Monoclonal Antibody cA2 to Tumor Necrosis Factor α for Crohn's Disease

Targan SR, for the Crohn's Disease cA2 Study Group (Cedars-Sinai Med Ctr, Los Angeles; et al)

N Engl J Med 337:1029-1035, 1997 5–9

Background.—Tumor necrosis factor α (TNF-α) seems to play a role in the pathogenesis of Crohn's disease, and thus antibodies to TNF-α might

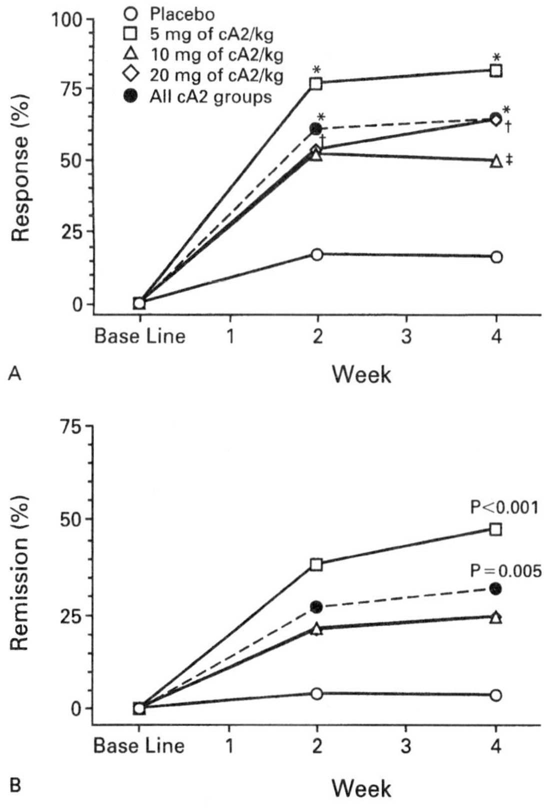

No. of Patients Evaluated

Placebo	25	24	24
5 mg of cA2/kg	27	26	27
10 mg of cA2/kg	28	23	28
20 mg of cA2/kg	28	28	28
All cA2 groups	83	77	83

FIGURE 1.—Rates of clinical response and remission after a single infusion of cA2 or placebo. Clinical remission was defined as a score of less than 150 on the Crohn's Disease Activity Index and a score of 170 to 190 on the Inflammatory Bowel Disease Questionnaire. The *asterisks* ($P < 0.001$), *daggers* ($P < 0.01$), and *double dagger* ($P < 0.05$) indicate a significant difference from placebo. (Reprinted by permission from *The New England Journal of Medicine* from Targan SR, for the Crohn's Disease cA2 Study Group: A short-term study of chimeric monoclonal antibody cA2 to tumor necrosis factor α for Crohn's disease. *N Engl J Med* 337:1029-1035. Copyright 1997, Massachusetts Medical Society. All rights reserved.)

help in treating the disease. These authors studied the effectiveness of chimeric monoclonal antibody cA2 (infliximab) in treating patients with active Crohn's disease.

Methods.—The subjects were 108 patients with Crohn's disease who had not responded to medical treatment. Crohn's Disease Activity Index (CDAI) scores were between 200 and 400 (on a scale of 0 to about 600, with 600 representing the most severe illness), indicating moderate to severe disease. Patients were randomized into 4 groups to receive either placebo (n = 25; 15 men and 10 women; mean age, 38.5 years) or cA2 at doses of 5 mg/kg (n = 27; 14 men and 13 women; mean age, 37 years), 10 mg/kg (n = 28; 13 men and 15 women; mean age, 39.3 years), or 20 mg/kg (n = 28; 13 men and 15 women; mean age, 36 years). Drugs were infused over 2 hours, and clinical and immunologic responses were assessed for 12 weeks after administration. Clinical response was defined as a reduction in the CDAI score of 70 points or more without a concomitant change in medications. Remission was defined as a reduction in the CDAI score to less than 150.

Findings.—At 4 weeks, clinical responses in the patients receiving 5, 10, or 20 mg/kg of cA2 were significantly higher than in those receiving placebo (81%, 50%, and 64% vs. 17%) (Fig 1). Similarly, at 12 weeks, clinical responses in the patients receiving 5, 10, or 20 mg/kg of cA2 were significantly higher than in those receiving placebo (48%, 29%, and 46% vs. 12%). At 4 weeks, significantly more of the patients receiving cA2 achieved remission than did patients receiving placebo (33% vs. 4%). At 12 weeks, however, there was no significant difference in remission rates between the cA2 and placebo groups (24% vs. 8%). The frequency of adverse effects (mainly headache, nausea, and upper respiratory tract infection) did not differ between the cA2 and placebo groups, with rates between 60% and 79%.

Conclusions.—In these patients with moderate to severe Crohn's disease that was refractory to other medical therapies, a single infusion of cA2 quickly and significantly improved the clinical response for up to 12 weeks. In all, 65% of the patients receiving cA2 experienced either a clinical response or remission. The 5 mg/kg dose of cA2 was more effective than larger doses.

▶ This landmark article ushers in a new era for the treatment of Crohn's disease. Infliximab is the first of a number of biotech agents that are based on translating the tremendous advances in bench research in inflammation and immunology into useful medications. However, the article raises as many questions as it answers. Even questions concerning infliximab's mechanisms of action need to be investigated to yield further insights into Crohn's disease as well as to improve therapy further. Central issues in the practical use of this promising agent remain, particularly with regard to its long-term efficacy and toxicity as well as the subgroup of patients for whom this therapy should be reserved. The dosing regimen needs clarification as well. Although in this study three different doses were tested and 5 mg/kg appears preferable, the groups are small and available data suggest that whereas more is not necessarily better, some patients may require higher doses. This issue is being addressed in ongoing studies. Although the side effect profile appears generally low, an identified risk of immune alterations (lupuslike reactions, infectious complications, delayed hypersensitivity reactions) exists. Other issues need to be better understood as experience with this medication grows; for instance, the significance of human antichimeric antibodies (HACA or antibodies to the TNF antibody) is uncertain. Concern over lymphoma in relation to the medication might or might not be warranted but ought not be dismissed at this point altogether. Given the relatively small number of patients studied with the drug, a cautious approach is warranted. This article, in conjunction with the similarly impressive study of infliximab in fistulous disease, has brought rapid FDA approval, but numerous issues remain to clarify our use of this medication. The most pressing questions concern the selection of patients for use now inasmuch as results of studies of long-term efficacy are several years away. At this point, use of infliximab ought to be reserved for patients with moderate to severe disease in whom other therapies have failed or as a bridge to initiating azathioprine/6-MP therapy. Approval by the FDA is for short-term therapy only, and re-treatment raises significant other problems best guided by a highly conservative approach as well.

G. Aliperti, M.D.

Mesalamine in the Maintenance Treatment of Crohn's Disease: A Meta-analysis Adjusted for Confounding Variables

Cammá C, Giunta M, Rosselli M, et al (Consiglio Nazionale delle Richerche, Palermo, Italy; Univ of Palermo, Italy)

Gastroenterology 113:1465-1473, 1997 5–10

Background.—The benefits of mesalamine for the maintenance of Crohn's disease remission have not been established definitively. The efficacy of mesalamine in maintaining such remission was further investigated in a literature review.

Methods and Findings.—Fifteen randomized, controlled studies involving a total of 2,097 patients were analyzed. Mesalamine treatment significantly decreased the risk of a symptomatic relapse. In a postoperative setting, the pooled risk difference was significant; however, it was not significant in a medical setting. A multivariate model predicted that the probability of symptomatic relapse would decline significantly with mesalamine therapy, by increasing the proportion of patients with ileal disease, prolonged disease duration, and operatively induced remission.

Conclusions.—This literature review indicates that mesalamine may be recommended for maintaining Crohn's remission. The benefits occur primarily in the postoperative setting, in patients with ileitis, and in patients with a prolonged duration of disease.

The Safety of Mesalamine in Human Pregnancy: A Prospective Controlled Cohort Study

Diav-Citrin O, Park Y-H, Veerasuntharam G, et al (Hosp for Sick Children, Toronto; Univ of Toronto)

Gastroenterology 114:23-28, 1998 5–11

Background.—Mesalamine, a first-line drug in the treatment of inflammatory bowel disease, is commonly used in women of childbearing age. However, little is known about its safety during pregnancy.

Methods.—One hundred sixty-five women exposed to mesalamine during pregnancy were prospectively enrolled in the study and followed up. One hundred forty-six women had been exposed to this agent in the first trimester. Pregnancy outcomes were compared with those in a matched control group.

Findings.—Major malformations occurred in 0.8% of the infants in the mesalamine group and in 3.8% of infants in the control group. The mesalamine group had an increase in the rate of preterm deliveries as compared with the control group (13% vs. 4.7%, respectively), a decline in mean maternal weight gain during pregnancy as compared with the control group (13.1 vs. 15.6 kg, respectively), and a reduction in the infants' mean birth weight as compared with the control group (3,253 vs. 3,461 g, respectively). The 2 groups did not differ in maternal obstetric histories, live birth rates, miscarriages, pregnancy terminations, ectopic pregnancies, delivery method, or incidences of fetal distress.

Conclusions.—When used at the recommended dose, mesalamine apparently does not represent a major teratogenic risk in humans. However, continuing surveillance of pregnancy outcomes after exposure to mesalamine is warranted.

A Comparison of Budesonide and Mesalamine for Active Crohn's Disease

Thomsen OØ, for the International Budesonide–Mesalamine Study Group (Univ of Copenhagen; et al)

N Engl J Med 339:370-374, 1998 5–12

Introduction.—A chronic inflammatory disorder of the bowel whose cause is unknown, Crohn's disease is often treated with glucocorticoids such as prednisolone and prednisone. These drugs, however, can cause moon face, hirsutism, and acne. A highly potent topical anti-inflammatory agent with lower systemic activity than conventional glucocorticoids is budesonide. It was found to be significantly more effective than placebo in inducing remission of active Crohn's disease affecting the ileum and ascending colon. In patients with mild to moderately active Crohn's disease, slow-release formulations of mesalamine that facilitate delivery of the drug to the small intestine are often used as first-line treatment, although results in controlled studies were conflicting.

Methods.—There were 182 patients with Crohn's disease who were randomly assigned to receive 9 mg of budesonide (93 patients) daily or 2 g of mesalamine twice daily (89 patients) for 16 weeks in a double-blind, multicenter trial. The patients had scores of 200 to 400 on the Crohn's Disease Activity Index, and higher scores indicate greater disease activity.

Results.—In the budesonide group, the rate of remission after 8 weeks of treatment was 69%, and in the mesalamine group, the rate of remission was 45%. After 16 weeks of treatment, the rate of remission for the budesonide group was 62%, and for the mesalamine group, it was 36%. In the budesonide group, 77 patients completed the 16 weeks of treatment, whereas, in the mesalamine group, 50 patients completed 16 weeks of treatment. In the 2 groups, the numbers of patients with adverse events were similar, but fewer severe adverse events occurred in the group assigned to budesonide therapy. In 67% of the patients treated with budesonide, the morning plasma cortisol value was normal, whereas 83% of the patients treated with mesalamine had normal morning plasma cortisol values. Normal increases in cortisol in response to cosyntropin occurred in 90% of the budesonide group and in 100% of the mesalamine group.

Conclusion.—A controlled-ileal-release formulation of budesonide was more effective in inducing remission than a slow-release formulation of mesalamine in patients with active Crohn's disease affecting the ileum, the ascending colon, or both.

▶ Mesalamine (5-aminosalicylic acid) is the first-line drug for patients with both Crohn's disease and ulcerative colitis. Unfortunately, there is a 40% rate of symptomatic relapse over 2 years in patients with Crohn's disease. Cammá et al. (Abstract 5–10) confirmed mesalamine's efficacy for Crohn's disease by a meta-analysis study. Overall, mesalamine is effective, but the risk of symptomatic relapse was reduced mainly in patients with ileitis, those with surgically induced remission, and those with prolonged disease duration. Because Crohn's disease occurs in younger individuals, it is evident that we will have to decide whether we should continue mesalamine therapy during a patient's pregnancy. Diav-Citrin et al. (Abstract 5–11), in a prospective, controlled cohort study, found that mesalamine does not represent a major teratogenic risk when used in clinically recommended doses in humans. It is hoped that its use will control active inflammatory bowel disease during pregnancy, which is associated with low birth weight, higher rates of prematurity, and perinatal complications.

Patients with more severe inflammatory bowel disease are frequently treated with prednisone; however, because of its side effects such as moon face, hirsutism and acne, its use in younger individuals may be limited. Thomsen et al. (Abstract 5–12) compared budesonide, which is a potent topical glucocorticoid with lower systemic activity than conventional glucocorticoids, to mesalamine in patients with active Crohn's disease. Budesonide had fewer side effects than systemic glucocorticoids, was more effective for patients with Crohn's disease, and had half the dropout rate for uncontrolled symptoms. Therefore, in patients with Crohn's disease, we need to initiate mesalamine and continue its use during a patient's pregnancy, and, in patients with severe disease, we should probably embrace budesonide when it becomes available in the U.S. market.

J.S. Barkin, M.D.

Intra-abdominal and Pelvic Abscess in Crohn's Disease: Results of Non-invasive and Surgical Management

Jawhari A, Kamm MA, Ong C, et al (St. Mark's Hosp, Harrow, England)
Br J Surg 85:367-371, 1998 5–13

Background.—Ten percent to 30% of patients with Crohn's disease have intra-abdominal and pelvic abscesses. The clinical characteristics and outcomes of patients with such abscesses secondary to Crohn's disease were investigated.

Methods.—Thirty-six patients with Crohn's-related intra-abdominal or pelvic abscess seen between 1991 and 1994 were included in the analysis. Their medical records were reviewed and data on management and outcomes obtained.

Findings.—Fifteen patients were considerd candidates for initial percutaneous drainage. Drainage was technically possible in 8 patients and failed in 4. In 2 patients, this procedure yielded good long-term outcomes. Another patient had a recurrence after 3 years. Twenty-eight patients underwent surgery. Only 4 required a stoma. Twelve had complications. At the 3-month follow-up assessment, 22 of the 36 patients were in remission.

Conclusion.—Intra-abdominal abscesses in patients with Crohn's disease are associated with high morbidity. Percutaneous drainage can be done in selected patients without increasing morbidity, sometimes resulting in the resolution of abscess.

► The use of percutaneous drainage of intra-abdominal abscesses to allow improved resection and improved operative outcome is supported by this article from St. Mark's Hospital in England. This policy follows very closely the policy used in many colorectal surgery units in the United States. The main difference between this report and our policy of treatment at Washington University is our use of total parenteral nutrition and bowel rest along with percutaneous drainage. In doing so, the pericolic and peri-intestinal inflammation are markedly reduced, and a resection becomes much easier. The abdominal cavity is easily approached and the resection is limited to only the primarily affected intestine rather than the intestine secondarily inflamed by purulent disease.

The authors even present a small group of patients who avoided surgery even though the inflammatory bowel disease persisted. This is something to consider for future study because there is no indication of the type of patient likely to respond to the use of percutaneous drainage and medical therapy as primary therapy.

J.W. Fleshman, Jr., M.D.

Oral Contraceptive Use and Smoking Are Risk Factors for Relapse in Crohn's Disease

Timmer A, and The Canadian Mesalamine for Remission of Crohn's Disease Study Group (Univ of Calgary, Alberta, Canada)

Gastroenterology 144:1143-1150, 1998 5–14

Background.—Lifestyle factors are known to affect the prognosis of Crohn's disease. This prospective study assessed the effects of smoking and oral contraceptive (OC) use on clinical relapse rates.

Methods and Findings.—One hundred fifty-two patients were included in the study. Patients were followed for 48 weeks or until relapse. Relapse occurred in 40%. In a univariate analysis, outcomes were unfavorable for women, current smokers, and OC users. Reduced risk of relapse was associated with recent surgery. A Cox model indicated a 2.1 hazard ratio for current smoking vs. never smoking, a 3.0 hazard ratio for OC use, and a 2.1 hazard ratio for medical compared with surgical induction of remission as predictors of relapse. The risk of relapse was not increased in former smokers. Sex, age, length of remission, disease location, and disease duration were nonsignificant predictors (Figs 1-3).

Conclusion.—Smoking and OC use are associated with an increased risk of relapse in patients with Crohn's disease. Women with Crohn's disease who are using OCs should be advised against smoking. The use of OCs by such patients should be reviewed on an individual basis.

▶ The relationship between smoking, OCs, and Crohn's disease is an interesting one. For surgeons, the issue is how to prevent postoperative recurrence of disease in patients. Proactive administration of prophylactic pentasa

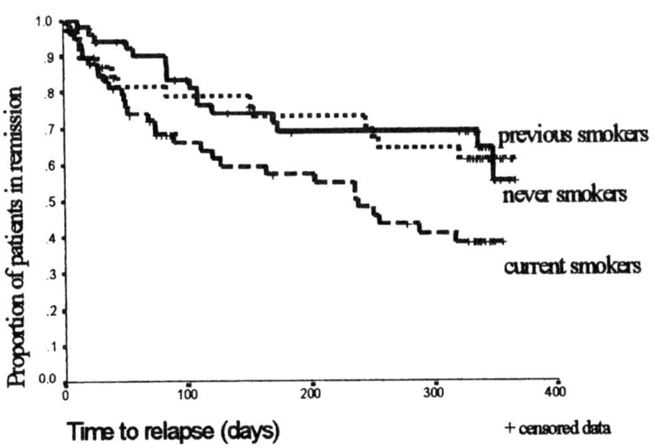

FIGURE 1.—Kaplan-Meier survival curves for relapse by smoking status. (Courtesy of Timmer A, and The Canadian Mesalamine for Remission of Crohn's Disease Study Group: Oral contraceptive use and smoking are risk factors for relapse in Crohn's disease. *Gastroenterology* 144:1143-1150, 1998.)

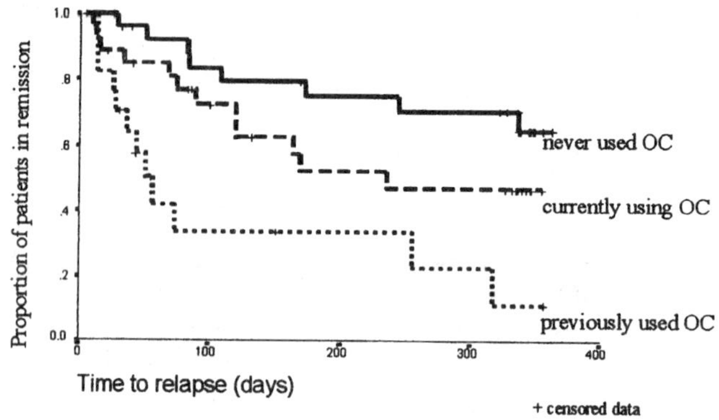

FIGURE 2.—Kaplan-Meier survival curves for relapse by oral contraceptive (*OC*) use. (Courtesy of Timmer A, and The Canadian Mesalamine for Remission of Crohn's Disease Study Group: Oral contraceptive use and smoking are risk factors for relapse in Crohn's disease. *Gastroenterology* 144:1143-1150, 1998.)

may reduce the risk of recurrence. However, simple maneuvers such as avoiding smoking and OCs may be as effective. This paper suggests that we should be more conscientious regarding lifestyle issues in this group of patients.

J.W. Fleshman, Jr., M.D.

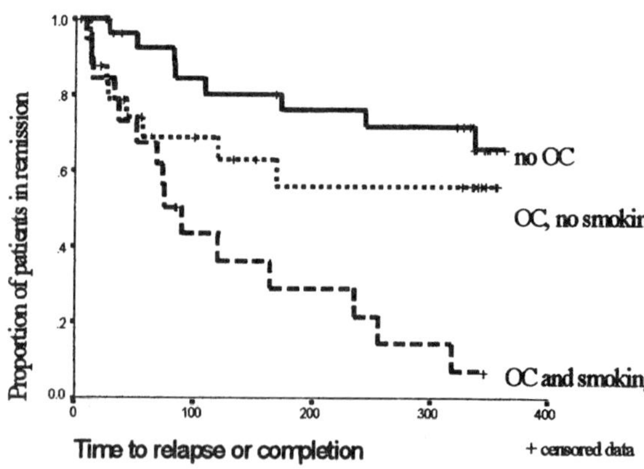

FIGURE 3.—Combined effect of smoking and use of oral contraceptives (*OCs*). (Courtesy of Timmer A, and The Canadian Mesalamine for Remission of Crohn's Disease Study Group: Oral contraceptive use and smoking are risk factors for relapse in Crohn's disease. *Gastroenterology* 144:1143-1150, 1998.)

Laparoscopy for Inflammatory Bowel Disease: Pros and Cons
Sardinha TC, Wexner SD (Cleveland Clinic Florida, Fort Lauderdale)
World J Surg 22:370-374, 1998 5–15

Background.—Laparoscopic surgery can offer significant relief to many patients with inflammatory bowel disease (IBD), although its role in the treatment of colorectal malignancies is still under investigation. The advantages and disadvantages of the laparoscopic management of IBD were studied.

Methods and Findings.—Reports published since 1992, when laparoscopic surgery for IBD was first described in print, were reviewed. The several studies published between 1992 and 1997 indicated that laparoscopy offers significant advantages over laparotomy in patients with terminal ileal Crohn's disease or anal Crohn's disease in need of fecal diversion. These benefits included reduced pain, length of hospital stay, and disability. In addition, cosmesis was improved, and symptomatic postoperative adhesions were reduced. These benefits were achieved with no increase in morbidity or cost. Conversely, laparoscopy for restorative proctocolectomy in patients with mucosal ulcerative colitis was associated with an increased operative time and incidence of intraoperative and postoperative complications compared with laparotomy.

Conclusion.—The literature demonstrates that laparoscopic coloretal surgery can be beneficial in the treatment of terminal ileal Crohn's disease. However, it cannot be recommended for routine use in the treatment of mucosal ulcerative colitis.

▶ This is a review of the existing literature to 1997 using a meta-analysis approach to evaluate the use of laparoscopic approaches to Crohn's disease and ulcerative colitis. The conclusion made by the authors—that patients with Crohn's disease may benefit from a laparoscopic approach—is, I feel, very appropriate. Our experience has been similar and, in fact, we have shown that the approach is possible in patients with complicated ileocolic disease, including phlegmon, abscess, or fistula. Unfortunately, the early experience with ulcerative colitis has been less than good, and the authors do not recommend this approach for patients with ulcerative colitis. New techniques and more experience may change this recommendation over time.

J.W. Fleshman, Jr., M.D.

Strictureplasty for Crohn's Disease: Techniques and Long-term Results
Hurst RD, Michelassi F (Univ of Chicago)
World J Surg 22:359-363, 1998 5–16

Background.—Strictureplasty is being used increasingly for the treatment of symptomatic intestinal strictures in patients with Crohn's disease.

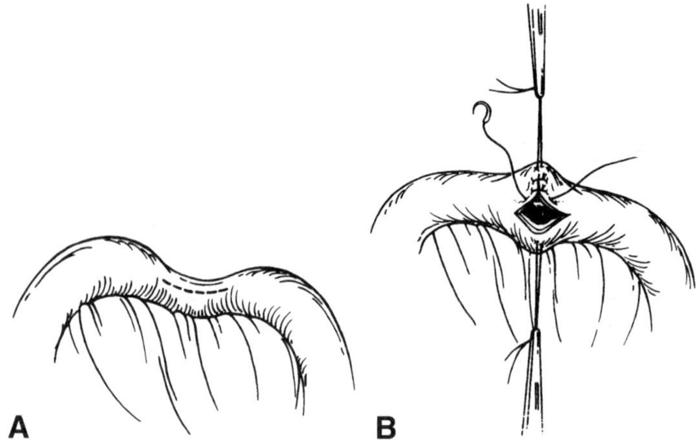

FIGURE 1.—Heineke-Mikulicz strictureplasty for short stenosis. (From Hurst RD, Michelassi F: Strictureplasty for Crohn's disease: Techniques and long-term results. *World J Surg* 22:359-363, copyright 1998 by Springer-Verlag. Courtesy of Fazio VW, Galandiuk S, Jagelman DG, et al: Strictureplasty in Crohn's disease. *Ann Surg* 210:621, 1989. With permission from Lippincott-Raven.)

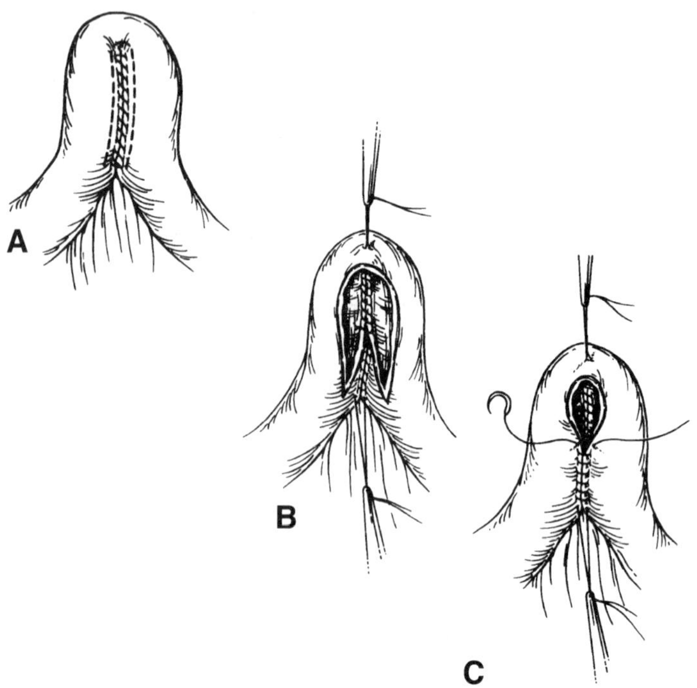

FIGURE 2.—Finney strictureplasty for stenosis longer than 7 to 8 cm. (Courtesy of Hurst RD, Michelassi F: Strictureplasty for Crohn's disease: Techniques and long-term results. *World J Surg* 22:359-363, copyright 1998 by Springer-Verlag.)

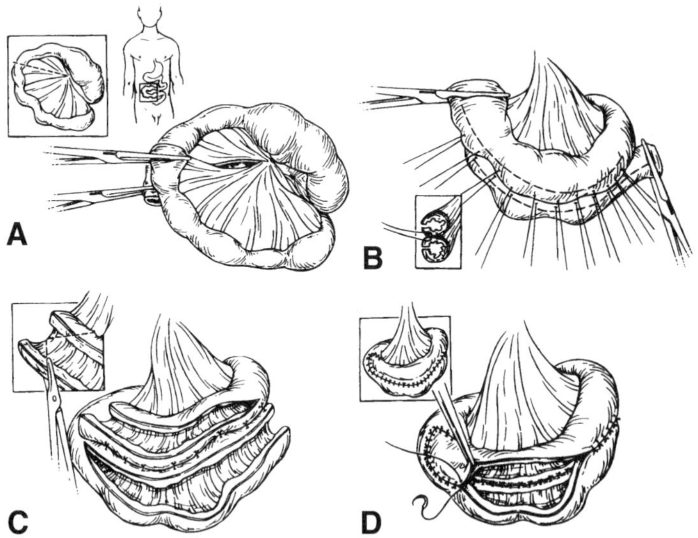

FIGURE 3.—Side-to-side isoperistaltic enteroenterostomy for stenosis and skip lesions of combined length of up to 30 cm. (From Hurst RD, Michelassi F: Strictureplasty for Crohn's disease: Techniques and long-term results. *World J Surg* 22:359-363, copyright 1998 by Springer-Verlag. Courtesy of Michelassi F: Side-to-side isoperistaltic stricturoplasty for multiple Crohn's strictures. *Dis Colon Rectum* 39:345, 1996. With permission of Williams & Wilkins.)

This study determined the overall clinical outcomes of strictureplasty for Crohn's disease at 1 institution.

Methods and Findings.—Fifty-seven patients with Crohn's disease undergoing 60 surgeries with a total of 109 strictureplasties between 1989

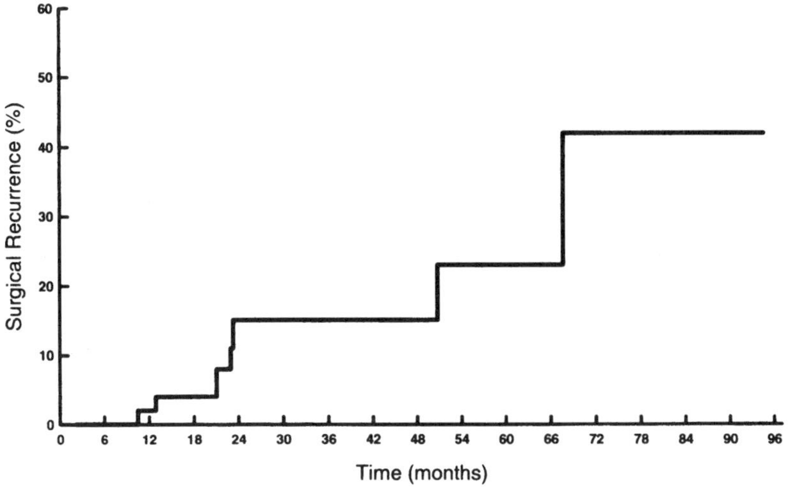

FIGURE 4.—Kaplan-Meier estimate of the rate of intra-abdominal recurrence requiring operation after intestinal strictureplasty. (Courtesy of Hurst RD, Michelassi F: Strictureplasty for Crohn's disease: Techniques and long-term results. *World J Surg* 22:359-363, copyright 1998 by Springer-Verlag.)

and 1997 were studied. At 30 days, morbidity was 12%. Complications were less common in patients undergoing elective procedures than unscheduled procedures. Crohn's disease recurrences necessitating surgery occurred in 7 patients after a mean 38 months of follow-up. The estimated cumulative recurrence rates at 2 and 5 years were 15% and 22%, respectively. Recurrence developed at the site of the previous strictureplasty in only 5 patients (Figs 1-4).

Conclusion.—Strictureplasty is a safe, effective procedure, providing long-term palliation in selected patients with Crohn's disease. In this series, the perioperative complication rates were comparable to those associated with standard surgery. In addition, recurrences were not excessive.

► Strictureplasty has been used since the early 1980s. The large series from Birmingham, England popularized the use of this technique for patients with Crohn's disease.[1] The group from the University of Chicago has produced an excellent series using this technique to treat isolated, narrowing, and small segments of active disease within the small intestine and even the ascending colon. This technique can be performed with low morbidity and mortality and a reasonable leak rate. As seen in Figure 4, the recurrence rate of the disease is no greater than if resection had been performed. Surgeons should be aware of the risk of cancer at the stricture site. A biopsy is recommended at the time of strictureplasty to avoid missing a flat, hidden cancer in the thickened wall of the stricture. This article includes excellent drawings of 3 techniques for performing strictureplasty, including a Heineke-Mikulicz, a Finney, and a side-to-side isoperistaltic enteroenterostomy.

J.W. Fleshman, Jr., M.D.

Reference

1. Sharif H, Alexander-Williams J: The role of strictureplasty in Crohn's disease. *Int Surg* 77:15, 1992.

Absence of Linkage Between Inflammatory Bowel Disease and Selected Loci on Chromosomes 3, 7, 12, and 16

Rioux JD, Daly MJ, Green T, et al (Whitehead Inst/Massachusetts Inst of Technology, Cambridge; McGill Univ, Montreal; Univ of Toronto; et al)

Gastroenterology 115:1062-1065, 1998 5–17

Background.—Four potential sites for inflammatory bowel disease (IBD) susceptibility genes—on chromosomes 3, 7, 12, and 16—have been identified. Whether linkage analysis of an independently obtained group of siblings with IBD would provide further evidence of linkage between these previously reported loci and IBD was determined.

Methods.—One hundred sixty-one families from Toronto were studied. The families included 114 with Crohn's disease, 36 with ulcerative colitis, and 50 mixed IBD sibling pairs. The segregation of 21 microsatellite marker loci spanning the 4 putative IBD gene loci was analyzed.

Findings.—Multipoint linkage analysis yielded no evidence for linkage between IBD and each of the 21 marker loci examined. In all instances, the logarithm of odds scores were less than 0.8. Exclusion mapping analysis showed that these linkage data did not include values of λs ranging from 1.5 to 3.0, depending on the locus examined.

Conclusion.—In this population, the loci previously reported as representing IBD susceptibility loci were not linked to IBD. Considerably more linkage data are needed to define the full complement of genes that predispose to IBD.

American Families With Crohn's Disease Have Strong Evidence for Linkage to Chromosome 16 but Not Chromosome 12

Brant SR, Fu Y, Fields CT, et al (Johns Hopkins Univ, Baltimore, Md; Univ of Chicago; Johns Hopkins Hosp, Baltimore, Md)

Gastroenterology 115:1056-1061, 1998 5–18

Background.—Two European genome-wide screens have identified 2 significant regions of linkage for inflammatory bowel disease (IBD), 1 on chromosome 16 (*IBD1*) and 1 on chromosome 12 (*IBD2*). In addition, 2 regions with suggestive levels of significance—chromosomes 3p and 7q—were identified. This study sought evidence of linkage to these regions in non-Jewish and Ashkenazi Jewish families multiplex for Crohn's disease in the United States.

Methods.—One hundred forty-eight affected relative pairs were genotyped with 10 to 14 highly polymorphic markers overlying each candidate region. Thirty-four percent were Ashkenazim. Nonparametric multipoint and 2-point linkage analyses were conducted.

Findings.—Significant evidence for linkage replication was obtained only for the chromosome 16 locus, *IBD1*, maximal at D16S769. Evidence was stronger among the Ashkenazim than among non-Jewish white populations. No significant evidence for replication on chromosome 12 was obtained. There was minimal evidence for extension of linkage evidence for the chromosome 3p and 7q regions.

Conclusion.—Significant evidence was found for the Crohn's disease susceptibility locus, *IBD1*, on chromosome 16 in this American population, especially the Ashkenazim. However, contrary to previous reports, no significant evidence was found for *IBD2* on chromosome 12.

Genetic Analysis of Inflammatory Bowel Disease in a Large European Cohort Supports Linkage to Chromosomes 12 and 16

Curran ME, Lau KF, Hampe J, et al (AxyS Pharmaceuticals Inc, La Jolla, Calif; Christian-Albrechts-Univ, Kiel, Germany; King's College of Medicine, London; et al)

Gastroenterology 115:1066-1071, 1998 5–19

Introduction.—Although the cause of inflammatory bowel disease (IBD) is unknown, epidemiologic data suggest a genetic basis. Recent studies have shown the existence of several IBD linkages, the significance of which must be determined in large patient series. This study sought to replicate previous reports of IBD linkages on chromosomes 12 and 16 in a large Northern European cohort.

Methods.—Individual IBD kindreds were identified by means of genotyping studies that used a total of 30 highly polymorphic microsatellite markers spanning chromosomes 12 and 16. A kindred consisted of at least 2 siblings with either Crohn's disease (CD) or ulcerative colitis (UC). A total of 359 affected sibling pairs were identified in 274 kindreds.

Results.—Linkage for both chromosomes 12 and 16 was identified by nonparametric statistical analyses. Two-point maximum logarithm of odds scores for chromosome 12 showed a peak at D12S303 for CD and at D12S75 for UC (logarithm of odds [LOD], 2.15 and 0.92, respectively). On multipoint analysis, a peak LOD of 1.8 was demonstrated for CD. On chromosome 16, linkage for CD was demonstrated at marker D16S415, whereas multipoint support peaked above markers D16S409 and D16S411 (LOD, 1.7).

Conclusions.—The results confirm previous studies showing linkage of IBD to chromosomes 12 and 16 in a large, independent cohort of European families. The findings suggest that important and common susceptibility genes for IBD are located in these regions and may be identified in future studies. The evidence suggests that genetic variants found on chromosomes 12 and 16 may play an important role in both CD and UC.

▶ The genetic basis of IBD, especially CD, is somewhat intuitive, but it is controversial at this point. The three articles reviewed (Abstracts 5–17 to 5–19) suggest that there is a difference between groups of patients with CD in terms of their genetic basis for their disease. The groups from Toronto, Europe, and Chicago and Baltimore, have produced varying results along these lines. Chromosomes 12 and 16 have been suggested as sites for genetic mutations responsible for IBD. The study from Toronto (Abstract 5–17) suggests that none of the loci that have been studied in the past on chromosomes 3, 7, 12, and 16 have actually been responsible for any of the IBD in Canada. On the other hand, the group from Europe (Abstract 5–19) suggests that there is linkage to chromosomes 12 and 16. The group from Chicago and Baltimore (Abstract 5–18) suggests that only chromosome 12 has influence over the IBD in the eastern United States. As one can see by the conflicting results, much work needs to be done to identify the true genetic basis for IBD. This seems to reflect the general confusion over the true cause of IBD and may reflect the existence of multiple diseases that are responsible for a complex group of symptoms and thus a "lumped" set of diseases called CD and UC.

J.W. Fleshman, Jr., M.D.

Analysis of MHC Class II DP, DQ and DR Alleles in Crohn's Disease

Cariappa A, Sands B, Forcione D, et al (Massachusetts Gen Hosp, Boston)
Gut 43:210-215, 1998 5–20

Introduction.—The presence of activated inflammatory T-helper cells in Crohn's disease suggests an important role of HLA class II molecules. However, there have been no genotyping studies of all MHC class II alleles in white patients with Crohn's disease. Complete molecular typing of the HLA class II DPB, DQB, and DRB alleles was performed in such patients.

Methods and Results.—For the typing studies, a polymerase chain reaction-sequence specific oligonucleotide–based approach was used. Fifty-eight white patients with Crohn's disease were studied, along with 93 healthy, ethnically matched controls. Crohn's disease was not significantly associated with any DPB or DQB alleles. The researchers used stringent genotyping criteria to investigate a previously noted DRB3*0301 and DRB1*1302 association in Crohn's disease. The DRB3*0301/DRB1*1302 haplotype was found in 21% of the patients with Crohn's disease vs. 5% of the controls, with a corresponding relative risk of 4.59.

Conclusions.—A complete molecular typing study identifies an HLA DRB3*0301/DRB1*1302 haplotype as the only significant MHC class II association in white patients with Crohn's disease. This is the strongest reported association of any locus—MHC or non-MHC—with Crohn's disease. The theory that it represents a real MHC class II susceptibility haplotype is supported by the finding of specific susceptibility alleles in Japanese patients with Crohn's disease.

► The search for a genetic basis for Crohn's disease is very important. This study from Massachusetts General Hospital suggests that there is a relationship between the major histocompatibility class II alleles DRB3 and DRB1 and Crohn's disease. The defect may influence T lymphocyte function and, in this way, reflect a portion of the clue to the true etiology of Crohn's disease. However, this finding will need to be confirmed by other groups. There is strong evidence from Japan that this is the case.

J.W. Fleshman, Jr., M.D.

Presence of Adherent *Escherichia coli* Strains in Ileal Mucosa of Patients With Crohn's Disease

Darfeuille-Michaud A, Neut C, Barnich N, et al (Centre Hospitalier Universitaire, Lille, France)

Gastroenterology 115:1405-1413, 1998 5–21

Objective.—Several lines of evidence suggest that bacteria, perhaps especially *Escherichia coli*, play a pathogenic role in Crohn's disease (CD). Various *E. coli* strains differ in their virulence properties. The bacterial virulence of *E. coli* strains from the ileal mucosa of patients with CD was studied.

Methods.—The study included ileal mucosa specimens from 50 patients with CD and 13 controls. Within the CD group, *E. coli* strains were recovered from resected chronic ileal lesions in 20 patients and from the neoterminal ileum after surgery in 19 patients with and 11 without endoscopic recurrence of CD. Bacterial adhesion, an important virulence factor of *E. coli*, was evaluated in vitro with the use of intestinal cell lines. Other virulence factors were determined by means of DNA hybridization and polymerase chain reaction assays.

Results.—A total of 136 strains for patients and controls were evaluated, with focus on the most virulent strain for both groups. The genes encoding for *E. coli* virulence in cases of acute enteric disease were not found in any of the strains studied. Eighty-five percent of strains from chronic CD lesions and 79% of strains from early recurrent lesions showed mannose-resistant adhesion to differentiated Caco-2 cells. This characteristic was present in only 33% of the control strains. Synthesis of α-hemolysin producing a cytolytic effect was noted in 22% of the strains from chronic and early CD lesions, compared with none of the control strains.

Conclusions.—The *E. coli* strains colonizing early and chronic CD ileal lesions appear to lack the virulence of strains associated with acute enteric disease. However, the results suggest that *E. coli* strains from patients with CD may adhere to differentiated intestinal cells and synthesize an α-hemolysin to disrupt the intestinal barrier. This combination of virulence factors might permit the bacterium to colonize the intestinal epithelium, damage intestinal cells, and contribute to inflammatory disease.

▶ The pathogenesis of Crohn's disease may depend on environmental factors, such as bacteria within the gastrointestinal tract. This article from France suggests that a specific, as yet undescribed, *E. coli* strain may produce an α-hemolysin, which causes cells to respond to its presence and develop a disease very similar to Crohn's disease. Although this is an experimental study of in vitro cells, the theory is very enticing and certainly bears some consideration. There have been studies that suggest that the intestinal barrier is decreased in patients with Crohn's disease and that transmural transport is increased also. The α-hemolysin may be the source of the intestinal barrier disruption and provide a source for the etiology of ongoing inflammatory response. This finding certainly fits in with some of the current theories and will be important to watch in the future.

J.W. Fleshman, Jr., M.D.

Ulcerative Colitis

An Interleukin 12–Related Cytokine Is Up-regulated in Ulcerative Colitis But Not in Crohn's Disease

Christ AD, Stevens AC, Koeppen H, et al (Harvard Med School, Boston; Univ of Chicago)

Gastroenterology 115:307-313, 1998 5–22

Purpose.—The proinflammatory cytokine interleukin-12 (IL-12) may play a pathogenetic role in inflammatory bowel disease (IBD). Recent studies have reported on the Epstein-Barr virus–induced gene 3 (EBI3), a glycoprotein that might function in an IL-12-related pathway. Expression of EBI3 messenger RNA (mRNA) was studied in colonic mucosa from normal controls and from patients with ulcerative colitis (UC) or Crohn's disease.

Methods and Findings.—Colonic tissue samples were analyzed by quantitative polymerase chain reaction for EBI3 mRNA and by immunohistology and Western blotting for EBI3. The mRNA was detected in control and Crohn's disease tissue. However, elevated EBI3 mRNA was detected only in patients with active UC. In these specimens, the level of EBI3 was significantly correlated with histologic activity and T-cell infiltration scores. Lamina propria was found to contain EBI3-positive cells shaped like macrophages. Western blotting confirmed the presence of EBI3 protein.

Conclusions.—The novel IL-12 related cytokine EBI3 is expressed by cells similar to macrophages in normal and Crohn's disease intestine. Expression of EBI3 is up-regulated in active UC, but not in active Crohn's disease. EBI3 may be an important target for immunomodulating therapy in IBD.

► Major advances in understanding the nature of inflammation in IBD have focused on the cytokine profiles distinguishing UC from Crohn's disease. The identification of 2 distinct subsets of T helper cells (T_h1 and T_h2)—particularly in murine models—which produce separate groups of cytokines. The divergent responses may explain fundamental differences between UC and Crohn's disease. The pivotal steps and cytokines responsible for inducing the different pathways have not been fully elucidated. Further insight into the nature of the varied response was offered in this study, which identified a novel hemapoietin receptor family member (EBI3) that may function as an IL-12 antagonist. IL-12, increased in Crohn's disease, may influence the development of a Th1 response. Its putative antagonist, EB13, may direct the inflammation toward a Th2 type cytokine production. In addition to providing support for the divergent inflammatory responses in UC and Crohn's disease, this study identifies possible pivotal cytokines that may serve as promising targets to provide more rational therapy in IBD.

G. Aliperti, M.D.

Is Colonoscopic Surveillance Reducing Colorectal Cancer Mortality in Ulcerative Colitis? A Population Based Case Control Study

Karlén P, Kornfeld D, Broström O, et al (Karolinska Inst, Stockholm)

Gut 42:711-714, 1998 5–23

Background.—Patients with ulcerative colitis (UC) are at increased risk of death from colorectal carcinoma. Thus, for patients with chronic extensive disease, colonoscopic surveillance programs are recommended. However, the effect of such programs on reducing the colorectal cancer mortality rate in these patients has not been proved. Thus, these authors used a population-based, case-control study to evaluate the effectiveness of colonoscopic surveillance in preventing death from colorectal cancer in patients with UC.

Methods.—The population from which cases and controls were drawn consisted of 4,664 patients with a diagnosis of UC in Stockholm County between 1955 and 1984 or in the Uppsala Health Care Region between 1965 and 1983. All patients were 10 years old or older and their UC had been diagnosed 5 years or more earlier. The cases consisted of 40 patients (26 men and 14 women) who had died of colorectal cancer but who did not have a diagnosis of colorectal cancer before the diagnosis of UC. The controls consisted of 102 patients (52 men and 50 women) matched for gender, age, and extent of disease at diagnosis and for duration of disease. Medical records were examined to determine details about the colonoscopic surveillance of cases and controls.

Findings.—At least 1 surveillance colonoscopy had been performed in 2 of 40 cases (5%) and in 18 of 102 controls (17.6%). Two or more surveillance colonoscopies had been performed in 1 case (2.5%) but in 12 controls (11.8%). Furthermore, on comparison of individual cases and matched controls, 10 of the controls (10.2%) underwent colectomy within the 5 years before colorectal cancer was diagnosed in the case patient.

Conclusions.—Surveillance colonoscopy appears to provide protection against death due to colorectal cancer in patients with UC. Although the number of cases and controls was small, controls who underwent 1 or more surveillance colonoscopies had a relative risk of 0.29 compared with cases, and controls who underwent 2 or more surveillance colonoscopies had a relative risk of 0.22. In addition, the fact that 10% of the controls underwent colectomy within 5 years of the case patient's cancer diagnosis further suggests that surveillance colonoscopy reduces the risk of colorectal cancer mortality in these patients.

▶ Colonoscopic surveillance is universally advocated in patients with UC because of the associated increased risk of cancer and the assumption that the identification of dysplasia as an indication of concurrent or likely cancer will reduce mortality in these high-risk patients. However, supportive evidence of the utility of this approach is not extensive, despite the general embracing of surveillance screening by the gastroenterology community. Large randomized controlled trials will never be undertaken for ethical reasons. To explore this question further through a novel approach, a population-based, nested case-control study supports colonoscopic screening. Although a tentative finding lacking in statistical significance, perhaps in part because of the relatively small sample size, the study noted a more pronounced protective effect with two or more surveillance colonoscopies, suggesting a "dose response." Patient compliance, need for aggressive persistence with screening programs on the part of physicians, and the inconsistencies in biopsy protocols may limit the effectiveness of this approach and make it more difficult to prove efficacy, but screening is a critical element in the care of these patients.

G. Aliperti, M.D.

Sialyl-Tn Antigen as a Marker of Colon Cancer Risk in Ulcerative Colitis: Relation to Dysplasia and DNA Aneuploidy

Karlén P, Young E, Broström O, et al (Karolinska Inst, Stockholm; Mount Sinai School of Medicine, New York; Huddinge Univ, Stockholm; et al)

Gastroenterology 115:1395-1404, 1998 5–24

Purpose.—Long-standing, extensive ulcerative colitis (UC) carries an increased risk of colorectal cancer. Malignant transformation to colorectal cancer—both sporadic and UC-related cases—is correlated with expression of the mucin-associated carbohydrate antigen sialyl-Tn (STn) and with DNA aneuploidy. The topographic and temporal relationship of STn expression to aneuploidy and neoplasia was studied in patients with long-standing UC.

Methods.—The study included 26 patients in a colonoscopic cancer surveillance program. All had a confirmed diagnosis of extensive UC, which had been present for more than 8 years. At serial colonoscopies or colectomies, a total of 1,691 mucosal specimens were prospectively collected. Expression of STn was assessed by immunohistochemical methods. Dysplasia and aneuploidy were assessed as well.

Results.—Six patients undergoing colectomy for dysplasia showed STn expression in 47% of the specimens, compared with 7% of the specimens from 6 well-matched patients undergoing surgery for medically intractable UC. Expression of STn was just 6% in 7 patients who never had any dysplasia or aneuploidy. Whether or not dysplasia was present, expression of STn was independent of aneuploidy. There were 5 patients with aneuploidy but without dysplasia; 4 of these showed STn expression before the development of aneuploidy.

Conclusions.—Neoplastic transformation in patients with long-standing, extensive UC is independently associated with expression of STn antigen and aneuploidy. Both markers are correlated with progressive degrees of dysplasia and occur earlier than dysplasia. The results suggest that STn may be a useful indicator, along with dysplasia and aneuploidy, of risk of neoplastic transformation of the colorectal mucosa.

▶ Screening of patients with UC for risk of colon cancer is an inexact science. Dysplasia is helpful but not 100% reliable, and cancer can develop even though colonoscopic screening is undertaken. The use of aneuploidy in the areas of dysplasia may indicate an increased risk of developing cancer. STn antigen is detected by monoclonal antibody immunohistochemistry. The combination of STn and aneuploidy may help predict the higher risk of developing colorectal cancer in the setting of ulcerative colitis.

J.W. Fleshman, Jr., M.D.

Differential Diagnosis of Dysplasia-associated Lesion or Mass and Coincidental Adenoma in Ulcerative Colitis

Suzuki K, Muto T, Shinozaki M, et al (Tokyo Univ)

Dis Colon Rectum 41:322-327, 1998 5–25

Introduction.—Patients with ulcerative colitis are regarded as being at high risk of colorectal cancer. Epithelial dysplasia is an important risk factor, but the clinical significance of "dysplasia-associated lesion or mass" (DALM), as seen at colonoscopy, is unclear. This study evaluated the ability of colonoscopy to differentiate between DALM and coincidental adenoma in patients with ulcerative colitis.

Methods.—The investigators reviewed 346 patients with ulcerative colitis who underwent colonoscopy over a 16-year period. Of 27 patients with macroscopic neoplasia, 16 had DALM and 11 had adenoma. Colonoscopic criteria for these findings were the presence and absence, respectively, of dysplasia in the flat mucosa adjacent to elevated lesions. The results of biopsy and polypectomy were related to the findings in the surgical specimens. Outcomes affecting the differential diagnosis between DALM and adenoma were assessed as well.

Results.—Colonoscopic biopsy detected DALM in 13 of 27 patients. DALM was found in the surgical specimens of all 10 patients undergoing colectomy. Two patients in whom biopsy revealed adenoma were found to have unsuspected DALM at surgery. The other 12 patients had clinical and colonoscopic evidence of adenoma, leading to excision of the macroscopic lesions at colonoscopy. The polypectomy specimen confirmed adenoma in 11 cases; the other specimen was DALM.

Compared with adenoma, the finding of DALM was associated with a younger patient, a longer duration of ulcerative colitis, and more extensive disease. The DALM appeared plaquelike in 46% of the cases, sessile in 46%, and pedunculated in 7%. In contrast, 94% of the adenomas were sessile or pedunculated. Mean lesion size was 1.8 cm for DALM vs. 0.5 cm for adenoma.

Conclusions.—In patients with ulcerative colitis, the colonoscopic distinction between DALM and adenoma can be made by biopsy to detect dysplasia in the flat mucosa adjacent to macroscopic neoplastic lesions. Age, duration of disease, extent of disease, tumor size, and colonoscopic appearance of the tumor all affect the differential diagnosis. These variables may help in making the preoperative diagnosis of macroscopic neoplastic lesions in patients with ulcerative colitis.

▶ The impact or implications of an adenoma in patients with ulcerative colitis is still undetermined. The presence of a DALM, however, has been shown to be truly predictive of cancer in these individuals. The existence of an adenoma in the patient with a long-standing ulcerative colitis may or may not imply premalignant change requiring an operation. This article is somewhat helpful in identifying those individuals who have a true adenoma that has no implication of future cancer. If a lesion is pedunculated, less than 1 cm in size, and is in an area that is unaffected by the colitis, it can be assumed to be an adenoma and treated by polypectomy and follow-up. However, if high-grade dysplasia is found with the polyp, or in the mucosa adjacent, this should be assumed to be a DALM and the patient requires colectomy. These lesions are usually greater than 1 cm in size and have an irregular appearance suggestive of potential malignancy. This controversy will continue until there is a clear definition of adenoma in the setting of ulcerative colitis and until the issue of the implications of low-grade vs. high-grade dysplasia are resolved.

Current recommendations suggest that any question of high-grade dysplasia or premalignant lesion should result in colectomy for these individuals, because the outcome is very poor if the cancer is greater than stage II in patients with ulcerative colitis. This paper, once again, illustrates that it is difficult to distinguish between an early-grade lesion and an advanced cancer in patients with ulcerative colitis, for one third of the patients had stage III disease.

J.W. Fleshman, Jr., M.D.

Is Ileal Pouch–Anal Anastomosis Really the Procedure of Choice for Patients With Ulcerative Colitis?

Jimmo B, Hyman NH (Univ of Vermont, Burlington)

Dis Colon Rectum 41:41-45, 1998 5–26

Background.—Previous reports have suggested that ileal pouch–anal anastomosis (IPAA) is now the procedure of choice for the treatment of ulcerative colitis. This procedure is generally regarded as improving quality of life; however, there are relatively few data to support this assertion. The quality of life of patients undergoing IPAA was compared with that of patients undergoing total proctocolectomy with ileostomy (TPC).

Methods.—The study included 67 patients undergoing elective surgery for ulcerative colitis. All operations were performed over a 5-year period by a single surgeon. The patients received complete information about both procedures before choosing between IPAA and TPC. Fifty-five opted for IPAA and 12 for TPC. Age, sex, and complications—including pouchitis—were compared between groups. The results were assessed in terms of functional outcomes and patient satisfaction. Quality of life was assessed with the use of a modified Inflammatory Bowel Disease Questionnaire.

Results.—Mean age was 31 in the IPAA group vs. 52 in the TPC group, and mean follow-up was 3 vs. 2 years, respectively. The 2 groups were otherwise similar. The complication rate was 49% in the IPAA group, compared with 8% in the TPC group, the most common complication being pouchitis. The 2 groups were similar in terms of patient satisfaction; none of the patients wished they had chosen the other procedure. The results were similar on the Inflammatory Bowel Disease Questionnaire, both overall and within categories.

Conclusions.—For patients with ulcerative colitis, both IPAA and TPC offer high satisfaction rates. Quality-of-life scores are similar with the 2 options, but TPC avoids the higher complication rate and longer recovery time of IPAA. Most patients choose to accept these risks; patients who select TPC over IPAA may be more focused on eliminating the colitis symptoms, with less concern over their appearance. They are older but otherwise similar to patients opting for IPAA.

► The issue of procedure choice for patients with ulcerative colitis remains controversial. The authors of this article have readdressed this question in a retrospective way with some inherent biases built into the study. Since patients were not randomized, the patients obviously chose the procedure of choice that fit their lifestyles and mind sets. Therefore, no direct comparison between permanent ileostomy and the pelvic pouch procedure can be drawn, and one must consider the issues of a patient's pride when evaluating the procedure. In fact, in the past there have been evangelical disciples of particular procedures who have tried to convert other patients to their procedure and way of life. Unfortunately, this evangelistic effort has been used by businessmen and surgeons to increase the number of cases in their series. This article does not have those same problems, but certainly the data must be viewed with a very critical eye. I agree with the authors that patients who undergo a total proctocolectomy and ileostomy should be allowed to feel good about their choice and that the procedure should remain an option for patients with ulcerative colitis. I also agree that patients choosing the total proctocolectomy with ileostomy should not be dissuaded from their choice because the authors have essentially proven that these patients can have a good quality of life that is equal to that of those who have chosen the pelvic pouch procedure. However, I am confident that, in a randomized prospective trial, the patients who undergo pelvic pouch procedure, if assigned to that arm rather than a total proctocolectomy and ileostomy, will certainly end up with a higher quality-of-life rating. Therefore, this should not be used to support returning to a mind-set that equates total proctocolectomy and ileostomy with pelvic pouch procedure for ulcerative colitis.

J.W. Fleshman, Jr., M.D.

Long-term Treatment of Ulcerative Colitis With Ciprofloxacin: A Prospective, Double-blind, Placebo-controlled Study

Turunen UM, Färkkilä MA, Hakala K, et al (Univ of Helsinki; Bayer AG, Gothenburg, Sweden)

Gastroenterology 115:1072-1078, 1998 5–27

Purpose.—The bacterial flora of the bowel are believed to play a pathogenic role in ulcerative colitis (UC), although no study has demonstrated persistence of any single pathogen as a major cause of inflammatory bowel disease. Antibiotic treatment for UC has been studied, but with inconsistent results. Ciprofloxacin was studied for its ability to induce and maintain remission in patients with UC, in combination with conventional therapy.

Methods.—The study included 83 patients with moderate to severe UC who responded poorly to conventional treatment with steroids and mesalamine. There were 58 men and 25 women (mean age, 34 years). The patients were randomized to receive either ciprofloxacin, 500 to 750 mg twice daily, or placebo. Treatment continued for 6 months, in combination with a high but decreasing dose of prednisone and maintenance therapy with mesalamine. Conventional therapy continued for another 6 months. The patients underwent clinical evaluation and colonoscopy at baseline and after 3, 6, and 12 months of treatment. Treatment failure was defined as both symptomatic and endoscopic failure to respond.

Results.—Patients in the ciprofloxacin group were less than half as likely to experience treatment failure in the first 6 months as patients in the placebo group: 21% vs. 44%. In the 6 months after termination of treatment with the study drug, failure rates were about 30% in both groups. The 2 groups were similar in cumulative prednisone dose. Patients receiving ciprofloxacin had significantly better endoscopic and histologic results at 3 months, although there was no significant difference by 6 months.

Conclusions.—Adding ciprofloxacin to conventional therapy with mesalamine and prednisone significantly lowers the treatment failure rate in patients with ulcerative colitis. The main benefit of ciprofloxacin may be limited to the period of active disease or steroid treatment, although more study is needed to define the optimal duration of treatment. Ciprofloxacin may be most beneficial in patients whose UC is relapsing despite steroid therapy.

► The addition of antibiotics to a regimen of steroids and anti-inflammatory drugs has certain attractions. Certainly, among patients with acute fulminant colitis, antibiotics have been used to initially restore homeostasis in acutely ill, questionably septic, individuals. This treatment may have been having a therapeutic affect on the ulcerative colitis itself, according to this article from Finland. It is interesting that ciprofloxacin helped achieve remission in a group of patients who were resistant to steroid therapy. The etiologic implications are also very interesting, since altering the bacterial flora can reduce the inflammatory response. Larger studies are needed to confirm the effect of the ciprofloxacin, but the results are certainly promising and one would hope to see follow-up on this issue.

J.W. Fleshman, Jr., M.D.

Effect of Surgery on Health-Related Quality of Life in Patients With Inflammatory Bowel Disease: A Prospective Study

Thirlby RC, Land JC, Fenster LF, et al (Virginia Mason Med Ctr, Seattle)
Arch Surg 133:826-832, 1998 5–28

Objective.—Health-related quality of life (HRQL) has become an important outcome measure for patients with chronic disease. Previous studies have examined the effects of medical or surgical interventions on HRQL in patients with inflammatory bowel disease (IBD). However, these studies have generally used disease-specific quality-of-life instruments. The generic Health Status Questionnaire (HSQ) was used to assess the HRQL impact of surgery in patients with IBD.

Methods.—The prospective study included 63 patients with IBD (38 men and 25 women; average age, 41 years). Thirty-six had Crohn's disease, and 27 had chronic ulcerative colitis. Each patient completed the HSQ before and every 3 months after surgery for IBD. For patients with Crohn's disease, this surgery consisted of resection with or without stricturoplasty for intractable disease. For most patients with ulcerative colitis, surgery consisted of ileoanal anastomoses with an ileoanal reservoir. The effects of surgery on HRQL were assessed, and the results were compared with those of the general population and of patients with other chronic diseases.

Results.—Before surgery, the patients with IBD had HRQL scores significantly lower than those of the general population on all 8 scales of the HSQ. Scores were also lower than for patients with diabetes or asthma. After surgery, HRQL improved significantly in both groups of patients with IBD, with scores similar to those of the general population on most HSQ scales. The improvement in HRQL was significantly greater for younger patients.

Conclusions.—Surgical treatment is associated with significant improvement in the low baseline HRQL scores of patients with IBD. Before surgery, HSQ scores are even lower than those of patients with other chronic diseases; afterward, scores improve to levels similar to those of the general population. The results support the use of early surgery for many patients with symptomatic IBD. Further studies using both disease-specific and generic HRQL data will permit valid conclusions regarding the value of surgery for IBD.

▶ This article addresses the issue of the effect of surgery on HRQL in patients with IBD. Unfortunately, there are two groups of patients in the study—patients with ulcerative colitis and patients with Crohn's disease. These 2 patient groups are difficult to lump together because they have very different disease outcomes. This is an excellent first effort in evaluating patients with a chronic, unrelenting disease process who achieve improvement after a surgical procedure. As the authors clearly state in their own conclusion, this needs to be used to evaluate the benefit of early surgery in patients with this type of disease. I congratulate the authors on an excellent first effort, and I look forward to the future comparison of the HRQL questionnaire data, comparing patients treated medically over a long term with those given early surgical treatment.

J.W. Fleshman, Jr., M.D.

Health-Related Quality of Life in Swedish Patients With Ulcerative Colitis

Hjortswang H, Ström M, Almer S (Linköping Univ, Sweden)

Am J Gastroenterol 93:2203-2211, 1998 5–29

Introduction.—Advances in treatment have improved the long-term outcome of ulcerative colitis. However, this disease still carries a significant burden in terms of inconvenience and hidden suffering. Health-related quality of life (HRQOL) was assessed among patients with ulcerative colitis.

Methods.—The study included an unselected population of 211 Swedish patients with ulcerative colitis. The investigators collected data on demographic and disease-related factors. They assessed HRQOL by means of 2 well-validated instruments: the disease-specific Rating Form of Inflammatory Bowel Disease Patient Concerns (RFIPC) and the generic Sickness Impact Profile (SIP). To these were added some complementary questions regarding information needs, medication, side effects, and well-being. Information on disease activity was collected from a variety of sources, including symptom cards, laboratory tests, and endoscopy. The effects of coexisting disease were analyzed as well.

Results.—The SIP indicated some form of functional impairment in 51% of the patients. Most of this was in the psychological and social areas, less so in the physical domain. On the RFIPC, the areas of greatest concern were those related to possible complications of the disease, such as the requirement for an ostomy appliance or surgery, the risk of cancer, loss of bowel control, uncertainty about the disease, and medication effects. Both HRQOL instruments gave higher scores for patients with active disease than for those in remission. Patients with coexisting diseases reported a large negative effect on daily living and overall HRQOL.

Conclusions.—Ulcerative colitis appears to negatively affect HRQOL in a number of ways. Subjective functional impairment occurs mainly in the psychological and social domains. Concerns and functional impairment are increased and well-being is decreased for patients with active disease compared with those in remission. However, this Swedish population appears to enjoy better HRQOL than patients in other western countries previously studied with the same questionnaires.

► The authors have performed a comprehensive evaluation of the impact of ulcerative colitis on a consecutive group of patients in a fairly uniform environment. It is interesting that we now have the capability of documenting "sick patients." Although it seems somewhat redundant to perform the paperwork and data collection, this is a very useful technique for comparing two modalities of treatment for the same disease. The task now is to compare patients with ulcerative colitis followed up a long period of time and treated medically with patients treated early in the course of their disease with an operation to restore their rectal function. When the pelvic pouch procedure and long-term medical therapy are compared, one would hope that there will be a clear difference that will help us decide whether a patient should be referred early or late for surgery.

J.W. Fleshman, Jr., M.D.

Ulcerative Colitis Has an Aggressive Course After Orthotopic Liver Transplantation for Primary Sclerosing Cholangitis

Papatheodoridis GV, Hamilton M, Mistry PK, et al (Royal Free Hosp, London)
Gut 43:639-644, 1998 5–30

Introduction.—Many patients with primary sclerosing cholangitis (PSC) have inflammatory bowel disease (IBD), particularly ulcerative colitis. When these patients undergo liver transplantation, the immunosuppressive therapy given for the transplant would be expected to improve the course of IBD. However, previous reports suggest that IBD has a variable course after liver transplantation. Most patients show no change or improvement, with a possible increase in the risk of colorectal cancer. The practice of withdrawing steroids in the early period after transplantation may influence IBD activity. This prospective study evaluated the course of IBD in patients undergoing liver transplantation for PSC, with no long-term steroids included in the maintenance immunosuppressive regimen.

Methods.—The 7-year study included 30 patients undergoing liver transplantation for PSC who survived longer than 12 months. The recipients were 26 men and 15 women, mean age 40. In 18 patients (60%) ulcerative colitis had been diagnosed before liver transplantation. Two of these patients had undergone previous colectomy. Colonoscopy was performed before and after transplantation in each patient. Mean follow-up was 38 months. Maintenance immunosuppression consisted of cyclosporin or tacrolimus, with or without azathioprine.

Results.—Compared with the course of ulcerative colitis at up to 5 years before transplantation, the posttransplant course was judged the same in half of the patients and worse in the other half. In 12 patients, the course of IBD had been quiescent before transplantation; 8 of these continued to have a quiescent course after transplantation. Of 4 patients with active ulcerative colitis before transplantation, all had a worsening course after transplantation. Of the 12 patients who were free of IBD before transplantation, new-onset ulcerative colitis developed in 3. None of the patients had colorectal cancer during follow-up.

Conclusions.—This study examines the course of IBD in patients undergoing liver transplantation for PSC without long-term steroid therapy as part of their immunosuppressive regimen. If these patients have pre-existing ulcerative colitis, it may follow an aggressive course after transplantation. New-onset ulcerative colitis may develop in patients with no previous history of IBD. In contrast to previous reports, this study finds a low risk of colorectal cancer.

▶ The course of ulcerative colitis after orthotopic liver transplantation, in the setting of primary sclerosing cholangitis, is often very aggressive. The treatment should also include aggressive use of steroids. The management of the ulcerative colitis may indicate an operation in these circumstances, since these patients are severely immunocompromised and should probably have early operation if there is a possibility of sepsis.

Of importance is the lack of development of colorectal cancer in the group of patients from London who were followed up for almost 10 years. This has been a concern for the management of these patients. Preoperative colonoscopy to screen the colon for the presence of active ulcerative colitis is very important because the pre-existing ulcerative colitis has an aggressive course and needs therapy.

J.W. Fleshman, Jr., M.D.

Irritable Bowel

Selected Symptoms Associated With Sexual and Physical Abuse History Among Female Patients With Gastrointestinal Disorders: The Impact on Subsequent Health Care Visits

Leserman J, Li Z, Drossman DA, et al (Univ of North Carolina, Chapel Hill)
Psychol Med 28:417-425, 1998 5–31

Background.—Women who have suffered physical or sexual abuse report more medical symptoms (particularly gastrointestinal and pelvic disorders) and functional disability. The physical and somatic symptoms more likely to be experienced by these women were determined, as was whether these symptoms prompt more health care visits.

Methods.—The study participants were 239 women (mean age, 39.4 years; mean level of education, 14.0 years; 83.7% white) who were being treated at a gasteroenterology clinic. Each participant completed an interview that addressed her sexual and physical abuse history. The severity of the abuse was graded on a scale of 0 (none) to 6 (forced intercourse with serious injury and 4 or more life threats). Participants were also assessed for 30 somatic symptoms and their functional disability. During the year after the interview, participants completed questionnaires about the number of health care visits they had made; 196 participants provided complete follow-up data.

Findings.—Half the participants (50.6%) reported some type of sexual or physical abuse; severity scores were moderate in 33.5% and high in 17.1%. Most of the women who had been abused (83%) had experienced their last life threat 5 or more years earlier. Compared with women who had not been abused, women who had been abused were significantly more likely to experience symptoms related to panic (especially shortness of breath, palpitations, numbness or tingling, or blurred or double vision; odds ratios, 2.35 to 2.49), depression (especially difficulty sleeping and tiredness or fatigue; odds ratios, 2.78 and 2.26, respectively), musculoskeletal disorders (especially frequent headaches, muscle aches, and ear or eye pain; odds ratios, 2.05 to 3.32), genitourinary disorders (especially pelvic pain, painful intercourse, vaginal discharge/itching, or low sexual desire; odds ratios, 2.4 to 4.25), skin disorders (especially rashes or itching; odds ratio, 2.18), and respiratory disorders (especially a stuffy or runny nose or sore throat/fever; odds ratios, 1.66 and 1.52, respectively). Women who had been abused were also significantly more likely to have gained weight. Furthermore, during the year after the interview, compared with women reporting no abuse, women who reported severe abuse made a median of 8 more health care visits, and women who reported moderate abuse made a median of 3 more health care visits. Regression analysis indicated that the severity of abuse history, the number of medical symptoms, and the extent of functional disability accounted for almost a third (30%) of the variance in health care visits.

Conclusions.—Half of these women with gastrointestinal complaints reported a history of physical and/or sexual abuse, and abused women were significantly more likely to experience somatic symptoms not related to the gastrointestinal tract. Furthermore, women who had been abused made significantly more health care visits than their unabused counterparts, even 5 or more years after their last life threat. Thus, physical and sexual abuse is associated with substantial emotional, physical, and medical costs even many years after the abuse occurs.

Level of Chronic Life Stress Predicts Clinical Outcome in Irritable Bowel Syndrome

Bennett EJ, Tennant CC, Piesse C, et al (Royal North Shore Hosp, Sydney, Australia)

Gut 43:256-261, 1998 5–32

Background.—In most patients with irritable bowel syndrome (IBS) and functional dyspepsia (FD), life stress contributes to the onset and exacerbation of symptoms. However, the strength of this effect is not clear. The relationship of chronic life stress to subsequent symptom intensity over time was assessed prospectively.

Methods.—One hundred seventeen consecutive outpatients meeting modified Rome criteria for IBS were interviewed at study entry and 6 and 16 months later. Life stress and symptom intensity measures were determined from the interview data, and the potency of the chronic life stress threat in the preceding 6 months or more was assessed, along with the severity and frequency of IBS and FD symptoms in the following 2 weeks.

Findings.—A long-term life stress threat strongly predicted subsequent symptom intensity. Life stress explained 97% of the variance on the symptom intensity measure over 16 months. None of the patients exposed to even 1 long-term, highly threatening stressor improved clinically during the 16 months. All improvements occurred in the absence of such stressors.

Conclusions.—In patients with IBS and FD, severe and long-term life stress threats have a powerful, consistent effect on symptom intensity over time. The level of the long-term life stress threat predicts the clinical outcome in most patients with these gastrointestinal disorders.

▶ These 2 articles (Abstracts 5–31 and 5–32) again reinforce our understanding that the mind and the gut are related. Irritable-bowel–type symptoms either disappear or improve after resolution of major life stress problems that may include (1) fear of illness, (2) chronic severe stress, whether it is family, job, or financially related, and (3) lack of control or fulfillment in the patient's life.

Dr. Drossman's group (see Abstract 5–31) strengthens our understanding that sexual and physical abuse are associated with indicators of poor health, reporting of medical symptoms, and functional disability. These events lead victims to seek health care later in life for a variety of symptoms. Unfortunately, we as health care providers may not explore both of these issues with our patients but, instead, focus on their multitude of complaints. Overall, we must be comfortable with our attempts to find out about these problems as well as to address the underlying problem. This approach will benefit our patients and decrease their use of health care resources.

J.S. Barkin, M.D.

The Appendix

Computed Tomography of Superior Mesenteric Vein Thrombosis Following Appendectomy

Schmutz GR, Benko A, Billiard JS, et al (Centre Hospitalier Universitaire, Caen, France; Univ of Sherbrooke, Canada)

Abdom Imaging 23:563-567, 1998 5–33

Objective.—Several different conditions can lead to pylephlebitis, or thrombophlebitis of the portal vein. Morbidity and mortality are high with this condition although they can be prevented by antibiotic and anticoagulant therapy. Rarely, suppurative thrombophlebitis of the superior mesenteric vein (SMV) will develop in a patient with appendicitis. Cases of thrombosis after appendectomy (but apparently unrelated to the initial appendicitis) have not been reported. Six cases of postappendectomy SMV are reported.

Patients.—Over a 5-year period, SMV thrombosis developed in 6 patients shortly after appendectomy. The patients were 5 men and 1 woman, ages 18 to 63 years. All patients were free of signs of SMV thrombosis at the time of their operations, and remained free of symptoms for longer than 2 weeks after appendectomy. Symptoms included fever in 3 patients, diffuse abdominal pain in 3, and diarrhea in 2. All patients had an elevated blood sedimentation rate and white blood cell count, with negative blood cultures. Two had elevated liver function test results. In 4 of 6 patients, the initial appendicitis was complicated. Postappendectomy abscess was suspected in 3 cases, pancreatitis in 2, and acute cholecystitis in 1. All patients underwent CT scanning.

Findings.—Postcontrast CT showed an enlarged SMV with enhancement of the vascular wall and intraluminal clot. One patient had thrombus extending to the portal vein, with areas of low attenuation in the liver corresponding to hepatic infarcts. Concomitant conditions predisposing to SMV thrombosis were idiopathic hypersplenism in 1 patient and chronic liver disease in another.

Discussion.—SMV thrombosis is a possible cause of abdominal symptoms after appendectomy. This complication may be more likely in the patient with a perforated appendix or with coagulation abnormalities. Early CT is needed to make the diagnosis of SMV thrombosis and to rule out abscess and other postoperative complications. This experience permits no conclusions about the value of early anticoagulant therapy for patients with SMV thrombosis.

▶ Acute appendicitis rarely results in thrombophlebitis of the mesenteric vein after a prolonged, complicated course or even after simple appendectomy, but it does occur in a significant number of patients. This result is uniformly significant in those patients in whom this problem develops. The symptoms and signs of SMV thrombosis are nonfocal and nonspecific. Only a high index of suspicion leads to an accurate diagnosis. This report of a small series of 6 patients from France and Canada reveals the usefulness of CT scanning in making the diagnosis of SMV thrombosis. In each of the patients, 3 criteria were fulfilled on CT scan. Enlargement of the thrombosed vein, an intraluminal clot, and a sharply defined contrast-enhanced wall were all present. CT scan was much better than ultrasonography. The entity of SMV thrombosis should be considered in patients who continue to have a prolonged, unrelenting course from appendicitis. Only a high index of suspicion will help patients survive.

J.W. Fleshman, Jr., M.D.

Diagnostic Laparoscopy in 1043 Patients With Suspected Acute Appendicitis

Moberg A-C, Ahlberg G, Leijonmarck C-E, et al (Univ Hosp of Malmö, Sweden; St. Göran Hosp, Stockholm; Akershus Central Hosp, Norbyhagen, Norway)

Eur J Surg 164:833-840, 1998 5–34

Purpose.—The diagnosis of acute appendicitis continues to be a challenging problem. Laparoscopy provides a new diagnostic tool for patients with suspected acute appendicitis. A prospective study of diagnostic laparoscopy for suspected acute appendicitis was performed, including assessment of the complications of laparoscopy and the effects of leaving an apparently normal appendix in place.

Methods.—Of 2,034 patients operated on for suspected acute appendicitis, 1,043 underwent diagnostic laparoscopy. If laparoscopy showed acute appendicitis, it was up to the surgeon to decide whether appendectomy would be performed laparoscopically or by open surgery. Macroscopically normal appendixes were not removed, even if no other intra-abdominal disease was apparent. Morbidity and mortality rates were assessed, along with the patients' clinical characteristics, diagnoses, length of hospital stay, and readmission rate.

Results.—Appendectomy was performed in 819 patients. Sixty-one percent of these procedures were done laparoscopically and 39% by open means. The complication rate was 10%. In 211 patients, diagnostic laparoscopy was the only procedure performed. This group included 181 women, 86 of whom had gynecologic disorders. Among patients undergoing diagnostic laparoscopy only, the complication rate was 2%. At 2 years' follow-up, none had required readmission for appendectomy. Thirteen patients underwent open procedures for other reasons, most commonly gynecologic disorders or diverticulitis. Four elderly patients died, for an operative mortality rate of 0.4%

Conclusions.—This study demonstrates the safety of diagnostic laparoscopy as a single procedure in patients with suspected acute appendicitis. This procedure is especially recommended in fertile women. When appendicitis is present, either perforated or unperforated, laparoscopic appendectomy can be performed. The results suggest that macroscopically normal appendixes need not be removed.

Abdominal Sonography Screening of Clinically Diagnosed or Suspected Appendicitis Before Surgery

Chen S-C, Chen K-M, Wang S-M, et al (Natl Taiwan Univ Hosp, Republic of China; Cathay Gen Hosp, Taiwan, Republic of China)

World J Surg 22:449-452, 1998 5–35

Background.—More accurate diagnostic tests for acute appendicitis are needed. Abdominal sonography has given promising results, but its screening accuracy has never been rigorously tested. A prospective trial of abdominal sonography for preoperative diagnosis of acute appendicitis was performed.

Methods.—The study included 191 patients with a clinical diagnosis or suspicion of appendicitis. The patients were 114 men and 77 women (mean age, 39 years.) All patients underwent abdominal sonography, performed by a staff surgeon with experience in this diagnostic procedure. A 3.75 MHz curved-array transducer with a graded compression technique was used for the sonography. Sonographic criteria for appendicitis were a noncompressible appendix, an anteroposterior diameter of 7 mm or greater, an appendicolith, interrupted continuity of the echogenic submucosa, or localized periappendiceal fluid collection. Each scan was classified as showing appendicitis or other diseases or as normal.

Results.—The sonographic diagnosis was appendicitis in 83% of the patients and other diseases in 9%; findings were normal in 8%. Sonography altered the diagnosis and treatment for 14% of the patients with clinically diagnosed appendicitis and 20% of those with clinically suspected appendicitis. There was 1 false negative examination. Ninety-one percent of the patients undergoing appendectomy had pathologically confirmed appendicitis. Sonography prevented 32 negative appendectomies. Its diagnostic sensitivity was 99%, with a specificity of 68%, an accuracy of 92%, a positive predictive value of 91%, and a negative predictive value of 97%.

Conclusions.—Abdominal sonography is a valuable test for the preoperative diagnosis of acute appendicitis. When sonography is negative, it is always a true negative. If sonography is positive, the differential diagnosis includes a normal and secondarily enlarged appendix. Sonography performed by an experienced surgeon is regarded as an essential preoperative examination for patients with clinically diagnosed or clinically suspected appendicitis.

▶ Accuracy in the diagnosis of appendicitis can prevent unnecessary operation and avoid complications of perforated appendicitis. The important features from these two articles (Abstracts 5–34 and 5–35) are the consecutive nature of the series and the diagnostic accuracy found. Diagnostic laparoscopy reveals the diagnosis of appendicitis 100% of the time and may avoid a resection if the appendicitis is not present. Unfortunately, diagnostic laparoscopy requires a general anesthetic. The article, which describes the use of ultrasonography, shows us that a reasonable accuracy can be achieved in a group of patients who have undergone preoperative ultrasonography of the right lower quadrant. Although the technique is operator-dependent, a surgeon can achieve reasonable results using ultrasonography in conjunction with clinical findings. In the article by Chen et al., 17% of the patients studied avoided an unnecessary appendectomy. The combination of laparoscopy and ultrasonography may be able to increase this percentage. The criteria for appendicitis on ultrasonography include an appendix greater than 7 mm in diameter, the presence of a fecalith, and periappendiceal fluid seen on the ultrasonogram. More stringent criteria and the use of Doppler ultrasonography may be able to increase the specificity along with the sensitivity of the test. In high-risk patients in whom a contrast study or diagnostic laparoscopy is not possible, Doppler ultrasonography may be a reasonable screening tool. In those patients in whom a diagnosis is still unclear, laparoscopy may be the next best step.

J.W. Fleshman, Jr., M.D.

Misdiagnosis of Primary Epiploic Appendagitis

Rao PM, Rhea JT, Wittenberg J, et al (Massachusetts Gen Hosp, Boston)
Am J Surg 176:81-85, 1998 5–36

Introduction.—Primary epiploic appendagitis (PEA) is an uncommon condition that is difficult to diagnose clinically and usually is recognized only at laparotomy. Normal appendices epiploicae can be identified on CT scans only when outlined by peritoneal cavity fluid (Fig 1). Recent reports have described the pathognomic CT appearance of appendageal inflammation (Fig 2). This study examined the rate of CT misdiagnosis of PEA, including its impact on patient management and use of hospital resources.

Methods.—The retrospective analysis included 660 CT scans performed over a 2-year period in patients with clinically suspected diverticulitis or appendicitis. Each scan was reviewed for the presence of strict radiologic criteria for PEA. These cases were reviewed to determine the clinical findings and course and for comparison with the original radiologic report. None of the scans was originally interpreted as showing PEA. The

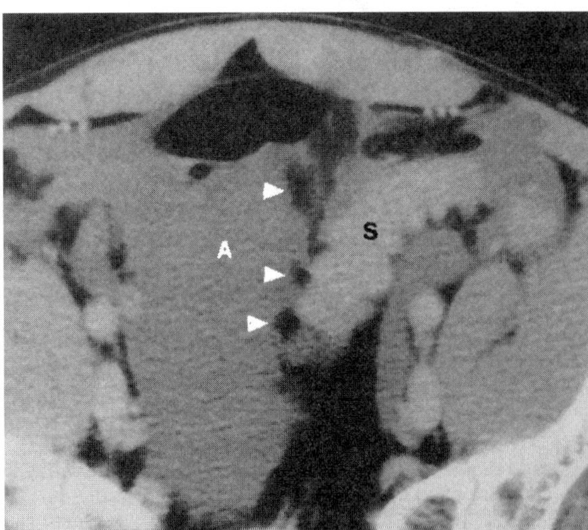

FIGURE 1.—Appendices epiploicae. CT scan in cirrhotic patient with ascites (*A*) outlining several normal appendices epiploicae (*arrowheads*) arising from sigmoid colon (*S*). (Courtesy of Rao PM, Rhea JT, Wittenberg J, et al: Misdiagnosis of primary epiploic appendagitis. *Am J Surg* 176:81-85. Copyright 1998, with permission from Excerpta Medica Inc.)

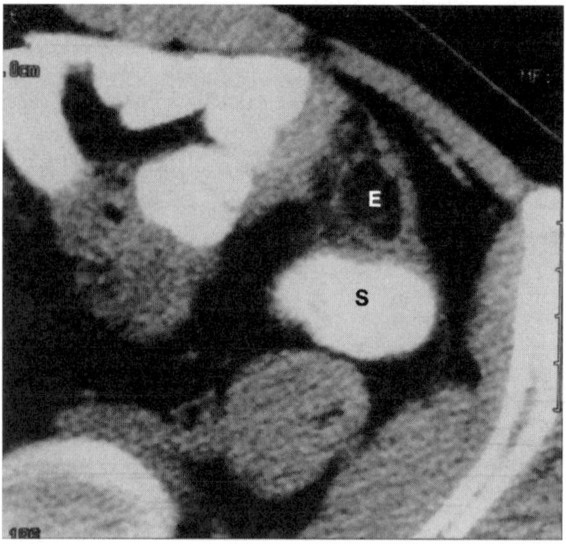

FIGURE 2.—Primary epiploic appendagitis. CT image shows oval-shaped, infarcted epiploic appendage 2 cm in maximum diameter (*E*), arising from sigmoid colon (*S*), with periappendageal fat stranding and visceral and parietal peritoneal thickening. (Courtesy of Rao PM, Rhea JT, Wittenberg J, et al: Misdiagnosis of primary epiploic appendagitis. *Am J Surg* 176:81-85. Copyright 1998, with permission from Excerpta Medica Inc.)

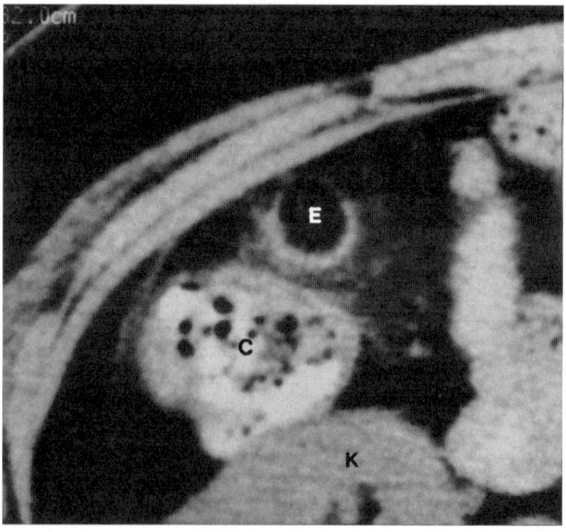

FIGURE 3.—Primary epiploic appendagitis. CT slice shows 2 cm, nearly round, infarcted epiploic appendage (*E*) arising from ascending colon (*C*), with periappendageal fat stranding and parietal peritoneal thickening. *Abbreviation: K*, right kidney. (Courtesy of Rao PM, Rhea JT, Wittenberg J, et al: Misdiagnosis of primary epiploic appendagitis. *Am J Surg* 176:81-85. Copyright 1998, with permission from Excerpta Medica Inc.)

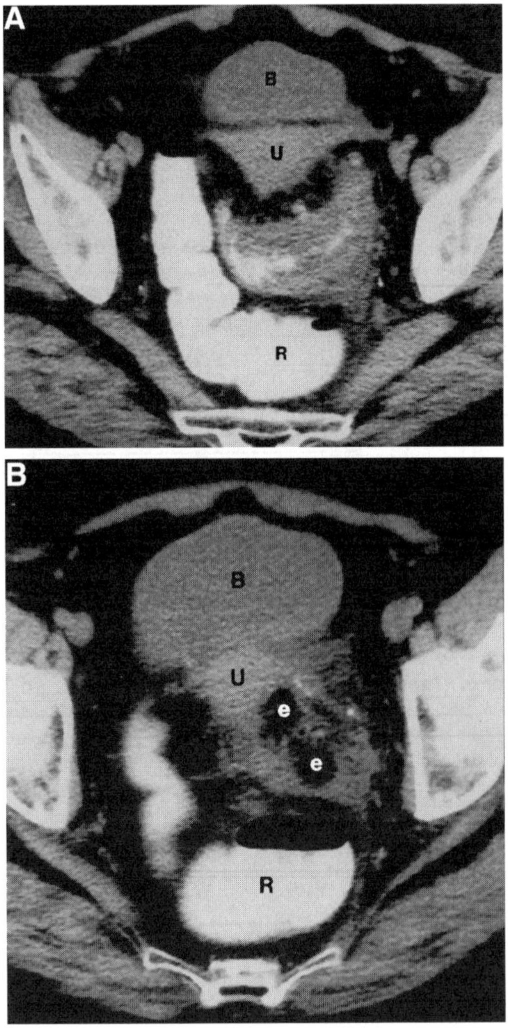

FIGURE 4.—Diverticulitis and secondary epiploic appendagitis. A, CT image through sigmoid colon shows luminal narrowing, wall thickening, multiple diverticula, and perisigmoid fat stranding, consistent with diverticulitis. B, Computed tomography image at lower level shows two intrinisically normal epiploic appendages (*e*), made visible by inflammatory fluid in pouch of Douglas. *Abbreviations: B*, bladder; *U*, uterus; *R*, rectum. (Courtesy of Rao PM, Rhea JT, Wittenberg J, et al: Misdiagnosis of primary epiploic appendagitis. *Am J Surg* 176:81-85. Copyright 1998, with permission from Excerpta Medica Inc.)

rate of radiologic misdiagnosis of PEA was determined, and its impact on patient management and costs was assessed.

Results.—A retrospective diagnosis of PEA was made in 7 cases, for a misdiagnosis rate of 2% (Figs 3 and 4). The patients were 7 men and 4 women, average age 46 years. Six of the 7 cases were misinterpreted as diverticulitis and 1 as appendicitis. The 7 patients stayed in the hospital for a mean of 4 days, with 6 receiving antibiotic therapy. Average cost of care

TABLE 1.—Clinical and CT Findings in Patients With Primary Epiploic Appendagitis

Clinical Signs and Symptoms	Percent Occurrence
Sudden onset abdominal pain	100
Focal abdominal pain	100
Worse with cough, stretch, deep breath	100
Rebound tenderness	91
Nausea/vomiting	27
Pain onset during exertion	18
Temperature >99.5°F (37.5°C)	18
White blood cell count >10,000/mm^3	18
Change in bowel habits	9
Computed tomography findings	
Oval-shaped mass lesion	100
Fat density	100
Paracolic lesion	100
Visceral peritoneal thickening	100
Periappendageal fat stranding	100
Parietal peritoneal thickening	82
Mass effect on adjacent bowel	18
Central high-attenuating dot	18

(Courtesy of Rao PM, Rhea JT, Wittenberg J, et al: Misdiagnosis of primary epiploic appendagitis. *Am J Surg* 176:81-85. Copyright 1998, with permission from Excerpta Medica Inc.)

for these patients was about $4,200. A correct initial diagnosis of PEA was made in 4 patients. Just 1 of these patients was admitted to the hospital overnight, and none received antibiotic therapy. Their average cost of care was about $1,200. Follow-up CT scans in 10 of the 11 patients showed resolution of PEA. All patients had resolution of their symptoms, with no recurrences at 6 months' follow-up (Table 1).

Conclusions.—Primary epiploic appendagitis is difficult to diagnose clinically but has a pathognomic CT appearance. The correct diagnosis avoids unnecessary treatment and associated costs. The diagnosis of PEA is easily made in patients undergoing CT scanning to confirm or exclude diverticulitis or appendicitis.

▶ The group from Massachusetts General Hospital once again provides a clear analysis of the use of CT scanning to evaluate patients with PEA and compares it with the evaluation of diverticulitis and appendicitis. The cost analysis, once again, reveals the CT scan to be very cost-effective. The diagnosis of primary appendagitis is very rare and occurs in fewer than 2% of patients evaluated for abdominal pain. The diagnosis of PEA is really one of exclusion and requires a high index of suspicion. It is normally treated nonoperatively and therefore is a cause for negative exploratory laparotomy for appendicitis or diverticulitis. The criteria for primary appendagitis are seen in the figures included in this review. An oval-shaped, infarcted epiploic appendage with periappendageal fat stranding and visceral and parietal peritoneal thickening are required for the diagnosis in this setting of an otherwise negative CT scan.

J.W. Fleshman, Jr., M.D.

Effect of Computed Tomography of the Appendix on Treatment of Patients and Use of Hospital Resources

Rao PM, Rhea JT, Novelline RA, et al (Massachusetts Gen Hosp, Boston)

N Engl J Med 338:141-146, 1998 5–37

Objective.—Approximately half the patients hospitalized for suspected appendicitis are ultimately given a diagnosis of some other condition. About 20% of appendicitis cases are missed, and 15% to 40% of patients undergo appendectomies unnecessarily. The accuracy of CT in helping to diagnose or rule out appendectomy was evaluated.

Methods.—A CT was performed on 100 consecutive patients (43 male), aged 6 to 75 years, admitted for suspected appendicitis. The CT results were compared with surgical findings, and final results were evaluated by clinical follow-up at 2 months in 41 patients. Treatment plans before CT were compared with actual treatment after CT. Use of hospital resources was analyzed retrospectively.

Results.—At surgery for appendicitis or other conditions, 53 patients had appendicitis and 47 did not. The CT results were positive in 53 patients, negative in 45, false positive in 1, and false negative in 1. These results demonstrated a level of 98% for sensitivity, specificity, positive predictive value, negative predictive value, and overall accuracy of the CT interpretations (Figs 1, 2). The CT results changed treatment strategies for 59 patients, including prevention of unnecessary appendectomy in 13, admission for observation in 18, admission for observation before appendectomy in 21, and admission for observation before diagnosis by CT of other medical conditions in 11. Prevention of unnecessary appendectomy in 13 patients resulted in a savings of $47,281 in surgical and allied costs and in a savings of 50 hospitalization days ($20,250) (Table 4). After deducting the cost of 100 CT scans ($22,800), the resulting savings per patient was $447.

Conclusion.—Routine CT scans of patients with suspected appendicitis decreases unnecessary surgery and reduces the use of hospital resources, resulting in a saving of $447 per patient.

► This use of CT scan as a screening test for patients with appendicitis may be cost effective when used to determine the admission and performance of operations in patients with symptoms suggestive of appendicitis. The article shows a large savings if CT scan is utilized in all patients coming to the emergency room complaining of symptoms suggestive of appendicitis. While the study is well-designed with clear end points and a strong conclusion based on outcomes and measures, it must be viewed with some skepticism. If patients with clear cases of appendicitis, such as the young male under the age of 20 with right lower quadrant pain, are eliminated from the routine CT scan, even more money could be saved. A judicious use of CT scanning in the emergency room, therefore, is more likely to produce good outcomes and cost effectiveness than to give carte blanche to order this otherwise expensive test.

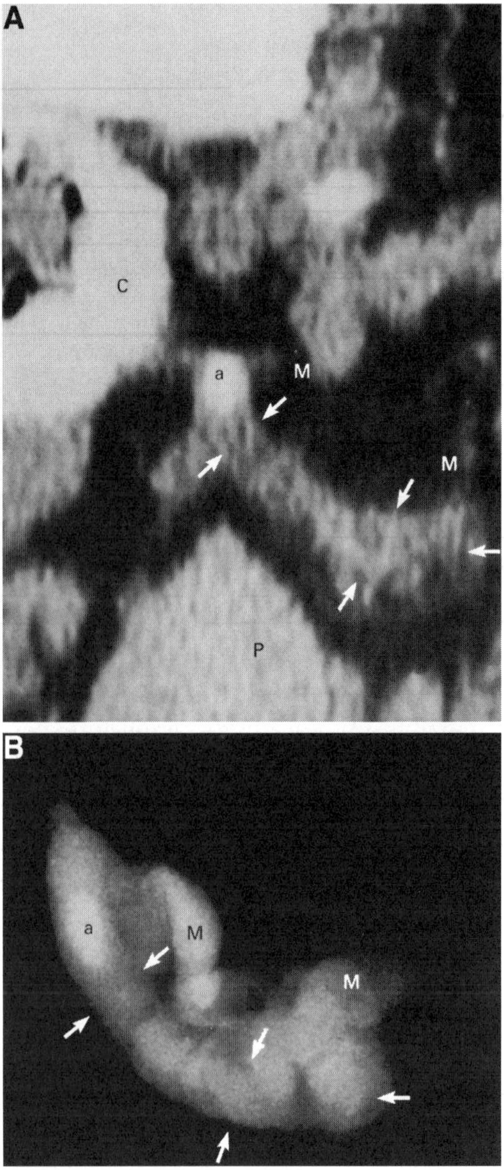

FIGURE 1.—Results of appendiceal CT in a 30-year-old man with suspected appendicitis and radiographic appearance of the specimen after appendectomy. **A,** coronally reformatted appendiceal CT scan showing an inflamed, unopacified appendix, 12 mm in diameter (*arrows*), with proximal appendolith (*a*). Also shown are the cecum (C), right psoas muscle (*P*), and appendiceal mesentery (*M*). **B,** radiograph of the inflamed appendix (*arrows*) and appendiceal mesentery after surgical removal. (Courtesy of Rao PM, Rhea JT, Novelline RA, et al: Effect of computed tomography of the appendix on treatment of patients and use of hospital resources. *N Engl J Med* 338:141-146, 1998. Reprinted by permission of *The New England Journal of Medicine*. Copyright 1998, Massachusetts Medical Society. All rights reserved.)

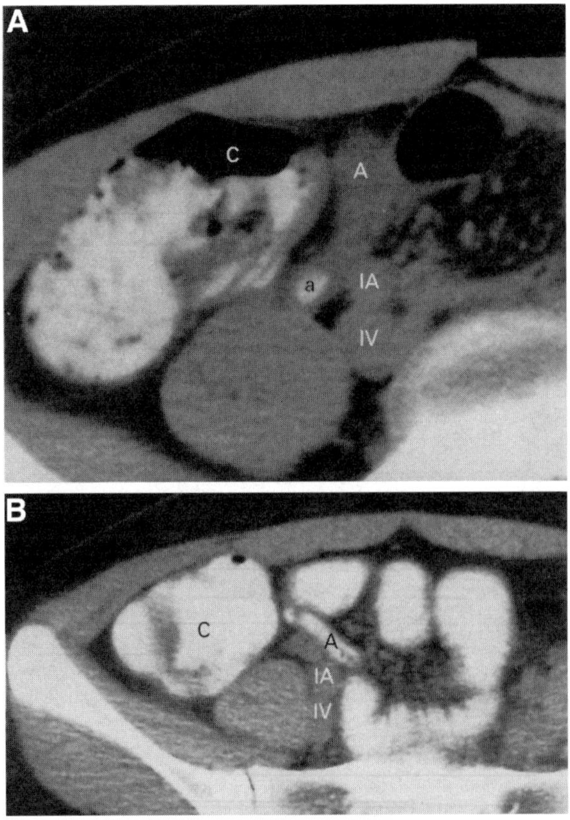

FIGURE 2.—Results of appendiceal CT in four patients. **A,** CT scan of a 17-year-old boy with suspected appendicitis. The axial image shows an inflamed, unopacified appendix, 15 mm in diameter (*A*), with proximal appendolith (*a*). Also shown are the cecum (*C*) and the common iliac artery (*IA*) and vein (*IV*). **B,** a 21-year-old woman with suspected appendicitis. The axial image shows a tubular, opacified normal appendix. **C,** CT scan of an 8-year-old girl with suspected appendicitis. The axial image at the level of the ascending colon (*AC*) shows clumped, enlarged mesenteric lymph nodes (*N*), a finding consistent with a diagnosis of mesenteric adenitis. Also shown are the aorta (*A*), inferior vena cava (*V*), right psoas muscle (*P*), and lumbar spine (*S*). **D,** a 39-year-old man with suspected appendicitis. the axial image shows a focally inflamed, right-sided, redundant loop of sigmoid colon (*S*), a finding consistent with a diagnosis of sigmoid diverticulitis. (Courtesy of Rao PM, Rhea JT, Novelline RA, et al: Effect of computed tomography of the appendix on treatment of patients and use of hospital resources. *N Engl J Med* 338:141-146, 1998. Reprinted by permission of *The New England Journal of Medicine*. Copyright 1998, Massachusetts Medical Society. All rights reserved.)

(*Continued*)

FIGURE 2 (cont.)

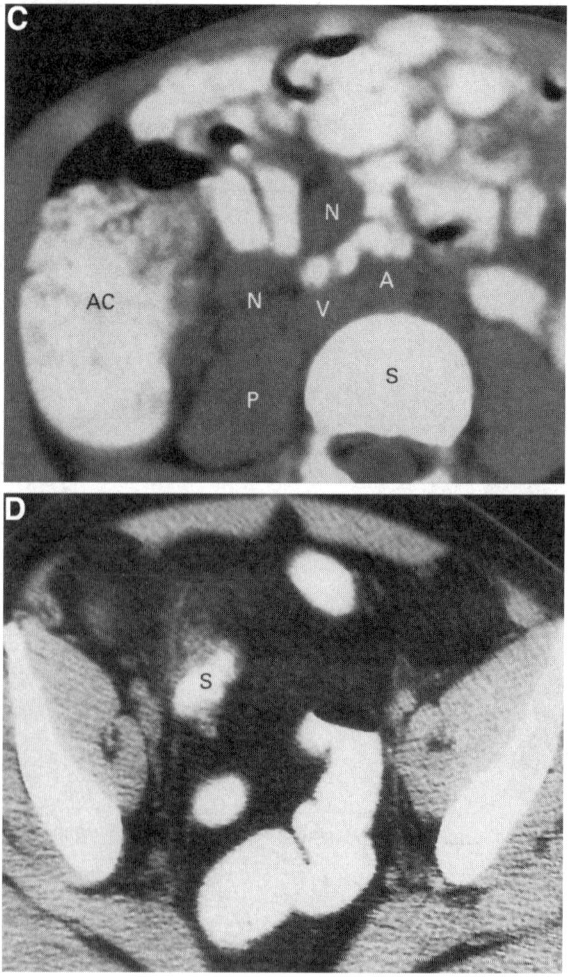

A helical "spiral" CT scan with contrast is necessary to achieve these results. State-of-the-art scanning is, therefore, mandatory if this technique is to be effective. As seen in the accompanying articles (ultrasonography and diagnostic laparoscopy), specificity and sensitivity can be very high in preoperative diagnostic testing. The combination of ultrasound, laparoscopy, and CT scanning should, therefore, continue to decrease the need for negative exploratory laparotomy and reduce the risk of complications of appendicitis.

J.W. Fleshman, Jr., M.D.

TABLE 4.—Effect of CT on Treatment and the Use of Resources for 100 Patients With Suspected Appendicitis

Treatment Change	No. of Patients	Savings or Costs per Patient (Dollars)	Total Savings or Costs (Dollars)
Savings			
Avoided unnecessary appendectomy	13	3,637	47,281
Avoided observation for 1 day before appendectomy	21	405	8,505
Avoided observation for 1 day before treatment for CT-diagnosed alternative condition	11	405	4,455
Avoided observation for 1 day before discharge	18	405	7,290
Costs			
Appendiceal CT examinations	100	228	22,800
Overall cost savings			44,731

(Courtesy of Rao PM, Rhea JT, Novelline RA, et al: Effect of computed tomography of the appendix on treatment of patients and use of hospital resources. *N Engl J Med* 338:141-146, 1998. Reprinted by permission of *The New England Journal of Medicine*.)

Colorectal Cancer and Other Neoplasms

MEDICAL

Aspirin Use and Colorectal Cancer: Post-trial Follow-up Data From the Physicians' Health Study

Stürmer T, Glynn RJ, Lee I-M, et al (Harvard Med School, Boston; Univ of Ulm, Germany)

Ann Intern Med 128:713-720, 1998 5–38

Introduction.—Observational studies have reported that the use of aspirin and other nonsteroidal anti-inflammatory drugs reduces colorectal cancer incidence or mortality. The Physicians' Health Study, however, found no association between aspirin and colorectal cancer after 5 years of low-dose aspirin. These authors extended this follow-up to a mean of 12 years.

Methods.—Two hypotheses were tested in the Physicians' Health Study: that the risk of cardiovascular disease is reduced by taking 325 mg aspirin on alternate days and that the incidence of cancer is decreased by taking 50 mg of β-carotene taken on alternate days. The aspirin arm of the trial was stopped early (January 1988) and the β-carotene arm continued until December 1995. Participants were male physicians aged 40 to 84 years. This analysis used all confirmed cases of colorectal cancer and all cases of colorectal cancer reported until October 25, 1995 (Fig 1).

Results.—Colorectal cancer was diagnosed in 341 participants, 173 in the aspirin group and 168 in the placebo group. Over 12 years of follow-up, assignment to low-dose aspirin was associated with a relative risk of 1.03 for colorectal cancer. When the aspirin arm of the trial was discon-

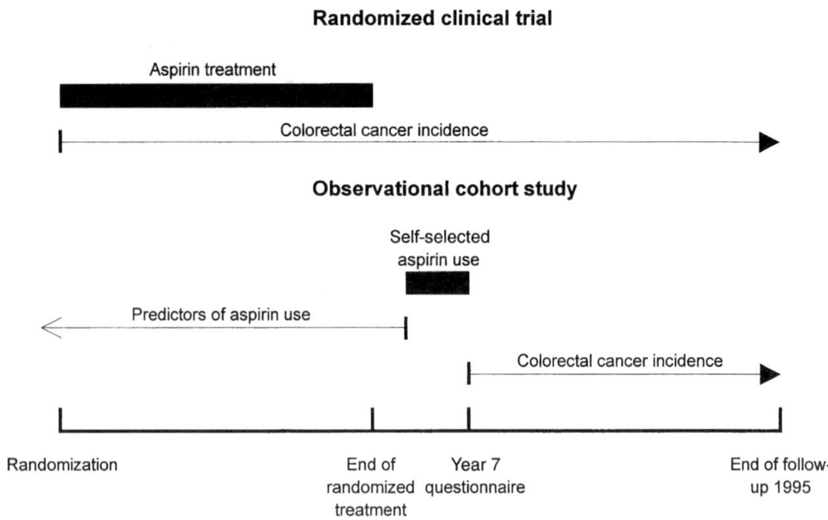

FIGURE 1.—Design of study of aspirin and colorectal cancer: post-trial follow-up from the Physician's Health Study. (Courtesy of Stürmer T, Glynn RJ, Lee IM, et al: Aspirin use and colorectal cancer: Post-trial follow-up data from the physicians' health study. *Ann Intern Med* 128:713-720, 1998.)

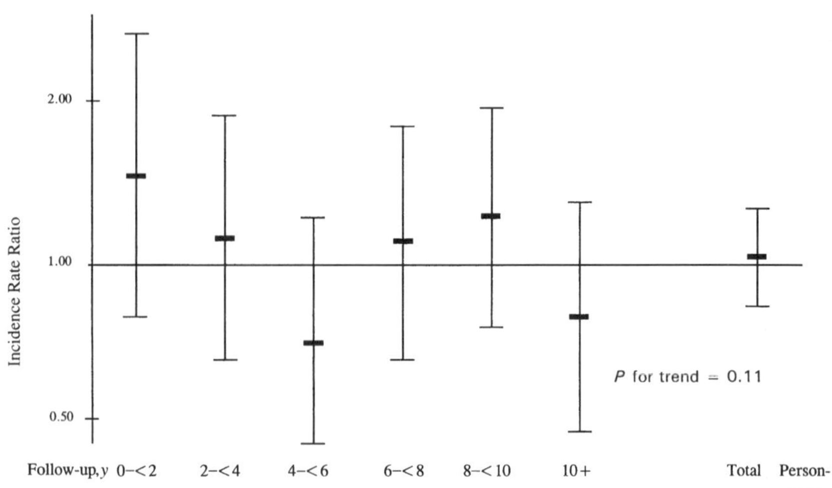

Patients, *n*								
Aspirin	25	29	22	31	38	28	173	129 387
Placebo	17	26	31	28	31	35	168	129 116

FIGURE 2.—Relative risk for colorectal cancer in the aspirin group compared with the placebo group. Bars represent 95% confidence intervals. (Courtesy of Stürmer T, Glynn RJ, Lee IM, et al: Aspirin use and colorectal cancer: Post-trial follow-up data from the physicians' health study. *Ann Intern Med* 128:713-720, 1998.)

tinued because of the beneficial effects on cardiovascular disease, participants could choose aspirin or placebo to take with the β-carotene. For those who used aspirin frequently after 1988, the relative risk for colorectal cancer was 1.07 (Fig 2).

Conclusion.—Both randomized and observational analyses of data from the Physicians' Health Study fail to show an association between the use of aspirin and the incidence of colorectal cancer. Clinicians should be cautioned about using aspirin or other nonsteroidal anti-inflammatory drugs for the primary prevention of colorectal cancer.

Nonsteroidal Antiinflammatory Drug Use and Reduced Risk of Large Bowel Carcinoma

Rosenberg L, Louik C, Shapiro S (Boston Univ, Brookline, Mass)

Cancer 82:2326-2333, 1998 5–39

Background.—The use of nonsteroidal anti-inflammatory drugs (NSAIDs) may reduce the incidence of large bowel carcinoma. The association between aspirin and nonaspirin NSAID use and the risk of large bowel carcinoma was further investigated.

Methods and Findings.—In this population-based, case-control study, data were obtained from 1,201 patients with large bowel carcinoma and 1,201 control participants matched by age, sex, and area of residence (Table 1). Regular NSAID use into the year before diagnosis was correlated with a significantly reduced relative risk estimate overall and among stage II to IV tumors (Table 3). Discontinued use of NSAIDs was not associated with risk reduction. The inverse association with regular, continuing use was observed across age and sex groups and in patients with both colon and rectal carcinoma. Similar inverse correlations were apparent for regular, continuing use of aspirin and nonaspirin NSAIDs. No significant evidence of an association between declining relative risk and increasing duration of use was found. Also, there was no trend across aspirin doses, which ranged from less than half a 325-mg tablet per day to 2 or more tablets per day. Discontinuing use of NSAIDs in response to symptoms of carcinoma did not appear to explain the inverse association, nor did bias related to the diagnosis of carcinoma (Table 4).

Conclusions.—These data support a causal association between NSAID use and a decrease in the incidence of large bowel carcinoma. Further studies are needed to define how the duration of use and the NSAID dose affect this incidence.

TABLE 1.—Characteristics of 1,201 Cases of Large Bowel Carcinoma and 1,201 Matched Community Controls

Factor	Cases No.	Cases (%)	Controls No.	Controls (%)	Factor	Cases No.	Cases (%)	Controls No.	Controls (%)
Male	686	(57)	686	(57)	Race				
Female	515	(43)	515	(43)	White	1132	(49)	1149	(96)
Age (yrs)					Religion				
< 40	29	(2)	29	(2)	Catholic	786	(65)	757	(63)
40-49	119	(10)	119	(10)	Protestant	356	(29)	355	(30)
50-59	342	(28)	342	(28)	Jewish	45	(4)	57	(5)
60-69	711	(59)	711	(59)					
Education (yrs)					Physical activity on the job				
< 12	215	(18)	148	(12)	Sedentary/light	565	(47)	566	(47)
12	456	(38)	487	(41)	Medium	475	(40)	463	(39)
13-15	224	(19)	221	(18)	Intense	156	(13)	153	(13)
16+	298	(25)	339	(28)					
Cholecystectomy	105	(9)	102	(8)	Moderate leisure-time physical activity				
Large bowel carcinoma in parent or sibling	195	(16)	101	(8)	None	392	(33)	303	(25)
					1-4 hrs/wk	365	(30)	433	(36)
					5+ hrs/wk	350	(29)	346	(29)
Vigorous leisure-time physical activity					Vegetable and fruit (servings/day)				
None	912	(76)	837	(70)	< 3	222	(22)	153	(17)
1-4 hrs/wk	167	(14)	216	(18)	3-4	418	(41)	304	(34)
5+ hrs/wk	75	(6)	95	(8)	5+	370	(37)	448	(50)
Alcohol (drinks/wk)					Fat intake (g/day)				
None	372	(31)	391	(33)	< 43	251	(25)	304	(34)
Former drinker	201	(17)	219	(18)	43-62	319	(32)	292	(32)
1-7/wk	310	(26)	331	(28)	63+	439	(43)	310	(34)
8-14/wk	129	(11)	121	(10)					
15+/wk	173	(15)	118	(10)					
Coffee (drinks/day)					Fiber intake (g/day)				
None	127	(11)	144	(12)	< 15	353	(35)	302	(33)
Former drinker	183	(15)	164	(14)	15-20	357	(35)	291	(32)
< 5/day	783	(65)	775	(65)	21+	299	(30)	313	(35)
5+/day	102	(8)	105	(9)					

*Totals on which percents are based vary.

(Courtesy of Rosenberg L, Louik C, Shapiro S: Nonsteroidal antiinflammatory drug use and reduced risk of large bowel carcinoma. *Cancer* 82:2326-2333.

TABLE 3.—Continuing and Discontinued Regular NSAID Use That Began 1+ Year Before Index Date Among 1,201 Cases of Large Bowel Carcinoma and 1,201 Matched Community Controls According to Age, Gender, and Cancer Site

	NSAID Use	Cases	Controls	Relative Risk* Estimate (95% Confidence Interval)
Age (yrs)				
< 50	None	111	115	1.0†
	Continuing	8	14	0.6 (0.2-1.4)
	Discontinued	18	16	1.2 (0.6-2.6)
50-69	None	695	629	1.0†
	Continuing	193	257	0.7 (0.6-0.8)
	Discontinued	101	101	0.9 (0.7-1.2)
Gender				
Female	None	348	327	1.0†
	Continuing	73	88	0.8 (0.6-1.1)
	Discontinued	62	67	0.9 (0.0-1.3)
Male	None	458	417	1.0†
	Continuing	128	183	0.6 (0.5-0.8)
	Discontinued	57	50	1.0 (0.7-1.6)
Site				
Colon	None	539	744	1.0†
	Continuing	136	271	0.7 (0.6-0.9)
	Discontinued	81	117	1.0 (0.7-1.3)
Rectum	None	264	744	1.0†
	Continuing	64	271	0.6 (0.5-0.9)
	Discontinued	37	117	0.9 (0.6-1.4)

Abbreviation: NSAID, nonsteroidal anti-inflammatory drug.
*Adjusted for age and gender.
†Reference category.
(Courtesy of Rosenberg L, Louik C, Shapiro S: Nonsteroidal antiinflammatory drug use and reduced risk of large bowel carcinoma. *Cancer* 82:2326-2333. Copyright © 1998 American Cancer Society. Reprinted by permission of Wiley-Liss, Inc., a subsidiary of John Wiley & Sons, Inc.)

TABLE 4.—Continuing Regular Use of Aspirin-containing Drugs That Began 1+ Year Before the Index Date, According to the Duration of Use and the Dose of Aspirin

Aspirin Use	Cases	Controls	Relative Risk* Estimate (95% Confidence Interval)
No use of any NSAID	806	744	1.0†
Continuing use: total years of use	150	203	0.7 (0.5-0.9)
< 2	18	26	0.6 (0.4-1.2)
2	32	29	1.0 (0.6-1.7)
3-4	28	56	0.5 (0.3-0.7)
5-9	36	47	0.7 (0.4-1.1)
10-14	17	24	0.7 (0.4-1.2)
15+	17	20	0.8 (0.4-1.5)
Aspirin dose (per day)			
< 162.5 mg	17	30	0.5 (0.3-1.0)
162.5-324 mg	28	31	0.8 (0.5-1.4)
325 mg	66	93	0.6 (0.5-0.9)
326-649 mg	9	14	0.6 (0.2-1.4)
650 mg +	16	23	0.6 (0.3-1.2)

Abbreviation: NSAID, nonsteroidal anti-inflammatory drug.
*Adjusted for age and gender.
†Reference category.
(Courtesy of Rosenberg L, Louik C, Shapiro S: Nonsteroidal antiinflammatory drug use and reduced risk of large bowel carcinoma. *Cancer* 82:2326-2333. Copyright © 1998 American Cancer Society. Reprinted by permission of Wiley-Liss, Inc., a subsidiary of John Wiley & Sons, Inc.)

Chemoprevention of Spontaneous Intestinal Adenomas in the Adenomatous Polyposis Coli *Min* Mouse Model With Aspirin

Barnes CJ, Lee M (Univ of Texas, Health Science Ctr, San Antonio; Veterans Affairs Med Ctr, San Antionio, Tex)

Gastroenterology 114:873-877, 1998 5–40

Introduction.—Human epidemiologic data and rodent models of colon cancer have shown that aspirin and other nonsteroidal anti-inflammatory drugs (NSAIDs) may inhibit the development of colon cancer. A mouse model of familial adenomatous polyposis was used to determine whether aspirin significantly inhibits gastrointestinal tumor formation.

Methods.—Nine male and 9 female C57BL/6J +/+ (control) mice and 9 male and 9 female C57BL/6J *Min* mice were fed either a control AIN-76A diet or one supplemented with 250 or 500 parts per million of aspirin over a 7-week period.

Results.—Gastrointestinal tumors developed in all *Min* mice and no control mice. Aspirin significantly diminished tumor multiplicity (number of tumors per animal) in the small intestines but not in the colon, from an average of 35.8 tumors per mouse in the control group to 16 and 18.5 tumors per mouse given 250 and 500 parts per million of aspirin, respectively (Table 1). The total tumor load, defined as the sum of tumor diameters per mouse, was significantly diminished from 93.2 mm to 40.4 and 45.0 mm with 250 and 500 parts per million of aspirin, respectively. A significant elevation of mouse serum salicylate concentrations in a dose-dependent manner was a result of aspirin suplementation of the control diet in both control and *Min* mice (Table 2). Prostaglandin E_2 formation, as expected, was significantly reduced with aspirin treatment in a dose-response manner (Table 3).

TABLE 1.—Effects of Aspirin on Min Mice Tumors

Tumor Distribution	Control (0 ppm)	Aspirin 250 ppm	Aspirin 500 ppm
Small intestine			
Proximal	8.0 ± 1.7	3.8 ± 0.6*	5.5 ± 0.7*
Middle	10.8 ± 2.6	3.3 ± 0.6*	5.2 ± 0.8
Distal	16.0 ± 2.0	8.3 ± 1.4*	7.0 ± 2.0*
Colon	1.0 ± 0.4	0.5 ± 0.2	0.8 ± 0.3
Total	35.8 ± 4.4	16.0 ± 2.3*	18.5 ± 2.4*

NOTE. Control and *Min* mice were fed either an AIN-76A diet without aspirin or one supplemented with 250 or 500 parts per million of aspirin for 7 weeks (n = 6 per group). Data are the mean ± SEM number of tumors per mouse (tumor multiplicity), presented by treatment group and intestinal region. The small bowel was arbitrarily subdivided into three sections of equal length (proximal, middle, and distal). No tumors were found in the control mice regardless of location or aspirin treatment (data not shown).

*significantly different from *Min* mice fed a diet without aspirin (within the same region of the intestine, P < 0.05.

(Courtesy of Barnes CJ, Lee M: Chemoprevention of spontaneous intestinal adenomas in the adenomatous polyposis coli *Min* mouse model with aspirin. *Gastroenterology* 114:873-877, 1998.)

TABLE 2.—Effects of Aspirin on Serum Salicylate Levels in Mice

	Control (0 ppm)	Aspirin 250 ppm	Aspirin 500 ppm
C57BL/6J/+/+	0 ± 0*	1.06 ± 0.16†	1.68 ± 0.16‡
C57BL/6J/*Min*/+	0 ± 0*	2.18 ± 0.29†,§	2.70 ± 0.37‡,§

Note: Control and *Min* mice were fed either an AIN-76A diet without aspirin or one supplemented with 250 or 500 parts per million of aspirin for 7 weeks (n = 6 per group). Data are the mean ± SEM serum salicylate levels (mg/dL) in blood collected at the time of death detected using a commercial kit as previously described.

*O = undetectable.

†Significantly different from control (0) and 500-parts per million aspirin groups with the same genetic status, P<0.05.

‡Significantly different from control (0) and 250-parts per million aspirin groups with the same genetic status, P<0.05.

§Significantly different from corresponding normal mice treated with the same aspirin dose, P < 0.05.

Note: Control and *Min* mice were fed.

(Courtesy of Barnes CJ, Lee M: Chemoprevention of spontaneous intestinal adenomas in the adenomatous polyposis coli *Min* mouse model with aspirin. *Gastroenterology* 114:873-877, 1998.)

Conclusion.—These findings show for the first time that aspirin diminishes the formation of spontaneous intestinal tumors in mice with a genetic predisposition to development of these tumors. Adenomas were significantly reduced by aspirin treatment in the small intestine but not in the colon.

► A number of observational studies have linked the use of aspirin and NSAIDs with a decreased incidence of colorectal cancer and colorectal polyps. The precise mechanism of this postulated chemopreventive action remains unclear. However, several lines of evidence suggest that this class of drugs inhibits gastrointestinal tumors by inhibition of COX isozymes. Apoptosis has been suggested as an additional mechanism of inhibition of carcinogen-induced tumor formation, suggesting a prostoglandin-independent pathway through restoration of normal intestinal mucosal homeostasis, possibly by reducing cell proliferation or inducing apoptosis. The results of laboratory studies and of human observational studies seemed to point

TABLE 3.—Effects of Aspirin on Intestinal PGE_2 Formation

	Control (0 ppm)	Aspirin 250 ppm	Aspirin 500 ppm
C57BL/6J/+/+	13.1 ± 2.95	5.59 ± 1.33*	4.07 ± 1.14*
C57BL/6J/*Min*/+	8.63 ± 1.42	6.50 ± 2.26	1.57 ± 0.44*

Note: Control and *Min* mice were fed either an AIN-76A diet without aspirin or one supplemented with 250 or 500 parts per million of aspirin for 7 weeks (n = 6 per group). Data are means ± SEM of mucosal PGE_2 formation ($pg \cdot mg\ tissue^{-1} \cdot min^{-1}$) in normal-appearing small intestinal mucosa using a previously described method.

*Significantly different from control (0 ppm) group with the same genetic status, P < 0.05.

(Courtesy of Barnes CJ, Lee M: Chemoprevention of spontaneous intestinal adenomas in the adenomatous polyposis coli *Min* mouse model with aspirin. *Gastroenterology* 114:873-877, 1998.)

toward a reversed association of use of aspirin and NSAIDs with colon cancer. The article by Stürmer (Abstract 5–38) is the first randomized trial attempting to define the association prospectively and reports no decrease in incidences of colorectal cancer in physicians randomized to the use of aspirin. The author states that low doses of aspirin used in the short treatment period (5 years, end of follow-up 12 years) may account for the null findings. In addition, a bias might have been introduced by precluding from randomization physicians who chose not to take aspirin regularly. The second report (Abstract 5–39), a population-based, case-control study by Lynn Rosenberg, on 1,201 incident cases of colorectal cancer and 1,201 matched controls suggests a protective effect of NSAIDs against large-bowel carcinoma. The third study (Abstract 5–40), in experimental *Min* mice with a germ line mutation in *APC*, concludes that high doses of aspirin are effective chemopreventive agents in a mouse model of spontaneous intestinal tubal formation. The accent in this study is on the high dose of aspirin as opposed to the duration of treatment.

It is too early to recommend that physicians prescribe aspirin solely for the purpose of preventing colorectal neoplasia. Additional studies designed both to determine a minimum effective aspirin dose and to assess the putative actions of aspirin are warranted. Prolonged case-controlled studies or randomized trials in human subjects are desirable, although the difficulty and the cost of such trials because of the length of the observation period needed are definite concerns.

G. Aliperti, M.D.

Acute Colonic Obstruction: Clinical Aspects and Cost-effectiveness of Preoperative and Palliative Treatment With Self-expanding Metallic Stents—A Preliminary Report

Binkert CA, Ledermann H, Jost R, et al (Kantonsspital Winterthur, Switzerland)

Radiology 206:199-204, 1998 5–41

Background.—Acute large bowel obstruction usually necessitates emergency surgery. A new technique to remove colonic obstruction involves placement of a self-expanding metallic stent. Stent placement has been performed primarily as a preoperative treatment prior to colon resection. The clinical aspects and cost-effectiveness of placement of self-expanding metallic vascular stents in patients with colonic obstruction were examined.

Study Design.—The study group consisted of 3 women and 10 men, aged 49 to 83 years, with acute large bowel obstruction. Ten patients were treated preoperatively, and in 3 patients with nonresectable tumors, stents remained as palliative treatment. All vascular stents (Wallstents), 16 mm in diameter and 56 mm in length when fully expanded, were used in all patients. Stent placement was performed in a conventional fluoroscopy room, with the patient under local anesthesia. The distal part of the

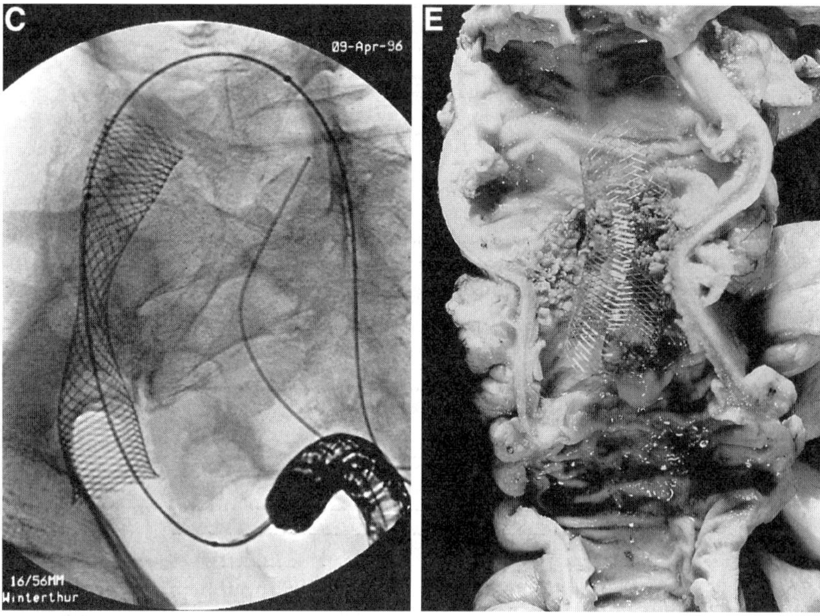

FIGURE 1.—Patient 1. Carcinoma of the distal sigmoid. C, fluoroscopic image obtained immediately after deployment depicts the self-expanding metallic stent with a waisted shape. E, photograph of pathologic specimen shows the self-expanding stent, which bridges the colon cancer. (Courtesy of Binkert CA, Ledermann H, Jost R, et al: Acute colonic obstruction: Clinical aspects and cost-effectiveness of preoperative and palliative treatment with self-expanding metallic stents—A preliminary report *Radiology* 206:199-204, 1998. Radiological Society of North America.)

obstruction was located endoscopically, and biopsy was performed. The stenosis was traversed with a guide wire, and the stent was then advanced over the guide wire under fluoroscopic guidance (Fig 1). Stents did not impair malignancy staging by CT. Cost-effectiveness of stent placement was analyzed by comparing total costs of preoperative stent placement and follow-up surgery with total costs of surgical treatment alone, at the same hospital.

Findings.—Stent placement was successful in 12 of the 13 patients with acute large bowel obstruction in this series. One patient had a very narrow stenosis that could not be passed. The remaining 12 patients recovered from mechanical obstruction. Single-stage surgery was possible in 8 of the 9 patients treated preoperatively. Dysfunction occurred in 2 long stenoses, with reocclusion at 2 and 6 weeks after stent placement. Overall, stent placement resulted in a 19.7% reduction in total costs, due to shorter hospitalization and lower complication rates. In those patients with colon cancer treated preoperatively, there was a 28.8% cost reduction.

Conclusions.—These preliminary results suggest that placement of a self-expanding metallic stent is safe, minimally invasive, and cost-effective for treatment of acute colonic obstruction. Cost reduction was attributable to reduced hospitalization and complication rates. This study will continue to investigate the benefit of stent placement for palliative indications.

Malignant Colorectal Obstruction: Treatment With a Flexible Covered Stent

Choo IW, Do YS, Suh SW, et al (Sung Kyun Kwan Univ, Seoul, Korea; Samsung Biomedical Research Inst, Seoul, Korea; Inha Univ Hosp, Inchon, Korea)

Radiology 206:415-421, 1998 5–42

Introduction.—Acute obstruction of the large bowel by primary colorectal carcinoma is a surgical emergency with a higher mortality rate than that of elective procedures (17% vs. 7.7%). Most patients are traditionally treated with a 2-stage procedure. Nonsurgical treatment of colonic obstruction using uncovered expandable metallic stents has been reported. However, tumor ingrowth through the stent and re-obstruction of the colon have occurred. The usefulness of flexible covered stents was assessed in the treatment of 20 patients with acute colorectal obstruction secondary to malignant colorectal carcinoma.

Methods.—Patients underwent intubation of a flexible stent with fluoroscopic guidance with occasional endoscopic assistance. Two types of stents were used: type 1, completely covered; type 2, two thirds of the proximal part uncovered. Twelve of 15 patients with primary colorectal carcinoma underwent placement of a stent for presurgical decompression; 3 patients had a stent placed for palliative decompression. Stents were also placed for palliative decompression in 2 patients with recurrent colonic carcinoma.

Results.—Ninety percent of patients (18 of 20) experienced successful stent placement. Fifteen patients (75%) had resolution of symptoms within 24 hours. Eight patients had an uneventful elective single-stage surgery 5 to 7 days after stent placement. Two patients required tumor resection and colostomy. Eight patients experienced palliative decompression of the abdomen after stent placement. Because 4 (50%) of the type 1 stents migrated, type 2 stents were used thereafter.

Conclusion.—Flexible stents were effective in relieving acute colonic obstruction secondary to malignant rectosigmoid neoplasm. Most patients were able to undergo single-stage surgery. The stents provided palliative decompression in patients who had inoperable or disseminated disease.

Initial Clinical Experience With Colonic Stent Placement

Wholey MH, Levine EA, Ferral H, et al (Louisiana State Univ Med Ctr, New Orleans)

Am J Surg 175:194-197, 1998 5–43

Purpose.—Interest in the use of self-expandable metallic stents for the treatment of patients with colonic strictures and occlusions is growing. Stent placement permits colonic decompression and bowel preparation before a single-stage procedure and may serve as an elective primary anastomosis without requiring temporary colostomy. Use of colonic stents for the treatment of colonic obstruction is reported.

Patients.—Stents were placed in 10 patients with acute colonic obstruction. There were 6 men and 4 women; mean age, 65 years. The cause of the obstruction was benign in some patients and malignant in others; in 3 patients with extensive metastases, treatment was considered palliative only. Five lesions were located in the descending colon and 5 in the rectosigmoid colon. Each patient underwent placement of a self-expanding metallic stent under fluoroscopic guidance. The results were assessed by clinical follow-up until stent removal or death.

Results.—The technical success rate was 100%. In 9 of the 10 patients, clinical decompression was achieved within 6 hours. Standard mechanical bowel preparation and elective resection of obstructions were performed in 6 patients, whereas stent placement was considered palliative in 4 patients. Stent migration occurred in 4 cases; 1 patient died of procedure-related causes. Stents migrating to the rectum were easily reached and replaced under fluoroscopic guidance. None of the patients had perforations.

Conclusions.—Results with the use of metallic stents to relieve acute colonic obstruction are encouraging. Stent placement is a minimally invasive procedure that requires little patient preparation and provides rapid relief of symptoms. Stents can either be used for stabilization and bowel preparation before elective single-stage surgery or remain in place for long-term palliation. If the gastrointestinal tract can tolerate stents on a long-term basis, they may be useful for indications such as strictures caused by inflammatory bowel disease.

► Metallic stents have come of age for treatment of malignant stricture in the gastrointestinal tract. Such stents have become commonplace in the management of esophageal and biliary strictures (Abstracts 5–41 to 5–43). More recently, expandable metal stents have been used in the management of obstructing colon cancer. The procedure for placement of the metallic stent is minimally invasive and requires little preparation. The relief of symptoms is usually rapid. After relief of colonic obstructions, the patient can be stabilized with adequate bowel preparation, prior to an elective single-stage operation. If the disease is inoperable, stents may remain in place as a long-term palliative device. The results of the current theories are still preliminary. However, placement of the stents appears to be simple and to have a relatively low complication rate in this high-risk population. Reported complications are prior placement failure, perforation in 1% to 17% of cases, and migration in 4% to 23% of cases. Stent migration is usually acknowledged with another endoscopic procedure. One of the authors, Wholey, has used metallic stents in treating noncancerous inflammatory disease. I am not sure whether this indication will clinch consensus, unless operative management is done shortly thereafter.

G. Aliperti, M.D.

A Cost-effectiveness Analysis of Colorectal Screening of Hereditary Nonpolyposis Colorectal Carcinoma Gene Carriers

Vasen HFA, van Ballegooijen M, Buskens E, et al (The Netherlands Found for the Detection of Hereditary Tumors, Leiden; Leiden Univ, The Netherlands; Erasmus Univ, Rotterdam, The Netherlands, et al)

Cancer 82:1632-1637, 1998 5–44

Introduction.—It is now possible to identify carriers of the hereditary nonpolyposis colorectal carcinoma gene within a family. Among the general population in Western countries, it has been estimated that the prevalence of carriers is between 5 and 50 per 10,000. Carriers have an extremely high risk of developing colorectal carcinoma and need follow-up. The cost-effectiveness of large-scale surveillance programs has not been assessed. Future legislation and benefits packages offered by insurance companies would need such information. The costs and effects of colorectal carcinoma surveillance of carriers of a mutated mismatch repair gene was analyzed and compared with the cost of no colorectal carcinoma surveillance.

Methods.—A model was constructed to estimate the life expectancy and health care costs of using surveillance and not using surveillance. Surveillance consisted of colonoscopy every 2 to 3 years. The Dutch hereditary nonpolyposis colorectal carcinoma registry was used to derive estimates of the lifetime risk of developing colorectal carcinoma and the stage distribution of colorectal carcinoma for symptomatic patients. Finnish studies were used to derive the colorectal carcinoma stage specific relative survival rates as well as the effectiveness of surveillance in preventing or detecting cancer early. American studies were used to derive the costs of surveillance and treatment.

Results.—There was an increase in life expectancy of 7 years with the surveillance of gene carriers. The costs involved with surveillance under a wide range of assumptions are less than the costs involved when there is no surveillance.

Conclusion.—It appears that colorectal carcinoma surveillance of the hereditary nonpolyposis colorectal carcinoma gene carriers is more effective and less costly than no surveillance. For that reason, government agencies and health insurance organizations should support surveillance.

Aspirin and Nonsteroidal Anti-inflammatory Agents and Risk for Colorectal Adenomas

Sandler RS, Galanko JC, Murray SC, et al (Univ of North Carolina, Chapel Hill)

Gastroenterology 114:441-447, 1998 5–45

Background.—Research has shown that aspirin and nonsteroidal anti-inflammatory drugs (NSAIDs) protect against the development of colorectal cancer. Because adenomas are precursors to most colorectal cancers, the relationship of aspirin and NSAID use to colorectal adenomas was studied.

Methods.—Two hundred ten patients with adenomas and 169 individuals without adenomas were included in this case-control study. Data on medication use, diet, and lifestyle factors were obtained by telephone interviews.

Findings.—After adjustment for potential confounding variables, regular aspirin and NSAID users were half as likely to have adenomas than nonusers were. Regular users of these agents who had stopped medication use at least 1 year before colonoscopy were still protected, although the small number of participants makes this finding tentative. The protective effects of aspirin and NSAIDs were comparable.

Conclusions.—Aspirin and NSAID use appears to disrupt the progression of adenoma to carcinoma early in the sequence. Further research is needed to establish the most effective dose and duration, as well as the mechanism of action.

▶ The authors utilize an outcome model to estimate potential health effects and health care costs of 2 different strategies for management of carriers of the gene for hereditary nonpolyposis colorectal carcinoma. One strategy involved periodic surveillance, the other involved simple treatment for symptomatic disease. The findings of Abstract 5–44 are not surprising: early detection of cancer by surveying gene carriers led to increased life expectancy and considerable cost savings.

This well-designed case-control study (Abstract 5–45) quantified the benefit from the use of aspirin or NSAIDs to reduction of colon adenoma formation. All study participants, in both groups, underwent colonoscopy for indications associated with lower gastrointestinal bleeding. The introduction of this selection bias might reduce the significance of the results, which may be less applicable to the general population of asymptomatic patients with average risk. Physicians are faced with a difficult decision regarding selection of patients who may benefit from aspirin or NSAIDs for prevention of colorectal neoplasia. At this point, and without further studies, it would be difficult to recommend the use of this type of prophylaxis in patients with average risks.

G. Aliperti, M.D.

Medical Residents' Colorectal Cancer Screening May Be Dependent on Ambulatory Care Education

Borum ML (George Washington Univ, Washington, DC)

Dig Dis Sci 42:1176-1178, 1997 5–46

Background.—Although screening is a critical part of cancer prevention, studies suggest that physicians may not consistently comply with surveillance guidelines. Residency training can significantly affect future practice patterns. The current study assessed the colorectal cancer screening practices of internal medicine residents in 2 ambulatory care education programs at one university medical center.

Methods and Findings.—The medical records of patients aged 50 years or older were reviewed to compare residents' screening practices. The analysis indicated that residents who received multiple lectures in colorectal cancer surveillance or who were required to document the performance of screening on a medical record preventive care summary form performed significantly more rectal examinations, fecal occult blood tests, and flexible sigmoidoscopies than other residents.

Conclusions.—Residency training can have an important impact on future practice patterns. Thus, postgraduate education should involve multiple educational methods and reinforcement procedures to increase physician compliance with cancer screening.

► Colorectal cancer screening is a critical component of cancer prevention and early detection. Despite the widespread acceptance of published surveillance guidelines, research suggests that there might be variable adherence to recommendations. Lessons learned during residency training have a significant impact on subsequent practice patterns. It is therefore important that preventive care and surveillance practices be emphasized during postgraduate training. A vigilant education process can make a significant difference in the implementation of recommended screening techniques. This concept does not limit itself to residency programs but expands to established clinical practices where improved physician compliance with colorectal cancer surveillance can significantly assist in reducing morbidity and mortality from this curable disease.

G. Aliperti, M.D.

Endoscopic Screening of Relatives of Patients With Colorectal Cancer

Hunt LM, Rooney PS, Hardcastle JD, et al (Univ of Nottingham, England)
Gut 42:71-75, 1998 5–47

Background.—Relatives of patients with colorectal cancer are at increased risk of such disease. However, the reported neoplastic yield from screening the relatives has varied substantially among studies, depending on the age and strength of the family history of the individuals screened. The current study determined the neoplastic yield of endoscopic screening of first-degree relatives of patients with colorectal cancer by age and familial risk.

Methods and Findings.—Three hundred thirty individuals with a family history of colorectal cancer underwent endoscopic screening according to a certain protocol. Adenomas were detected in 12% of high-risk individuals screened mainly by colonoscopy. In 8%, adenomas were greater than 1 cm. Twenty-six percent of those with neoplasia had lesions at or proximal to the splenic flexure. Neoplasia was detected in 9.5% of persons at lower familial risk, screened mainly by 60 cm flexible sigmoidoscopy. Four percent of these had neoplasms exceeding 1 cm or cancer. Neoplastic yield was highest in the fourth and fifth decades of life in those at greatest risk and increased with age in those at lower risk.

Conclusions.—Colonoscopy appears to be the only satisfactory screening method for individuals who have 2 or more first-degree relatives with colorectal cancer or who have relatives in whom colorectal cancer developed at a young age. For those at lower risk, 60-cm flexible sigmoidoscopy may be adequate.

▶ Another study attempting to advise on the utilization of the most efficient means of screening for colorectal cancer in individuals at high risk. This study finds adenomas in 12% of individuals with 2 or more first-degree relatives in whom colorectal cancer developed at a young age. Of those with neoplasia, 26% had lesions at or proximal to the splenic flexure; thus, the recommendation to proceed with colonoscopy in this "high-risk" group. A different controlled study had found 48% of adenomas being proximal to the splenic flexure, compared with 25% in controls. On the basis of this difference, the author's recommendation that the 60-cm flexible sigmoidoscopy may be useful in those at lower levels of risk might be difficult to justify. Of course, the value of any screening program must be pragmatic, in that efficacy of outcomes needs to be balanced in the face of cost considerations. However, limitations of such studies due to sample selection and geographic-genetic-environmental variability do not allow the recommendation of a perfect screening strategy at this time.

G. Aliperti, M.D.

Family History of Colorectal Adenomatous Polyps and Increased Risk for Colorectal Cancer

Ahsan H, Neugut AI, Garbowski GC, et al (Columbia Univ, New York; Mount Sinai School of Medicine, New York)

Ann Intern Med 128:900-905, 1998 5–48

Background.—First-degree relatives of a patient with colorectal cancer are clearly at increased risk of colorectal cancer themselves. But is the risk of colorectal cancer increased for first-degree relatives of patients with colorectal adenoma? These authors addressed this question in a large cohort study.

Methods.—Colonoscopy was performed in 1,554 first-degree relatives of 244 patients with newly diagnosed colorectal adenoma and in 2,173 first-degree relatives of 362 controls with normal endoscopic findings. Data were adjusted for sex and race.

Findings.—Compared with first-degree relatives of controls, first-degree relatives of patients with colorectal adenoma were at significantly increased risk of colorectal cancer (relative risk [RR], 1.74). Parents and siblings were equally at risk (RR, 1.58 for both). However, first-degree relatives of patients with colorectal adenoma were not at higher risk of other cancers. The younger the patient at diagnosis of colorectal adenoma, the greater the risk of colorectal cancer in first-degree relatives. For first-degree relatives of patients who were 50 years or less when the adenoma was diagnosed, the risk of colorectal cancer was 4 times greater (RR, 4.26) than in first-degree relatives of patients whose colorectal adenoma was diagnosed when they were older than 60 years.

Conclusions.—The risk of colorectal cancer is indeed increased in first-degree relatives of patients with newly diagnosed colorectal adenoma. The risk for relatives is particularly great if the patient is 50 years or less when the adenoma is diagnosed. Thus, first-degree relatives of patients with colorectal adenoma should be offered screening for colorectal cancer.

Colonoscopic Screening in First-degree Relatives of Patients With "Sporadic" Colorectal Cancer: A Case-Control Study

Pariente A, for the Association Nationale des Gastroentérologues des Hôpitaux and Registre Bourguignon des Cancers Digestifs (INSERM CRI 9505) (Centre Hospitalier, Pau, France; et al)

Gastroenterology 115:7-12, 1998 5–49

Background.—A screening policy for the first-degree relatives of patients with sporadic colorectal cancer has not been clearly defined. The risk of a colorectal adenoma in a cohort with 1 affected first-degree relative was determined.

Methods.—Four hundred seventy-six first-degree relatives of 195 patients with sporadic colorectal cancer were offered colonoscopy. The relatives ranged in age from 40 to 74 years. Each relative assessed was matched with 2 control research subjects by age, sex, symptoms, and medical center.

Findings.—The odds ratios in the 185 relatives assessed were 1.5 for adenomas, 2.5 for large adenomas, and 2.6 for high-risk adenomas. High-risk adenomas were more prevalent in relatives of index patients who were younger than 65 years and male and who had distal rather than proximal cancer.

Conclusions.—Patients with family histories of sporadic colorectal cancer are more likely to have high-risk adenomas than those without this family history. Such individuals need to be monitored more carefully than the general population, especially when the index patient is younger than 65 years old and male and has cancer on the left side.

► We have now realized the importance of colonoscopy screening for high-risk individuals. These include those with a history of inflammatory bowel disease or a family history of colorectal carcinoma, as the risk is increased by approximately twofold for subjects who have 1 first-degree relative with colorectal cancer.

Pariente et al. studied the risk of a colorectal adenoma, a precursor to colorectal cancer, in a cohort of individuals with only 1 affected first-degree relative with colorectal cancer. They were found to have an increased incidence of approximately 1.5 times for adenoma and a significant increase in the incidence of high-risk adenomas in relatives. In addition, this risk was higher if the index patient was a male below 65 years with distal rather than proximal cancer. We therefore need to add this history to our colonoscopy screening recommendations; we need to include first-degree relatives of patients with colon cancer, especially if the index patient was younger than age 65 years.

J.S. Barkin, M.D.

SURGICAL

Colon Cancer

Perioperative Blood Transfusions Reduce Long-term Survival Following Surgery for Colorectal Cancer

Edna T-H, Bjerkeset T (Innherred Hosp, Levanger, Norway)

Dis Colon Rectum 41:451-459, 1998 5–50

Introduction.—While being stored, white blood cells release bioactive substances. It has been suggested that these substances might be related to detrimental effects of perioperative blood transfusion. Reports vary regarding the effect of transfusion on the prognosis for patients with varying types of cancer. The association between blood transfusion and long-term outcome was evaluated in patients treated for colorectal cancer.

Methods.—Medical records from 336 patients who underwent colorectal cancer resections between 1980 and 1992 were reviewed for data regarding general health, surgery, risk factors for cancer recurrence, tumor localization, anemia on admission, irradiation of rectal carcinoma, TNM stage, and histologic differentiation of the tumor. Patients were followed up every 3 months in the first year after surgery, every 6 months during the second year, and every year thereafter until 5 years had elapsed. Median time of follow-up was 5.8 years (2 to 16.8 years) or until death. Median patient age was 70 years (range, 35 to 88 years).

Results.—Local recurrences with distant metastases were significantly more common in patients who received more than 2 units of blood. Risk factors significantly related to death by colorectal cancer were tumor stage (T stage and N stage), perforation of tumor, age, and the need for a blood transfusion. Transfusion of more than 2 units was independently and significantly correlated with death from colorectal cancer. Length of time of blood storage had no effect on prognosis. Age and American Society of Anesthesiologists group (but not blood transfusions) were significantly related to death in patients who died of diseases unrelated to colorectal cancer.

Conclusion.—There was an independent and significant relationship between perioperative blood transfusion and poor prognosis in patients with colorectal cancer. Length of time blood was stored was not a prognostic factor.

Association Between Transfusion of Stored Blood and Infective Bacterial Complications After Resection for Colorectal Cancer

Edna T-H, Bjerkeset T (Innherred Hosp, Levanger, Norway)

Eur J Surg 164:449-456, 1998 5–51

Objective.—Blood transfusion appears to influence prognosis in colorectal cancer. The association between blood transfusion and bacterial infections in the hospital after operations for colorectal cancer was examined in a retrospective cohort study in Norway.

Methods.—Of 446 patients (216 women), aged 35-99 years, who had a colorectal resection because of colorectal cancer, 290 received blood transfusions, and 101 of those received more than 3 units. The main outcome measure was the postoperative bacterial infection rate.

Results.—One or more bacterial infections developed in 112 patients (25%). Significantly more transfusion patients (91, 31%) than nontransfusion patients (21, 13%) had infections. Sixteen (62%) of the patients who died in the hospital had an infection. The median hospital stay was 9 days for patients without infection and 16 days for patients with infection. Risk factors for infection, according to multivariate analysis, included older age, rectal cancer, T stage, N stage, and blood transfusion. The risk of infection increased with the number of transfusion units received (odds ratio, 1.5 for 1 to 3 units and 3.1 for more than 3 units).

Conclusion.—Transfusion of stored blood is an independent risk factor for postoperative infection after resection for colorectal cancer.

► The group from Levanger, Norway, produced two articles (Abstract 5–50 and 5–51) regarding blood transfusion and outcome after resection for colorectal cancer. Both indicate an immune suppression effect from blood transfusions. The article on infective bacterial complications after blood transfusion indicates that filtered blood may improve this outcome. Although there is presumptive evidence that it is the white blood cells that cause immune suppression after transfusion, there is no clinical evidence that filtering reduces the adverse effect on cancer outcome. Certainly, common sense would dictate that reduction in blood transfusion is important in the treatment of all patients with cancer after major operations.

J.W. Fleshman, Jr., M.D.

Race, Treatment, and Survival Among Colorectal Carcinoma Patients in an Equal-Access Medical System

Dominitz JA, Samsa GP, Landsman P, et al (Veterans Affairs Med Ctr, Durham, NC; Duke Univ Med Ctr, Durham, NC; VA Puget Sound Health Care System, Seattle)

Cancer 82:2312-2320, 1998 5–52

Objective.—Colorectal cancer is the second most common fatal malignant disease in the United States. Cancer survival rates are higher among whites than among blacks. The use of surgery, radiation therapy, and chemotherapy in the treatment of colorectal cancer and 5-year survival rates were examined in a retrospective cohort study of white and black veterans in VA hospitals. For this study, the VA patient treatment file (PTF) and outpatient clinic files were used.

Methods.—Of 3,176 veterans with colorectal cancer, 569 (17.9%) were black. Likelihood of surgical resection, chemotherapy, radiation therapy, and death was analyzed statistically.

Results.—Black patients were less likely to have rectal cancer and more likely to have distal or unspecified disease. There were no differences with respect to therapy or 5-year survival rate between groups.

Conclusion.—When there is equal access to health care, there are no differences in survival or treatment between white and black patients with colorectal cancer.

► The VA system is a noneconomically oriented system when it comes to the treatment of its patients. Although there is some controversy over the quality of care in a system that does not have financial constraints and tends not to practice preventive care in a systematic way, the population is fairly ubiquitous. Therefore, a study looking at differences in outcome between races may be very telling. There is a very small difference in outcome between white and African-American patients who are treated for colorectal cancer within the VA system. This difference cannot be explained by tumor characteristics or disease status at the time of presentation. Further investigation is, therefore, warranted to identify any potential social reasons for this outcome.

J.W. Fleshman, Jr., M.D.

Randomized Trial of Surgery Versus Surgery Followed by Adjuvant Hepatic Arterial Infusion With 5-Fluorouracil and Folinic Acid for Liver Metastases of Colorectal Cancer

Lorenz M, for the German Cooperative on Liver Metastases (Arbeitsgruppe Lebermetastasen) (Johann Wolfgang Goethe Univ, Frankfurt am Main, Germany)

Ann Surg 228:756-762, 1998 5–53

Background.—Liver metastases develop in 40% to 50% of patients with colorectal cancer. The five-year survival rate after curative resection is only 25% to 30%; 60% of patients have intrahepatic recurrence at a median of 9 to 12 months. Postoperative intra-arterial infusion of 5-fluorouracil (5-FU) was used in an attempt to reduce intrahepatic recurrence and improve survival in patients undergoing resection of liver metastases from colorectal cancer.

Methods.—Two hundred twenty-six patients with colorectal liver metastases, stratified for number of metastases and primary tumor site, were included in the randomized, multicenter trial. The patients' median age was 61 years. All underwent resection of the hepatic metastases. In addition, the adjuvant therapy group (n = 113) received postoperative 5-FU, given by hepatic arterial infusion at a rate of 1,000 mg/m²/day for 5 days as a continuous 24-hour infusion. This group also received a short infusion of folinic acid, 200 mg/m²/day for 5 days. Survival was the main outcome measure. The findings at the first planned interim analysis, at which there were 219 evaluable patients, are described in this report.

Results.—Curative resection was achieved in 89% of the patients. At interim analysis, 91 patients had died; median survival was similar between groups: 34.5 months for the adjuvant therapy group and 40.8 months for the control group. Median survival time to progression was 14.2 and 13.7 months, respectively. On "as-treated" analysis, median survival was 44.8 months with adjuvant therapy vs. 39.7 months in the control group, while median survival time to progression was 44.8 vs. 23.3 months. However, the advantages of adjuvant therapy did not translate into a significant difference in survival. One fourth of the cycles of adjuvant 5-FU were associated with grade 3 or 4 toxicity, mainly stomatitis and nausea; nearly three fourths of patients were affected.

Conclusions.—For patients undergoing resection of colorectal cancer metastases to the liver, adjuvant hepatic arterial infusion of 5-FU/folinic acid does not appear to be beneficial, even on as-treated analysis. The confidence interval is consistent with a possible 15% reduction or a possible 100% increase in risk of death with adjuvant therapy. This study was terminated at the first planned interim analysis. Adjuvant intra-arterial therapy for colorectal liver metastases should be limited to controlled trials.

▶ This article is an interim analysis of the German Cooperative on Liver Metastasis randomized prospective trial comparing liver resection alone with liver resection and postoperative hepatic artery infusion of 5-FU and folinic acid for patients with liver metastases from colorectal cancer. Unfortunately, the trial shows that there is no difference between the two arms. However, there are some issues that may require a repeat study in the future. The preoperative staging was done by CT scan and angiography alone. There is no use of positron emission tomography scanning or other techniques to identify distant metastases. The chemotherapy group had a higher postoperative mortality rate, and there were a number of deaths due to the chemotherapy itself, suggesting that there may be some technical problem with the adjuvant therapy protocol. For now, however, the use of hepatic artery infusion for patients with hepatic metastases should be reserved for palliation in patients with symptoms who desire some form of treatment and in whom resection is not possible. The overall survival after hepatic resection is approximately 40% in this large group of study patients who were followed very closely postoperatively. This indicates that there is an advantage to hepatic resection for small numbers of metastases from colorectal cancer.

J.W. Fleshman, Jr., M.D.

Is Colonoscopy Needed for the Nonadvanced Adenoma Found on Sigmoidoscopy?

Schoen RE, for the Polyp Prevention Trial (Univ of Pittsburgh, Pa; et al)
Gastroenterology 115:533-541, 1998 5–54

Background.—The need for colonoscopy in patients with small tubular adenomas with low-grade dysplasia found on sigmoidoscopy has not been established. The prevalence and characteristics of proximal adenomas in patients with distal adenomas were studied.

Methods and Findings.—Nine hundred eighty-one patients with distal adenomas seen on index colonoscopy before randomization in the Polyp Prevention Trial were studied. A pathologically advanced distal adenoma of 1 cm or greater was detected in 46.9% of the patients, any proximal adenoma was in 21.5%, and an advanced proximal adenoma was detected in 4.3%. Six percent of patients with advanced distal adenomas had advanced proximal adenomas compared with only 2.9% of those with nonadvanced distal adenomas. Had colonoscopy not been performed in patients with nonadvanced distal adenomas, 36% of the advanced proximal adenomas would have been missed.

Conclusions.—A large proportion of the prevalent advanced proximal adenomas would be missed if colonoscopy were not done in patients with nonadvanced distal adenomas. Thus, colonoscopy is indicated in patients with nonadvanced distal adenomas on sigmoidoscopy.

▶ Increased use of flexible sigmoidoscopy as a screening examination for colorectal carcinoma has led to increased detection of small (≤ 10 mm in diameter) benign adenomatous polyps in the rectosigmoid of asymptomatic patients. While it is generally accepted that adenomas are neoplastic lesions considered to be the precursors to most colorectal cancers, the clinical importance of small adenomas found at sigmoidoscopy has been the subject of considerable debate. Some believe that adenomas of the rectosigmoid, of no matter what size, are markers for neoplastic change throughout the colon and thus recommend colonoscopy for these patients. Others feel that the probability of discovering an advanced proximal neoplasm is low, and therefore colonoscopy is not indicated. In an effort to limit costs, some large HMOs, such as Kaiser Permanente, are not routinely pursuing colonoscopy in individuals with tubular adenomas smaller than 1 cm found on flexible sigmoidoscopy.

The data from Schoen et al. support other recent studies finding a substantial prevalence (3%-7%) of advanced neoplasms (adenomas ≥ 10 mm in diameter, adenomas with a villous component or moderate-severe dysplasia, carcinoma in situ, or carcinoma) in the proximal colon of persons with nonadvanced adenomas in the rectosigmoid. The authors conclude, as have others, that colonoscopy should be offered to patients found to have an adenoma on screening flexible sigmoidoscopy, regardless of size or histologic type. However, as the true prevalence of isolated advanced proximal neoplasms (in the absence of distal neoplasms) in asymptomatic, average-risk persons remains unknown, it is unclear whether the absence of adenomas found on screening flexible sigmoidoscopy is reassuring. Hopefully, data from the Veterans Affairs screening colonoscopy study will help resolve this issue.

These controversies illustrate some of the issues involved in determining optimal colorectal cancer screening strategies. Given the risk of missed proximal neoplasms with fecal occult-blood testing and screening sigmoidoscopy, it may make more financial (and medical) sense to perform screening colonoscopy at age 50 and then risk-stratify persons based on the findings. Screening colonoscopy every 10 years is estimated to be as cost-effective as annual stool hemoccult plus screening sigmoidoscopy every 5 years, assuming screening begins at age 50 and is discontinued at age 85.

T.E. Read, M.D.

Relative Frequency of Upper Gastrointestinal and Colonic Lesions in Patients With Positive Fecal Occult-Blood Tests

Rockey DC, Koch J, Cello JP, et al (Duke Univ Med Ctr, Durham, NC; Univ of California, San Francisco)

N Engl J Med 339:153-159, 1998 5–55

Background.—Bleeding lesions anywhere in the gastrointestinal (GI) tract can produce a positive reaction on guaiac-based fecal occult-blood tests. However, the relative frequency of upper GI and colonic lesions is not known. The incidence of lesions in the GI tract of patients with positive guaiac-based fecal occult-blood tests was investigated.

Methods.—Two hundred forty-eight patients, aged 40 to 89 years, were studied. None had documented iron deficiency anemia or active GI bleeding. Standard guaiac-based tests were used to detect fecal occult blood.

Findings.—Lesions consistent with occult bleeding were detected in 48% of the patients. Seventy-one lesions were in the upper GI tract, and 54 were in the colon. Esophagitis was the most common upper GI lesion, occurring in 23 patients, followed by gastric ulcers in 14, gastritis in 12, and duodenal ulcers in 10. In a logistic regression analysis, upper GI tract symptoms were shown to be associated with the detection of lesions in the upper GI tract; the odds ratio was 2.6. The prevalence of lesions in the upper GI tract in patients with and without symptoms was greater than or equal to that of colonic lesions.

Conclusions.—Upper GI lesions were more common than colonic lesions in this group of patients with positive fecal occult-blood tests referred for further assessment. The population studied did not include patients with iron deficiency anemia or active bleeding.

A Systematic Review of the Effects of Screening for Colorectal Cancer Using the Faecal Occult Blood Test, Hemoccult

Towler B, Irwig L, Glasziou P, et al (Flinders Med Centre, Adelaide, Australia; Univ of Sydney, Australia; Univ of Queensland, Herston, Australia; et al)
BMJ 317:559-565, 1998 5–56

Background.—Colorectal cancer is a common cause of illness and death in the West. Much research effort has been expended to find a screening method that will detect this cancer at an early, curable stage. The ability of the fecal occult blood test, Hemoccult, to detect colorectal cancer was examined with meta-analysis.

Study Design.—The health literature was searched for controlled trials of colorectal cancer screening with the fecal occult blood test. Four randomized, controlled trials and 2 nonrandomized trials including over 400,000 patients were assessed. Data were extracted and analyzed using Meta-analyst version 0.991 for the effect of screening on colorectal cancer mortality.

Findings.—The quality of these clinical trials was generally good. Meta-analysis of the 4 randomized trials demonstrated that those in the screening group had a 16% reduction in colorectal cancer mortality risk on an intention-to-treat basis. When these results were adjusted for screening attendance, there was a 23% reduction in mortality risk. The results indicate that if a biennial Hemoccult screening program were offered to 10,000 people and if two thirds participated in at least 1 test, 8.5 deaths from colorectal cancer could be prevented over a 10-year period.

Conclusion.—Meta-analysis of several studies involving screening for colorectal cancer with Hemoccult demonstrates that Hemoccult screening would reduce colorectal cancer mortality. The cost of this screening, the community response to screening, and any adverse effects of screening remain to be elucidated.

▶ Several large, randomized, controlled trials have shown that annual or biannual testing for fecal occult blood with complete diagnostic evaluation of the colon for patients with a positive fecal occult blood test, primarily with colonoscopy, reduces mortality from colorectal cancer. However, a fecal occult blood test is a nonspecific examination that will fail to detect many small cancers and precancerous lesions. The study by Rockey et al. (Abstract 5–55) addresses the poor specificity of the test by demonstrating the inability of fecal occult blood testing to discriminate upper from lower gastrointestinal bleeding sources.

Although Rockey et al. detected advanced colorectal adenomas or carcinomas in 17% of all patients with a positive fecal occult blood test, they were not examining an asymptomatic, average-risk population. Specifically, they did not exclude patients for the following: a personal history of colorectal cancer, neoplastic polyps, inflammatory bowel disease, or a family history of colorectal cancer or polyposis. It is interesting to note that patients who had occult blood detected by digital rectal examination were more likely to have colonic neoplasms found on colonoscopy than those patients who had occult blood detected by screening home hemoccult tests. However, as the groups were not randomized, this finding may be the result of bias introduced because of the different patient populations.

The major drawback to using fecal occult blood testing as a screening technique for colorectal neoplasia (Abstract 5–56) is poor compliance. Only 38% to 60% of patients in large, randomized trials completed all the planned fecal occult blood tests, and use of fecal occult blood testing in the general population is estimated to be much lower. It may ultimately prove more effective to perform total colonic evaluation at 10-year intervals in asymptomatic, average-risk persons than to depend on yearly compliance with fecal occult blood testing, which is neither sensitive nor specific for early-stage colonic neoplasia.

T.E. Read, M.D.

A UK Training Programme for Nurse Practitioner Flexible Sigmoidoscopy and a Prospective Evaluation of the Practice of the First UK Trained Nurse Flexible Sigmoidoscopist

Duthie GS, Drew PJ, Hughes MAP, et al (Univ of Hull, England)
Gut 43:711-714, 1998 5–57

Background.—There is increasing demand in the United Kingdom for diagnostic flexible sigmoidoscopy. One potential method for meeting this demand is to train colorectal nurse practitioners in flexible sigmoidoscopy. The structure and a prospective evaluation of the first United Kingdom English Nursing Board–recognized nurse practitioner flexible sigmoidoscopist training program were presented.

Methods.—A multidisciplinary committee developed a structured program of study and practice involving a staged process of study, observation, withdrawals, and full procedures. Independent practice was permitted only when the clinical supervisor was satisfied with the trainee's competence. Independent nurse practitioner examinations were assessed with reference to barium enema, video recordings, and clinical follow-up.

Results.—One nurse practitioner has completed this program and independently examined 215 patients. Of these 215 examinations, 93% were judged successful and pathology was identified in 51%. The nurse endoscopist identified all significant pathology. There were no complications. No patients declined to be examined by a nurse.

Conclusion.—After completion of a comprehensive training program, nurse endoscopists are capable of performing flexible sigmoidoscopy safely and effectively.

► As flexible sigmoidoscopy is used more frequently as a screening examination for colorectal neoplasia, the demand for competent endoscopists will increase. Some nurse practitioners and physician assistants in the United States have been trained to perform screening flexible sigmoidoscopy.

Duthie et al. describe the British experience with a formalized training program for nurses, which used didactic sessions, practice on a colon model, supervised endoscopy, and, finally, independent endoscopy verified by barium enema examinations. Although barium enema is known to be less sensitive than endoscopy for small lesions, no large lesions were missed by the nurses.

Duthie et al. confirm that motivated nonphysician health care workers, with proper supervision and training, can achieve expertise in flexible sigmoidoscopy. The program they describe should be considered for all endoscopists in training, especially for primary care physicians who intend to perform flexible sigmoidoscopy in their practices, as they may receive less rigorous endoscopy training in residency than gastroenterologists or colon and rectal surgeons.

T.E. Read, M.D.

Adenoma Characteristics at First Colonoscopy as Predictors of Adenoma Recurrence and Characteristics at Follow-up

Van Stolk RU, for the Polyp Prevention Study Group (Cleveland Clinic Found, Ohio; et al)

Gastroenterology 115:13-18, 1998 5–58

Background.—Colorectal adenomas are common benign neoplastic lesions often detected in colonoscopy studies in Americans over the age of 50 years. Data from a chemoprevention trial were analyzed to assess whether baseline adenoma characteristics could be used to determine the risk of adenoma recurrence.

Study Design.—The Polyp Prevention Study involved 6 American clinical centers. Eligible patients had had a large-bowel adenoma removed during the previous 3 months, had had a complete colonoscopy, were judged polyp free, were younger than 80 years, and were in good health. The study design included a baseline colonoscopy, a 1-year clearing examination, and a final study examination 3 years later. Complete histologic data were available for 479 patients who formed the basis for the study. The number, size, histologic type, and degree of atypia of adenomas was identified from the baseline colonoscopy. These were then compared with the recurrent adenomas detected at the final colonoscopy.

Results.—By univariate analysis, the number of adenomas, the presence of tubulovillous-type adenomas, and severe atypia were all significantly associated with recurrence. By multivariate analysis, multiple adenoma recurrence was associated with the presence of at least 3 adenomas at baseline and at least 1 tubulovillous adenoma. There was no specific characteristic that was associated with high-risk polyp recurrence. Of those patients with less than 3 adenomas at baseline, 70% had no recurrence and only 3.3% of recurrent adenomas were of clinical significance.

Conclusion.—The number and type of adenomas at baseline colonoscopy significantly predicted adenoma recurrence at follow-up colonoscopy, but these recurrences were rarely clinically significant. Excluding those with genetic syndromes, most patients can safely wait at least 3 years for follow-up and those patients with less than 3 tubular adenomas are in a low-risk subgroup and could wait even longer.

► These data from the Polyp Prevention Study Group Trial support the findings of the National Polyp Study, indicating that patients undergoing colonoscopic polypectomy of benign adenomatous polyps can safely wait 3 years before undergoing repeat colonoscopy. In this study, the number of adenomas at initial colonoscopy was the strongest predictor of adenoma recurrence at follow-up colonoscopy, although villous histology and severe atypia also increased the risk of multiple adenomas at follow-up. The number of advanced adenomas found after a 3-year interval was very low, leading the authors to suggest that low-risk patients may be equally served by an interval longer than 3 years before their first follow-up examination.

Although making biological sense, given the long dwell time of adenomas prior to malignant degeneration, this hypothesis would need further evaluation before adoption by most clinicians. It should be noted that these recommendations do not apply to persons at risk for hereditary nonpolyposis colorectal cancer. Because of germline mutations in mismatch repair genes, these patients may have accelerated growth and malignant degeneration of adenomas and, thus, require shorter intervals between screening colonoscopies.

T.E. Read, M.D.

Benefits of Colonoscopic Surveillance and Prophylactic Colectomy in Patients With Hereditary Nonpolyposis Colorectal Cancer Mutations

Syngal S, Weeks JC, Schrag D, et al (Harvard Med School, Boston; Harvard School of Public Health, Boston)

Ann Intern Med 129:787-796, 1998 5–59

Background.—Colorectal cancer is the second most common cause of cancer-related death in the United States. In a subset of these patients, an increased risk of colorectal cancer is inherited through a single mutation. The most common hereditary colon cancer syndrome is hereditary nonpolyposis colorectal cancer. It is now possible to identify carriers of a mutated gene within a family, so carriers and their caregivers must make decisions about cancer risk–reduction strategies. A decision analysis was used to evaluate outcomes of various colorectal cancer prevention strategies for patients with a mutation in a gene associated with hereditary nonpolyposis colorectal cancer.

Study Design.—A Markov model was constructed using the decision analysis program, DATA, to compare different approaches to colorectal cancer prevention in carriers of a mutation for hereditary nonpolyposis colorectal cancer. The model follows a hypothetical cohort of 25-year-old patients over time, tracking annual incidence, progression, and mortality. Assumptions were based on data from published clinical studies.

Results.—All risk-reduction strategies yielded gains in life expectancy for carriers. Benefits ranged from 13.5 years for endoscopic surveillance to 15.6 years for prophylactic proctocolectomy, when compared with no intervention. The benefits of colectomy decreased with increasing age and were minimal if colectomy was performed at the time of colorectal cancer diagnosis. When health-related quality of life was considered, surveillance led to the largest quality-adjusted life expectancy benefit.

Conclusion.—Decision analysis was used to compare management strategies for carriers of mutations associated with hereditary nonpolyposis colorectal cancer. Although prophylactic colectomy at the age of 25 years led to the largest life expectancy, the benefits decreased with age or with cancer identification. When quality-of-life considerations were incorporated, surveillance appeared to be the preferred cancer prevention option. The choice between prophylactic surgery and surveillance is complex, and personal preferences play an important role.

Clinical Findings With Implications for Genetic Testing in Families With Clustering of Colorectal Cancer

Wijnen JT, Vasen HFA, Khan PM, et al (Leiden Univ Med Ctr, The Netherlands; Found for the Detection of Hereditary Tumors, Leiden, The Netherlands; Norwegian Radium Hosp, Oslo, Norway)

N Engl J Med 339:511-518, 1998 5–60

Background.—Hereditary nonpolyposis colorectal cancer is caused by germ-line mutations in 1 of 5 DNA mismatch repair genes: *MSH2*, *MLH1*, *PMS1*, *PMS2*, and *MSH6*. Little is known about the clinical risk factors that best predict mutations in these genes. Denaturing gradient gel electrophoresis with guanosine and cytidine extensions (GC clamping) was used to examine *MSH2* and *MLH1* mutations in 184 unrelated kindreds with familial clustering of colorectal cancers. Logistic regression analysis was used to compare clinical factors with the probability of a mutation.

Study Design.—Data on the 184 unrelated kindreds were collected by geneticists. Information was collected on the type, site, and number of cancers; age at diagnosis; and pathologic tumor characteristics. Of the 184 kindreds, 92 met the Amsterdam criteria for hereditary nonpolyposis colorectal cancer. Blood samples were collected, genomic DNA isolated, the polymerase chain reaction used for amplification, and denaturing gradient gel electrophoresis with GC clamping performed mutation analysis. Exons with altered migration patterns were sequenced and compared with those in the rest of the family to determine segregation with disease phenotype.

Results.—Mutations were detected in 47 of the kindreds (26%). Clinical factors found to be associated with these mutations were early age at diagnosis, occurrence of kindred endometrial or small intestine cancer, higher numbers of family members with colorectal or endometrial cancer, presence of multiple colorectal cancers or both colorectal and endometrial cancer in 1 family member, and fulfillment of the Amsterdam criteria. Multivariate analysis indicated that younger age at diagnosis, the Amsterdam criteria, and the presence of endometrial cancer in the kindred were independently associated with germ-line mutations. A logistic model for estimating the likelihood of germline mutations was devised.

Conclusion.—Logistic regression analysis was used to devise a simple method based on clinical findings for calculating the likelihood of detecting germline mutations in families suspected of having hereditary nonpolyposis colorectal cancer.

▶ Hereditary nonpolyposis colorectal cancer is an inherited disorder that predisposes patients to the development of colorectal cancer, with up to 75% of patients having the disease by age 65. Hereditary nonpolyposis colorectal cancer (HNPCC) is inherited in an autosomal dominant fashion and is the result of germline mutations in mismatch repair genes (genes that code for proteins responsible for correcting errors during DNA replication). The progression from adenoma to carcinoma appears to be accelerated in patients with HNPCC as compared with patients with sporadic cancers; thus, time intervals between recommended screening colonoscopies are short (1-3 years). There is a tendency for multiple colorectal cancers to develop, if patients with HNPCC and colorectal cancer undergo segmental colectomy, 30% to 50% will develop a second cancer in 10-15 years. Patients with HNPCC are also at high risk for cancers of other organs, especially the ovary and uterus.

At present, the diagnosis of HNPCC in a family is clinical, based on the Amsterdam criteria: colorectal cancer in 3 or more family members; 2 generations affected; 1 affected person a first degree relative, and 1 cancer diagnosed before age 50 years. These criteria were originally developed for research purposes, to standardize the definition of HNPCC. However, they fail to identify patients who may be affected with HNPCC but do not fit the strict criteria because of unknown or abbreviated family histories, as well as patients with a personal or family history of extracolonic malignancies associated with HNPCC. A recent National Cancer Institute working group acknowledged the shortcomings of the Amsterdam criteria as clinical guidelines and published recommendations for expanding the clinical suspicion of the disease to a broader range of patients.

Germline mutational analysis may assist in the management of at-risk family members in an HNPCC family. Although there exist at least 5 reported loci for germline mutations in mismatch repair genes that result in HNPCC, virtually all have been found in *MSH2* and *MLH1*. The penetrance of colorectal cancer in *MSH2* and *MLH1* mutation carriers is approximately 80% by age 80. Screening all patients with colorectal cancer and their relatives for these mutations is not cost effective; however, because the prevalence of these mutations in patients with sporadic cancer is low and the heterogeneity of the mutations in patients with HNPCC is great, necessitating exon-by-exon screening for an accurate molecular diagnosis.

Wijnen et al. have delineated the clinical features that will increase the chance of finding such a mismatch repair gene mutation in families with colorectal cancer: early age of onset of colorectal cancer; fulfillment of the Amsterdam criteria; presence in a kindred of a patient with cancer of the endometrium or small bowel; multiple colorectal cancers; or both colorectal and endometrial cancer. Software is available to calculate the probability of finding a mutation from the Web site of the International Collaborative Group on HNPCC (http://www.nfdht.nl). If the predicted probability is low, one may consider the less expensive method of analyzing the tumor for microsattelite instability, a phenotypic variant often associated with mismatch repair gene mutations.

Although much attention has been devoted to the identification of at-risk family members who have a high risk of colorectal cancer, it is also important to identify average-risk persons within an HNPCC family who could potentially avoid intensive colonoscopic screening. Some families who meet the clinical criteria for HNPCC, however, do not have an identifiable mismatch repair gene mutation. Given the potentially fatal outcome of delayed diagnosis, it is not yet clear what recommendations to give to these patients.

Although prospective, randomized trials are lacking, total abdominal colectomy with ileorectal anastomosis and endoscopic screening of the rectum should be strongly considered for patients with HNPCC and colon cancer and for select HNPCC-associated mutation carriers who have multiple adenomatous polyps. Patients with rectal cancer should be considered for total proctocolectomy. Select HNPCC-associated mutation carriers can be considered for prophylactic colectomy, although the benefit from this approach has not yet been tested. Syngal et al. present a decision analysis for a known 25-year-old mutation carrier and conclude that both intensive colonoscopic surveillance and prophylactic colectomy will lead to large gains in life expectancy (up to 15 years).

T.E. Read, M.D.

Postsurgical Surveillance of Colon Cancer: Preliminary Cost Analysis of Physician Examination, Carcinoembryonic Antigen Testing, Chest X-ray, and Colonoscopy

Graham RA, Wang S, Catalano PJ, et al (New England Med Ctr, Boston; Dana Farber Cancer Inst, Boston; Hosp of the Univ of Pennsylvania, Philadelphia)

Ann Surg 228:59-63, 1998 5–61

Background.—Monitoring of patients after surgery for colon cancer is performed to detect recurrent or metachronous disease. There is little information on the actual cost of such monitoring. The relative and absolute costs of monitoring patients after surgical resection for primary colon carcinoma were determined. These costs included physician examination, carcinoembryonic antigen assessment, chest radiographs, and colonoscopy.

Methods.—Of 1,356 patients who underwent surgical resection for primary colon carcinoma, 421 had recurrent disease and were included in this study. The cost of each test was based on 1995 Medicare reimbursement: \$65 for physician examination; \$28 for carcinoembryonic antigen assessment; \$46 for film and interpretation of chest radiographs; and \$409 for colonoscopy, including a 1-hour facility fee and a physician fee. Follow-up was defined as time to recurrence, or up to 5 years in patients who did not have recurrent disease. Patients were divided into 3 groups: nonrecurrent disease, recurrent but not resectable disease, and recurrent but resectable disease with curative intent. The mean cost of each test in detecting recurrent but resectable disease was determined.

Results.—Of 421 patients with recurrent disease, 96 had recurrent but resectable disease and underwent surgical resection. For these 96 patients, recurrent disease was first identified by carcinoembryonic antigen assessment in 30 patients, chest radiographs in 12 patients, colonoscopy in 14 patients, and other testing in 40 patients. Of these last 40 patients, 24 had symptoms. Routine physician examination did not identify resectable recurrent disease in any patient. The total cost of physician examination was just over \$418,600. For carcinoembryonic antigen assessment, the total cost was \$170,880, the detection rate was 2.2%, and the cost per recurrence was nearly \$5,700. For chest radiographs, the total cost was about \$120,935, the detection rate was 0.9%, and the cost per recurrence was nearly \$10,080. For colonoscopy, the total cost was about \$641,345, the detection rate was 1.0%, and the cost per recurrence was just over \$45,800.

Discussion.—These results show that carcinoembryonic antigen assessment was the most cost-effective test for identifying potentially curable disease in patients after surgical resection for primary colon carcinoma. Physician visits were useful for evaluating symptoms, but routine physician examination did not improve detection of recurrent disease.

▶ There is an increasing body of evidence that "routine" postresection surveillance for recurrent colorectal carcinoma does not improve detection of resectable disease or survival. Graham et al. report the Eastern Cooperative Oncology Group data regarding the cost effectiveness of various routine surveillance techniques in the detection of potentially resectable recurrent disease. Consistent with other reports, the authors found that routine physical examination in the absence of symptoms was virtually useless and that chest radiographs had an extremely low yield. Carcinoembryonic antigen testing was the most cost-effective method but was the first indicator of recurrence in only 31% of patients with potentially resectable disease.

Colonoscopy was predictably poor in detecting recurrent cancer, but was not evaluated with regard to its ability to detect metachronous adenomatous polyps. This report, as well as others documenting the futility of routine follow-up CT, may eventually sway clinicians to abandon routine follow-up surveillance tests in asymptomatic patients.

T.E. Read, M.D.

Effect of Perioperative Blood Transfusions on Recurrence of Colorectal Cancer: Meta-analysis Stratified on Risk Factors

Amato AC, Pescatori M (Clinica Villa Flaminia, Rome)

Dis Colon Rectum 41:570-585, 1998 5–62

Background.—Several articles have reported conflicting results about the effect of allogenic blood transfusion on tumor growth. The influence of perioperative blood transfusions on colorectal cancer recurrence was further explored in a review of the literature.

Methods and Findings.—One hundred thirty-one articles published through 1996 were identified, and 32 met inclusion criteria. A total of 11,071 patients participated in these studies. The results of 20 studies showed that perioperative blood transfusion had a detrimental effect. In 11 of 19 articles using multivariate analyses, perioperative blood transfusion was found to be an independent prognostic indicator. In pooled estimates of the effect of perioperative blood transfusions on colorectal cancer recurrence, patients given transfusions had an overall odds ratio of 1.68 of metastasis, with a rate difference of 0.13. These findings were confirmed after patients were stratified by disease site and stage. The effect of perioperative blood transfusion was dose related, regardless of timing and type, although there was some heterogeneity.

Conclusions.—The use of perioperative blood transfusion has been consistently associated with colorectal cancer recurrence. Further research is needed to determine whether this association is causal.

► There is borderline evidence that suggests that blood transfusion increases the likelihood of recurrence in patients undergoing surgery for colorectal cancer. This study uses a meta-analysis approach to analyze 32 original articles regarding 11,071 patients. With statistical analysis using odds ratios and rate differences, the authors were able to show a detrimental association between perioperative blood transfusion and colorectal cancer recurrence. This is probably adequate confirmatory evidence to suggest that, to limit the potential for immune suppression, every effort should be made to avoid transfusion in patients with colorectal cancer. In this setting, any blood products are significant. The only exception would be autologous blood or filtered leukocyte-poor blood. Any large studies in the future should include transfusion as a risk factor.

J.W. Fleshman, Jr., M.D.

Incidence of Hereditary Nonpolyposis Colorectal Cancer and the Feasibility of Molecular Screening for the Disease

Aaltonen LA, Salovaara R, Kristo P, et al (Univ of Helsinki; Perkin-Elmer Corp, Foster City, Calif; Ohio State Univ, Columbus; et al)

N Engl J Med 338:1481-1487, 1998 5–63

Background.—The polyposis syndromes and hereditary nonpolyposis colorectal cancer are genetic disorders that predispose patients to colorectal cancer. The polyposis syndromes have distinctive clinical features, whereas hereditary nonpolyposis colorectal cancer does not. However, a molecular characteristic of the latter is germ-line mutation of DNA mismatch-repair genes. Tumor specimens from 509 consecutive patients with colorectal adenocarcinomas were screened prospectively for DNA replication errors.

Methods.—Microsatellite-marker analyses of tumor DNA were performed to detect replication errors. DNA in normal tissue from patients with replication errors was also screened for the germ-line mutations of the mismatch-repair genes MLH1 and MSH2.

Findings.—Sixty-three patients (12%) had replication errors. Normal tissue specimens from 10 of these patients showed a germ-line mutation of MLH1 or MSH2. Nine of these 10 patients had a first-degree relative with endometrial or colorectal cancer. Seven of the patients were younger than age 50, and 4 had had colorectal or endometrial cancer previously.

Conclusions.—At least 2% of the patients in this series were found to have hereditary nonpolyposis colorectal cancer. Testing for replication errors is indicated in all patients with colorectal cancer meeting at least 1 of the following criteria: a family history of colorectal or endometrial cancer, age younger than 50, and a history of multiple colorectal or endometrial cancer. Patients with replication errors should have further analysis for germ-line mutations in DNA mismatch-repair genes.

► The group from Helsinki, Finland is very active in evaluating the detection of hereditary nonpolyposis colorectal cancer (HNPCC) in the general population in their country. This evaluation is possible because of a standardized database and registry. Their estimate that 2% of all patients with colorectal cancer in Finland had HNPCC is a much lower estimate than in the past. The authors looked at methods of screening, including molecular testing for mismatched-repair mutations in the general population of patients with colorectal cancer. The clinical criteria for HNPCC established at a consensus conference at the National Cancer Institute in Bethesda predicted the majority of patients having genetic defects of HNPCC. The use of these criteria to select patients who should have molecular genetic testing avoids expensive testing of every patient who had colon and rectal cancer. A focused screening is much more cost-effective and much more likely to yield positive results. The familiarity with these criteria is important. They include family history of colorectal or endometrial cancer, an age of less than 50 years, and a history of multiple colorectal or endometrial cancers. These should become part of the routine history data points in patients who have colorectal cancer. Unfortunately, the routine testing for microsatellite instability and mismatch-repair mutations is very expensive and not universally available. More testing is needed to clarify the role of this genetic screening in the treatment of colorectal cancer.

J.W. Fleshman, Jr., M.D.

Social Environment and Prognosis of Colorectal Cancer Patients: A French Population-based Study

Desoubeaux N, Herbert C, Launoy G, et al (Registre des Tumeurs Digestives du Calvados, Caen, France; CHU, Caen, France)

Int J Cancer 73:317-322, 1997 5–64

Background.—Social environment appears to influence survival in patients with colorectal cancer. The effects of social environment on patient survival were investigated in a well-defined French population.

Methods.—A total of 1,642 patients with colorectal cancer diagnosed between 1978 and 1987 were studied. Socioprofessional category, place of residence, and distance from place of residence to a specialized health care center were included in the analysis. The association among social environment, clinical variables, and survival was determined using 2 multivariate methods.

Findings.—Poorer prognosis was associated with farm work among male and female patients and with unemployment among male patients. Survival differences were not fully explained by variations in stage at diagnosis and in treatment.

Conclusions.—Consistent with previous research, this study shows that social environment in itself influences colorectal cancer prognosis. The survival differences noted could not be explained by variations in tumor stage at diagnosis or in treatment or by potential variations in co-morbidity associated with sex and age.

▶ These French authors have utilized their database on colorectal cancer and have based an analysis on socioeconomic status. Their findings are consistent with several other studies that suggest a lower socioeconomic status results in poorer survival. However, the unique finding here is that there is no correlation with lower economic status and stage of tumor; rather, survival correlates very well with socioeconomic status itself, regardless of stage or delay in presentation. The mechanism for this correlation is unclear, but it is an indicator that emphasis should be placed on screening in this lower socioeconomic population, since these individuals utilize more medical funds and suffer more from the inevitability of colorectal cancer.

J.W. Fleshman, Jr., M.D.

Monoclonal Antibody Therapy for Resected Dukes' C Colorectal Cancer: Seven-Year Outcome of a Multicenter Randomized Trial

Riethmüller G, Holz E, Schlimok G, et al (Ludwig-Maximilians-Universität München, Germany; Chirurgische Universitätsklinik Groβhadern München, Germany; Zentralklinikum Augsburg, Germany; et al)

J Clin Oncol 16:1788-1794, 1998 5–65

Background.—A previous 5-year study found that monoclonal antibody therapy improved survival for patients with resected Dukes' stage C colorectal cancer. However, there was no observed effect on the local relapse rate. The 7-year results in this group of patients are reported.

Methods.—The randomized trial included 189 patients with resected Dukes' C colorectal cancer and histopathologically confirmed curative resection. Patients were randomized with stratification by center, sex, tumor location, number of affected lymph nodes, and carcinoembryonic antigen concentration. Those assigned to active therapy received up to 900 mg of monoclonal antibody 17-1A: 500 mg postoperatively, followed by 4 monthly doses of 100 mg. Primary end points for the 7-year follow-up were overall survival and disease-free interval.

Results.—Mortality was 43% in the antibody group vs. 63% in the control group, a relative mortality reduction of 32%. Recurrence rate was 52% vs. 68%, a reduction of 23%. Recurrence-free interval and recurrence-free survival were both significantly better in the treatment group. At 7 years, 46% of patients in the antibody group were at risk, whereas only 29% of the control group were alive and recurrence free. Analysis of recurrence patterns suggested that 17-1A acted preferentially on isolated tumor cells, thus preventing outgrowth of distant metastases. It did not reduce the rate of local recurrences as the first sign of disease progression.

Conclusions.—Mature data show that postresection 17-1A antibody therapy reduces the rate of distant metastases in patients with Dukes' stage C colorectal cancer. Frequent minimal residual disease in patients with solid tumors is an indication for antibody therapy. Current studies are assessing the value of adding antibody to chemotherapy to attack dormant as well as proliferating, metastatic tumor cells. Some patients in this control group received radiation therapy, a source of bias that may account for the apparent difference in local recurrence rate.

▶ In the early 1980s, monoclonal antibodies were felt to be the treatment of the future for metastatic cancer. Colorectal cancer was one of the areas most enthusiastically investigated. However, only recently has therapy with monoclonal antibody to colorectal cancer been shown to be effective. This article from the multi-institutional trial in Germany suggests that a 30% reduction in recurrence and an improved survival can be accomplished by the use of postoperative repeat injections of high doses of a non-carcinoembryonic antigen monoclonal antibody in patients with stage III colorectal cancer. Follow-up at this time is 7 years, is considered mature, and now certainly suggests that this treatment is an option that should be pursued.

There are currently other studies, which are being sponsored by industry, looking at this mode of therapy. The transition to a truly human monoclonal antibody will need to be made, because the anti-mouse antibody response limits the amount of treatment that can be provided. When this transition has been accomplished, then monoclonal antibody therapy for colorectal cancer may become standard.

J.W. Fleshman, Jr., M.D.

Transanal Self-expanding Metal Stents as an Alternative to Palliative Colostomy in Selected Patients With Malignant Obstruction of the Left Colon

Turégano-Fuentes F, Echenagusia-Belda A, Simó-Muerza G, et al (Univ Gen Hosp 'Gregorio Marañón,' Madrid)

Br J Surg 85:232-235, 1998 5–66

Background.—In many patients with malignant obstruction of the left colon, palliative colostomy cannot be avoided. One experience with a series of patients with left-sided colon obstruction treated with transanal self-expanding metal stent (SEMS) placement for palliation was described.

Methods.—Eleven patients with malignant obstruction of the rectosigmoid region were treated. All patients had advanced pelvic disease, peritoneal carcinomatosis, and/or multiple parenchymatous metastatic disease. Wallstent esophageal endoprostheses were used. Interventional radiologists performed the procedure.

Findings.—Obstruction was relieved in 7 patients. Surgical intervention was prevented in 6 patients, 5 of whom died with an unobstructed colon 26 days to 7 months after SEMS placement. The procedure was unsuccessful in 4 patients, 3 of whom had emergency colostomy.

Conclusion.—Transanal SEMS placement is an attractive palliative procedure for relieving malignant obstruction in selected patients. This procedure can obviate the need for palliative colostomy.

► The SEMS has become an alternative to diverting colostomy in patients with low colonic or upper rectal cancers. This report of a series of patients in Spain gives examples of some of the pitfalls of this technique and some of the criteria for success. Low rectal tumors tend to be better palliated with laser ablation of tumor and opening of stenosis, as the stent will cause severe tenesmus. This has occurred in several patients, in my personal experience, and is a real issue in these individuals. The stent actually burrows into the wall of the rectum and may cause perforation at the distal end of the wire cage. Patients with lesions that cannot be cannulated with a wire passed through a flexible sigmoidoscope may be poor candidates for this technique. Certainly, the risk of perforation of the cancer into the abdominal cavity after placement of the stent in the colon is a possibility and has occurred in our experience.

This series of patients from Madrid suggests that two thirds of individuals with obstructing, or near obstructing, rectal sigmoid lesions are amenable to palliation with the SEMS, and, indeed, some of them may avoid an operation. This is a technique that should always be remembered when dealing with obstructing left-sided colon cancers.

J.W. Fleshman, Jr., M.D.

Conditional Survival Estimates in 34,963 Patients With Invasive Carcinoma of the Colon

Merrill RM, Henson DE, Ries LAG (Natl Cancer Inst, Bethesda, Md)

Dis Colon Rectum 41:1097-1106, 1998 5–67

Background.—Projected 5- and 10-year survival rates are usually made from the time of cancer diagnosis. Colon cancer survival rates conditional on patients having already survived for 1 or more years after diagnosis were reported.

Methods.—Population-based data were obtained from the Surveillance, Epidemiology, and End Results Program of the National Cancer Institute. The patients included had been given a diagnosis of cancer between 1983 and 1987 and were followed through 1994. The life table method was used to determine conditional survival rates.

Findings.—Survival rates for up to 10 years after diagnosis were computed by disease stage, sex, and race for patients with colon cancer surviving from 1 to 5 years after diagnosis. Survival rates were also determined by lymph node involvement (Figs 1-5).

Conclusion.—In this study, 5- and 10-year survival rates among patients with colon cancer who had already survived 1 to 5 years after diagnosis were calculated. Disease stage and race continue to significantly influence survival.

▶ This article looks at the survival of individuals who have already survived 1 to 5 years after operation for colorectal cancer. The bottom line is that stage, age, and race continue to affect the survival for the next 5 to 10 years. The survival curves from the Surveillance Epidemiology, and End Results program are interesting to look at and provide some data which are worth viewing in graph form.

J.W. Fleshman, Jr., M.D.

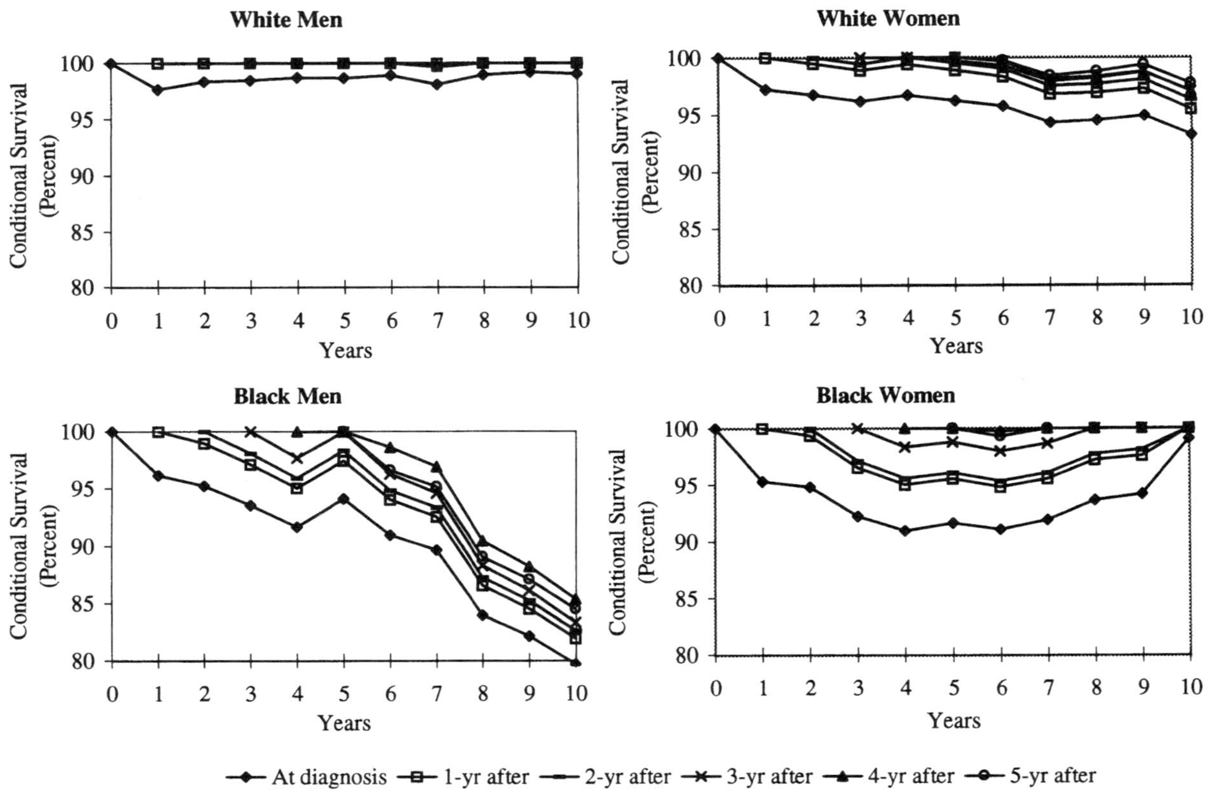

FIGURE 1.—Conditional survival for diagnosed stage I colon cancer cases in the Surveillance, Epidemiology, and End Results Program between 1983 and 1987 and followed through 1994. (Courtesy of Merrill RM, Henson DE, Ries LAG: Conditional survival estimates in 34,963 patients with invasive carcinoma of the colon. *Dis Colon Rectum* 41:1097-1106, 1998.)

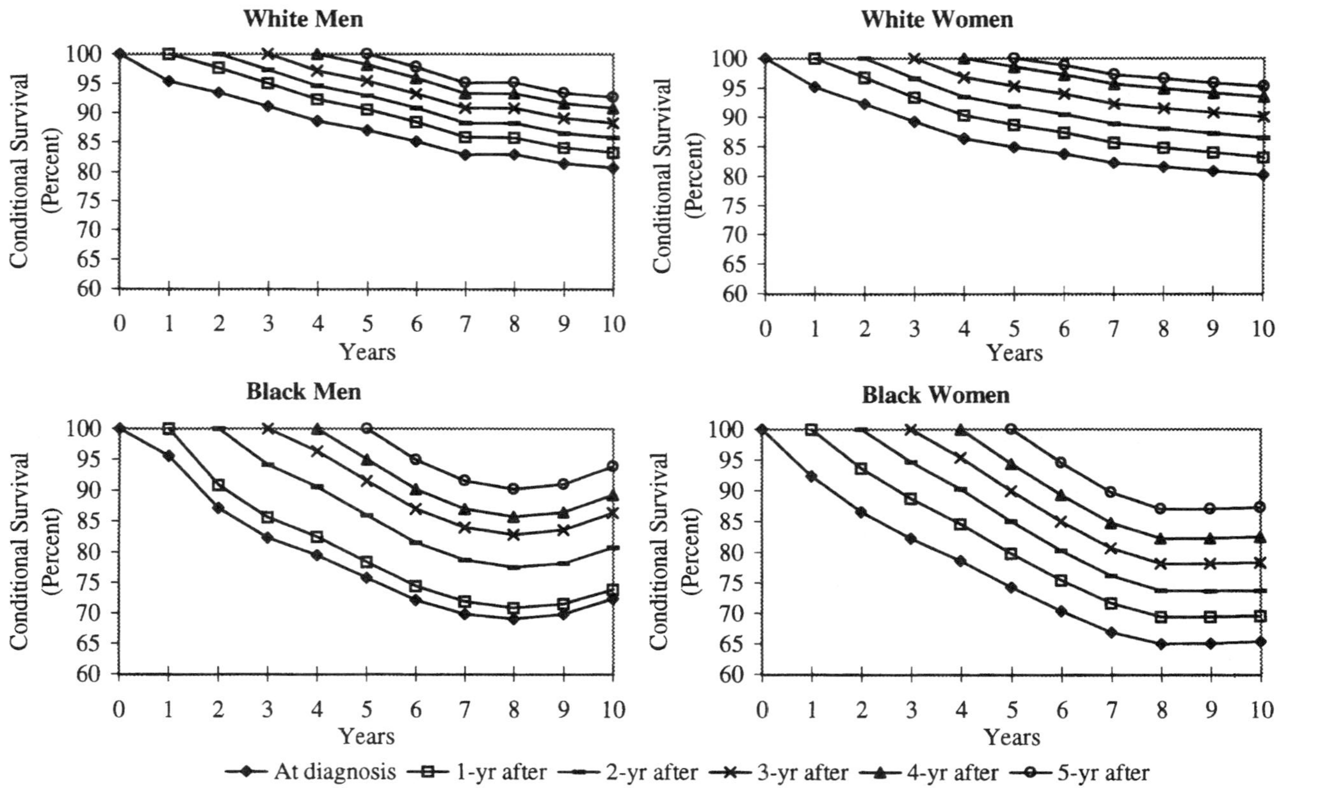

FIGURE 2.—Conditional survival for diagnosed stage II colon cancer cases in the Surveillance, Epidemiology, and End Results Program between 1983 and 1987 and followed through 1994. (Courtesy of Merrill RM, Henson DE, Ries LAG: Conditional survival estimates in 34,963 patients with invasive carcinoma of the colon. *Dis Colon Rectum* 41:1097-1106, 1998.)

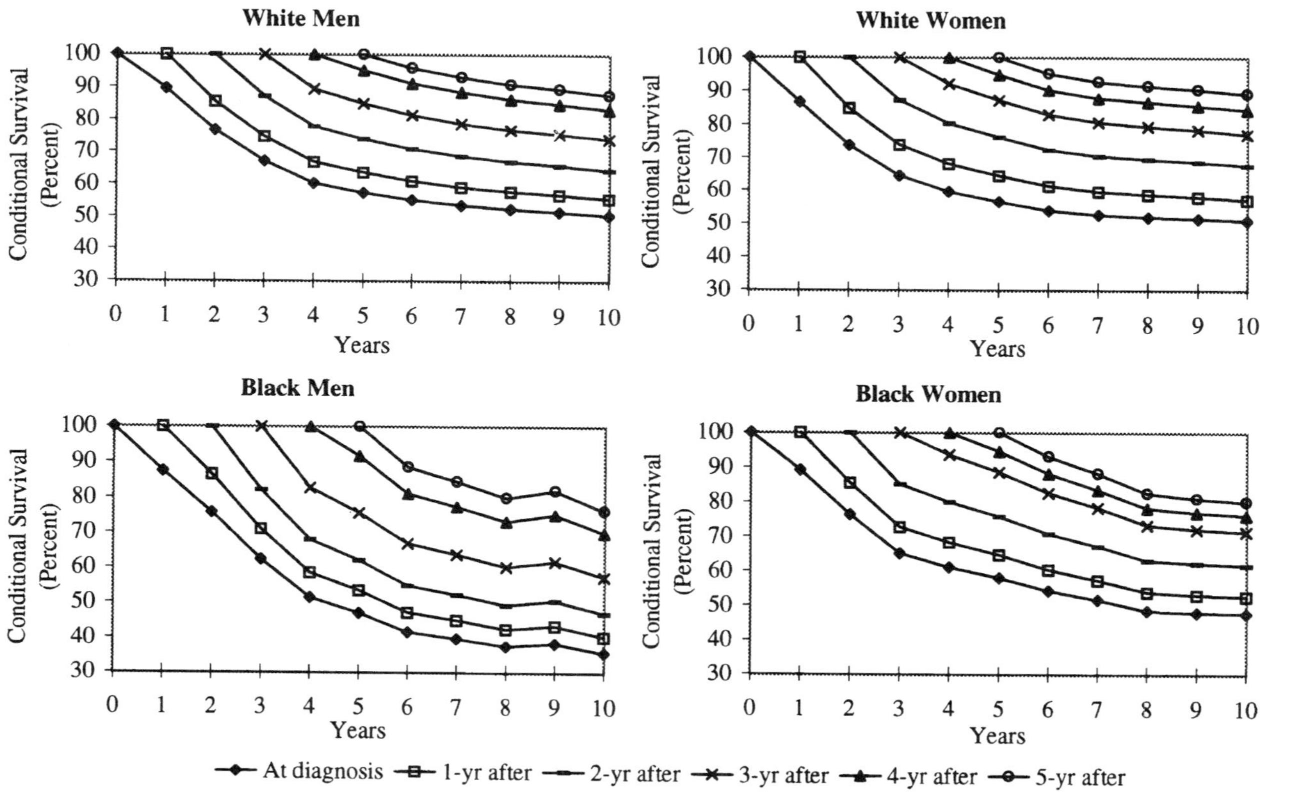

FIGURE 3.—Conditional survival for diagnosed stage III colon cancer cases in the Surveillance, Epidemiology, and End Results Program between 1983 and 1987 and followed through 1994. (Courtesy of Merrill RM, Henson DE, Ries LAG: Conditional survival estimates in 34,963 patients with invasive carcinoma of the colon. *Dis Colon Rectum* 41:1097-1106, 1998.)

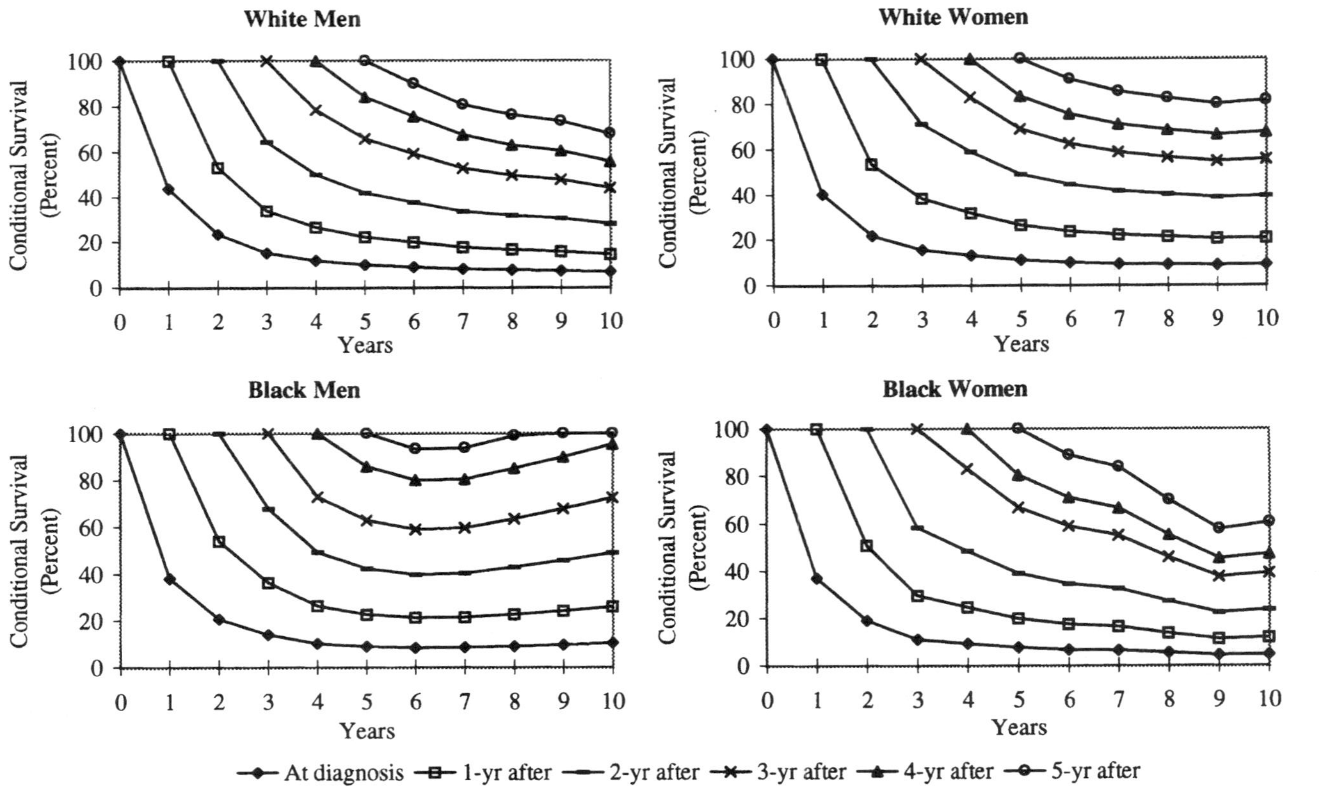

FIGURE 4.—Conditional survival for diagnosed stage IV colon cancer cases in the Surveillance, Epidemiology, and End Results Program between 1983 and 1987 and followed through 1994. (Courtesy of Merrill RM, Henson DE, Ries LAG: Conditional survival estimates in 34,963 patients with invasive carcinoma of the colon. *Dis Colon Rectum* 41:1097-1106, 1998.)

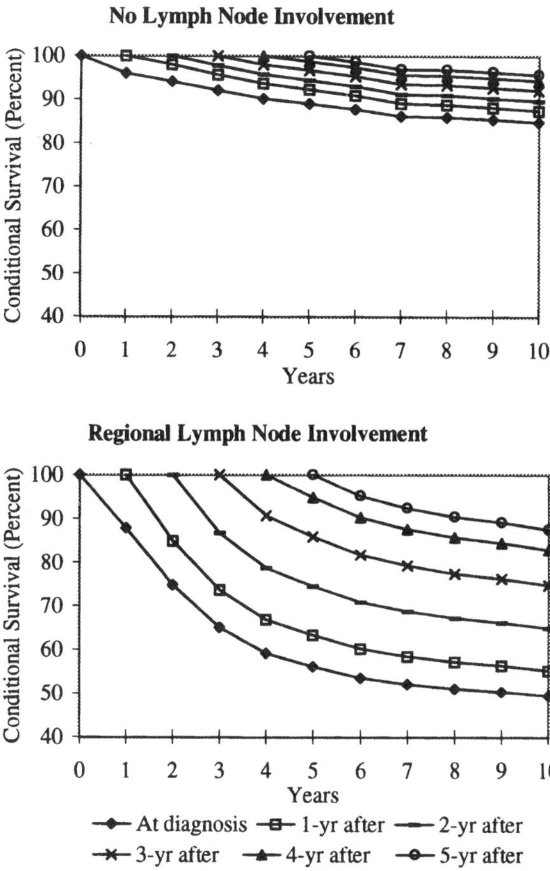

FIGURE 5.—Conditional survival for diagnosed colon cancer cases in the Surveillance, Epidemiology, and End Results Program between 1983 and 1987 and followed through 1994 by lymph node involvement. (Courtesy of Merrill RM, Henson DE, Ries LAG: Conditional survival estimates in 34,963 patients with invasive carcinoma of the colon. *Dis Colon Rectum* 41:1097-1106, 1998.)

Micrometastases and Survival in Stage II Colorectal Cancer

Liefers G-J, Cleton-Jansen A-M, van de Velde CJH, et al (Leiden Univ, The Netherlands)

N Engl J Med 339:223-228, 1998 5–68

Background.—Standard treatment of colorectal cancer includes adjuvant chemotherapy for patients with stage III but not stage II disease. However, 20% of those with stage II disease ultimately die of recurrent disease. Whether detection of micrometastases is useful for identifying patients with stage II disease who are at high risk for recurrence was studied.

Methods.—One hundred ninety-two lymph nodes from 26 consecutive patients with stage II colorectal cancer were analyzed using a carcinoembryonic antigen-specific nested reverse-transcriptase polymerase chain reaction. Five-year follow-up data on all patients were also obtained for analysis.

Findings.—Fifty-four percent of the patients had micrometastases in 1 or more lymph nodes. In this group of patients, the adjusted 5-year survival rate was 50% compared with 91% in the group of patients without micrometastases. Observed 5-year survival rates were 36% and 75% in the patients with and without micrometastases, respectively. The 2 groups were comparable in age, sex, tumor side, degree of tumor differentiation, and primary tumor diameter.

Conclusions.—Micrometastasis detection by reverse-transcriptase polymerase chain reaction amplification of carcinoembryonic antigen mRNA in lymph nodes from patients with stage II colorectal cancer may be of clinical value. The finding of micrometastases was associated with a significant decrease in the 5-year survival rate.

▶ This is a very important article that indicates that node-negative patients, i.e., stage II patients, may actually be stage III patients in over 50% of cases. The use of reverse-transcriptase polymerase chain reaction to detect carcinoembryonic antigen in lymph nodes in patients who have histologically negative lymph nodes may be clinically relevant. In this small series, over half of patients felt to have histologically negative lymph nodes were found to have micrometastases to lymph nodes after resection of colorectal cancer. This finding was clinically significant in that it was an independent, poor prognostic factor. These patients would, therefore, have otherwise been candidates for postoperative adjuvant chemotherapy. Disease-free survival and local control were lower in the group with micrometastases detected by reverse-transcriptase polymerase chain reaction of carcinoembryonic antigen. This article indicates that we may be closer to identifying a pure group of patients to perform adjuvant therapy trials and surgical trials. Larger studies using this technique will be required to identify its true place in the staging of patients with colorectal cancer. This technique is very labor intensive and may require some refinement before becoming clinically available, however.

J.W. Fleshman, Jr., M.D.

Intraperitoneal Exfoliated Cancer Cells in Patients With Colorectal Cancer

Hase K, Ueno H, Kuranaga N, et al (Self-Defense Forces Central Hosp, Tokyo)

Dis Colon Rectum 41:1134-1140, 1998 5–69

Purpose.—In patients undergoing laparoscopic surgery for colorectal cancer, recurrence at the site of trocar insertion may result from direct implantation of exfoliated cancer cells. Such recurrences are still rare, but may become more common. Factors associated with the presence of exfoliated cancer cells in the peritoneal cavity, including the prognostic significance of intraoperative peritoneal lavage with cytologic examination, were evaluated.

Methods.—The 2-year study included 140 patients undergoing peritoneal lavage cytology during surgery for colorectal cancer. Resection was curative in 88 patients and noncurative in 52. Washing cytology was performed once immediately after the peritoneal cavity was opened and again just before the abdomen was closed. Lavage was performed by instillation of 100 mL of saline solution into the peritoneal cavity, retrieved by suction irrigation. Papanicolaou, Giemsa, periodic acid-Schiff, and Alcian blue stains were used for cytologic examination.

Results.—The preresection results were positive in 15% of patients and the postresection results were positive in 9%. Overall, peritoneal cancer cells were detected, either preresection or postresection in 16% of patients. The positive cytology rate was 10% for patients undergoing curative resection. Several tumor characteristics were associated with tumor cell exfoliation into the peritoneal cavity: macroscopic peritoneal dissemination, liver metastasis, ascites greater than 20 mL, ulcerated tumors with indefinite borders, invasion into or beyond the serosal surface, semiannular or annular shape, and moderate to marked lymphatic invasion. For the curative resection group, the only factor strongly correlated with positive cytologic results was circumferential involvement.

Patients with positive cytologic results had worse outcomes. In the curative resection group, local recurrence risk was more strongly affected by the postresection cytology results than by the preresection cytology results. Patients with positive preresection cytology results had a higher local recurrence rate than patients with negative postresection cytology results, independent of the preresection cytology results. Recurrence developed in every patient found to have cancer cells in the peritoneal cavity at the end of surgery.

Conclusions.—Risk factors for cancer cell exfoliation into the peritoneal cavity during surgery for colorectal cancer are identified. The results may help to guide decisions regarding laparoscopic surgery. The long-term postoperative results are significantly associated with the results of peritoneal lavage cytology at the end of surgery. Even after curative resection, patients found to have free cancer cells in peritoneal lavage fluid may benefit from close follow-up, and possibly from adjuvant chemotherapy.

► Control of tumor contamination remains an important factor in cancer surgery. A surprisingly high percentage (15%) of these patients were positive for cells in the cytologic wash before resection of the colon cancer had taken place. This fact may influence the implantation of cells in laparoscopic treatment, as well as local recurrence in standard surgery. Interestingly, the incidence of distant and local recurrence was much higher (100%) in the group that had cells positive after the resection than in the group that had cells positive only before the resection. There may be some benefit to intraoperative lavage of the abdominal cavity to prevent implantation of free cells. Large annular lesions, lesions with intraperitoneal implantations, and poorly differentiated cancers have a higher incidence of exfoliated cells and, therefore, a higher incidence of distant recurrence. Once again, this is evidence that surgical technique definitely influences outcome.

J.W. Fleshman, Jr., M.D.

Young Age Is Not a Poor Prognostic Marker in Colorectal Cancer

Chung YFA, Eu K-W, Machin D, et al (Singapore Gen Hosp, China; Natl Med Research Council, Singapore, China)

Br J Surg 85:1255-1259, 1998 5–70

Background.—Colorectal cancer is largely a disease of older adults, but it can also affect younger patients. Previous studies have suggested that colorectal cancer has a poor prognosis, often attributed to delayed diagnosis, in young adults. However, most of these studies have included only small numbers of young adults, with no suitable comparison group. The incidence, characteristics, and prognosis of colorectal cancer in young patients were studied.

Methods.—The retrospective study included 110 patients with colorectal cancer who were younger than 40 years. The 62 men and 48 women (median age 35 years) represented 5.1% of all patients with colorectal cancer. They were compared with 2,064 older patients with colorectal cancer: 1,147 men and 917 women. Mode of presentation, stage at diagnosis, tumor characteristics, and survival were compared between groups. Mean follow-up was 32 months.

Results.—Twenty-one percent of the younger patients had predisposing malignant disease and a family history of colorectal cancer, compared with 2% of the older group. Change in bowel habits and rectal bleeding were frequent presenting symptoms; younger patients were more likely than older patients to complain of abdominal pain. The 2 groups were similar in disease stage at presentation, as well as in tumor site and characteristics. Younger patients had a somewhat higher incidence of mucinous/signet ring cell and poor-grade tumors. Five-year survival was about 55% in both groups, with no significant age-related differences with disease stages. Compared with those for patients aged 40 to 59 years, adjusted hazard ratios for survival were 1.3 for patients younger than 40, 1.4 for those aged 60 to 79, and 2.4 for those 80 and older.

Conclusions.—Colorectal cancer patients aged younger than 40 years are similar in tumor characteristics and survival to older patients with the same disease. However, there is evidence that patients under 40 may have a worse prognosis than those aged 40 to 59 years. Young patients are more likely to have a family history of colorectal cancer and other predisposing conditions, which underscores the need for aggressive screening, surveillance, and treatment for high-risk patients. Though the diagnosis of colorectal cancer in young patients is not different from that in older patients, it does require a high index of suspicion.

► The group from Singapore shows once again that there is no increase in aggressiveness of colorectal cancer in patients under the age of 40. This series is possible only because of a well-kept database in a colorectal surgery group in a large metropolitan hospital. Interestingly, there is an increase in familial inherited cancer within this group of patients. Polyposis coli, hereditary nonpolyposis colorectal cancer, and ulcerative colitis were all heavily represented in these young patients. Aggressive screening and high index of suspicion are the keys to managing young patients with colorectal cancer to improve their chances of survival.

J.W. Fleshman, Jr., M.D.

Prognostic Significance of Allelic Loss at Chromosome 18q21 for Stage II Colorectal Cancer

Carethers JM, Hawn MT, Greenson JK, et al (Univ of California, San Diego; Univ of Michigan, Ann Arbor; Ohio State Univ, Columbus)

Gastroenterology 114:1188-1195, 1998 5–71

Objective.—About one third of patients diagnosed with colorectal cancer have Dukes' stage B2 disease, in which survival is not improved by adjuvant chemotherapy. Previous studies have suggested that allelic loss of a portion of chromosome 18q and lack of expression of deleted in colorectal cancer (DCC) protein are adverse prognostic factors for stage II disease. This study examined the impact of allelic loss at the DCC gene locus on survival for patients with stage II colorectal cancer.

Methods.—The study included paraffin-embedded, formalin-fixed specimens from 70 patients with stage II colorectal cancer. Using DNA from these specimens, the investigators amplified 5 DNA microsatellite markers on chromosome 18q21, surrounding or located within the DCC gene locus. The markers included a DCC intragenic $(ta)_n$ microsatellite. Epidemiologic and survival associations were assessed without knowledge of the microsatellite data.

Results.—At an average follow-up of 63 months, 11 patients had died of colorectal cancer. Overall, 43% of tumors showed loss of heterozygosity of 18q21. This allelic loss was not a significant predictor of survival, after adjustment for other variables: hazard ratio was 1.17, with 1 95% confidence interval of 0.27 to 5.10.

Conclusions.—For patients with stage II colorectal cancer, loss of heterozygosity of 18q21 does not appear to be a significant prognostic factor. The findings do not support its use as a prognostic factor or its use in stratifying patients for chemotherapy. Though there may still be a candidate tumor-suppressor gene on chromosome 18q, its location is likely telomeric to that of DCC and other suspected tumor-suppressor genes.

► Loss of heterozygosity at the DCC gene locus on chromosome 18 has been suggested as a prognostic indicator for patients with colorectal cancer. This study by Carethers et al. confirms that the majority of patients with colorectal cancer have a loss of heterozygosity at 18q21, but fails to confirm the prognostic importance of the finding. The *smad4* and *smad2* genes may be targets for tumorigenesis and metastasis and may be related to the TGF-β receptor on tumor cells, but, according to the current data, have very little to do with survival disadvantage in patients with stage II colorectal cancer. Obviously, we are a long way from identifying all of the factors which influence and determine the development of colorectal cancer. The true role of chromosome 18 will eventually be found and more data will be necessary. Thus, prospective studies involving chromosomal analysis are very important for our future understanding of the genetics of colorectal cancer.

J.W. Fleshman, Jr., M.D.

Rectal Cancer

Prognostic Significance of Extranodal Microscopic Foci Discontinuous With Primary Lesion in Rectal Cancer

Ueno H, Mochizuki H, Tamakuma S (Natl Defense Med College, Saitama, Japan)

Dis Colon Rectum 41:55-61, 1998 5–72

Objective.—Because of increased morbidity after radical abdominopelvic dissection for rectal cancer, lesser operations are desirable for appropriate patients. Reliable predictors of cancer spread are needed. The clinical significance of extranodal, extramural cancer foci discontinuous with the primary rectal lesion, especially microscopic cancer foci, and their prediction measures are discussed.

Methods.—Resected specimens from 427 patients with rectal cancer were examined histologically. Patients who were not followed up for more than 3 years were excluded from the study.The prognostic significance of each form of cancer spread outside the rectum and the significance of microscopic permeation (mic) as an important predictor of intrapelvic local recurrence after curative operations were evaluated for 218 patients.

Results.—Mic was found in 96 patients (22.5%) and was morphologically classified as tumor scattering (28), vessel invasion (72), and neural invasion (28). Mic was associated with extrarectal tumor, large tumor nodules, and lymph node invasion. Compared with patients with mic, patients without mic had a worse survival rate. Patients with two types of mic had a worse survival rate than those with only one type of mic, and node-positive patients had a survival difference according to mic status. Because tumor nodules and metastatic lymph nodes can be detected by palpation and examined microscopically, they may be predictive indicators of mic.

Conclusion.—The presence of large tumor nodules and metastatic lymph nodes may predict the presence of microscopic disease and may aid in determining the extent of local disease.

▶ Pathologists have differed in their reporting of microscopic foci of tumor deposits within the perirectal fat after operative resection of rectal cancer.

The AJCC staging now includes a classification of N_3 for patients with extranodal perirectal fat implants. This paper from Saitama, Japan, confirms the poor prognostic indication of extranodal perirectal fat implants of rectal cancer. The poor prognosis holds even in patients who have lymph node metastases and extranodal implants (Figure 2,C). These small implants may respond to preoperative radiation, and their control may actually influence long-term survival. For this reason, it is difficult once again to accurately stage patients receiving preoperative radiation therapy since the small microscopic implants may have been present but influence outcome after radiation. Pathologic evaluation and staging remain an important feature of prognostication in the treatment of rectal cancer. Until biomarkers are available, these histologic and pathologic findings should be evaluated and recorded accurately in all communications.

J.W. Fleshman, Jr., M.D.

The Impact of 5-Fluorouracil and Intraoperative Electron Beam Radiation Therapy on the Outcome of Patients With Locally Advanced Primary Rectal and Rectosigmoid Cancer

Nakfoor BM, Willett CG, Shellito PC, et al (Harvard Med School, Boston)
Ann Surg 228:194-200, 1998 5–73

Background.—Innovative strategies for improving local control in patients with locally advanced primary rectal and rectosigmoid cancer have included the administration of 5-fluorouracil (5-FU)-based chemotherapy during preoperative external beam irradiation and the application of intraoperative electron beam radiation therapy (IOERT) to the tumor bed at the time of resection. The impact of these 2 modalities on the outcome of patients with locally advanced rectal cancer was investigated.

Methods.—Between 1978 and 1996, 145 patients with locally advanced rectal cancer underwent moderate- to high-dose preoperative irradiation followed by surgery. Ninety-three patients were given a bolus of 5-FU for 3 days during the first and last weeks of radiation therapy or a continuous infusion of 5-FU throughout irradiation. In 73 patients with persistent tumor adherence or residual pelvic disease, IOERT was administered to the surgical bed.

Findings.—Sphincter preservation, pathologic downstaging, and resectability rates did not differ with 5-FU use. However, patients receiving 5-FU during irradiation had significantly better 5-year actuarial local control and disease-specific survival rates than patients undergoing irradiation without 5-FU. In the group undergoing IOERT, local control and disease-specific survival were associated with the extent of resection. Patients undergoing complete resection and IOERT had a 5-year actuarial local control rate of 89% and a disease-specific survival rate of 63%. For patients undergoing IOERT for residual disease, these figures were 65% and 32%, respectively. The overall actuarial complication rate at 5 years was 11%.

Conclusions.—The use of 5-FU during external beam irradiation and IOERT is beneficial and well tolerated in patients with locally advanced rectal cancer. To improve outcomes, efforts are being aimed at intensifying the 5-FU chemotherapy regimen during irradiation and the use of maintenance chemotherapy postoperatively.

▶ The authors present a very large series of patients with locally advanced rectal cancer. Their data suggest that preoperative radiation and chemotherapy probably yield the most significant benefit to these patients. Although the complete response rate was no different between preoperative combined chemoradiation and preoperative radiation, the disease-free survival and local control rate were markedly improved. The use of intraoperative radiation therapy may or may not have an effect. Certainly, if gross residual disease is present, the long-term prognosis is poor. However, frozen sections and the supplementation of pelvic radiation with intraoperative radiation or brachytherapy or even postoperative external beam radiation may be appropriate in patients with close margins or even microscopically positive margins. These results once again give us reason to use preoperative chemoradiation in the treatment of rectal cancer to improve local control and disease-free survival. It would be difficult to perform a randomized, controlled trial comparing surgery alone with adjuvant therapy plus surgery. The use of intraoperative radiation therapy and postoperative radiation therapy may be addressed in randomized trials, but a trial to test the excellent results from the preoperative combined modality therapy in locally advanced disease does not seem to be ethically possible.

J.W. Fleshman, Jr., M.D.

The National Cancer Data Base Report on Patterns of Care for Adenocarcinoma of the Rectum, 1985-1995

Jessup JM, Stewart AK, Menck HR (Univ of Pittsburgh Med Ctr, Pa; American College of Surgeons, Chicago)

Cancer 83:2408-2418, 1998 5–74

Objective.—Trends in the patterns of care for patients with rectal adenocarcinoma treated in hospitals that submit data to the National Cancer Data Base were examined.

Methods.—Data solicited from 2,200 US hospitals yielded 5,850,000 patients with cancer. Adenocarcinomas of the rectum included 6,163 cases reported in 1985 to 1986, 15,402 cases reported in 1989 to 1990, and 21,169 cases reported in 1994 to 1995. Stage-specific survival outcomes, treatment regimens, relative survival rates, and expected survival rates were evaluated.

Results.—Stage I disease represented 37.1% of the cases diagnosed in 1985 to 1986 and 33.9% of those diagnosed in 1994 to 1995. The younger the patient, the more advanced the disease at diagnosis. Whereas surgery alone as the first course of therapy declined from 53.1% in 1985

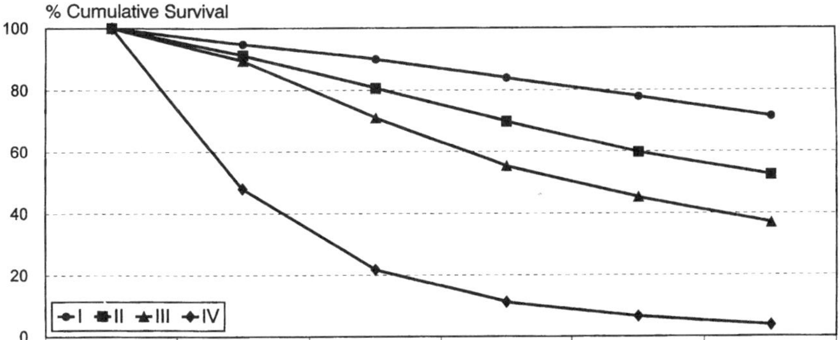

	0	1	2	3	4	5
I	100	94.8	89.9	83.9	77.8	71.5
II	100	91.2	80.6	69.8	59.7	52.4
III	100	89.4	71	55.3	45.1	36.9
IV	100	48	21.7	11.1	6.5	3.6

Years Following Diagnosis

FIGURE 3.—Relative survival by American Joint Committee on Cancer stage of disease, cases diagnosed in 1989-1990. (Courtesy of Jessup JM, Stewart AK, Menck HR: The National Cancer Data Base report on patterns of care for adenocarcinoma of the rectum, 1985-1995. *Cancer* 83:2408-2418. Copyright 1998 American Cancer Society. Reprinted by permission of Wiley-Liss, Inc., a subsidiary of John Wiley & Sons, Inc.)

to 1986 to 42.1% in 1994 to 1995 and the combination of surgery plus radiation declined from 25.6% to 8,4% over the same period, the use of surgery plus radiation and chemotherapy has increased from 5.9% in 1985 to 1986 to 19.5% in 1989 to 1990 and to 29.6% in 1994 to 1995.

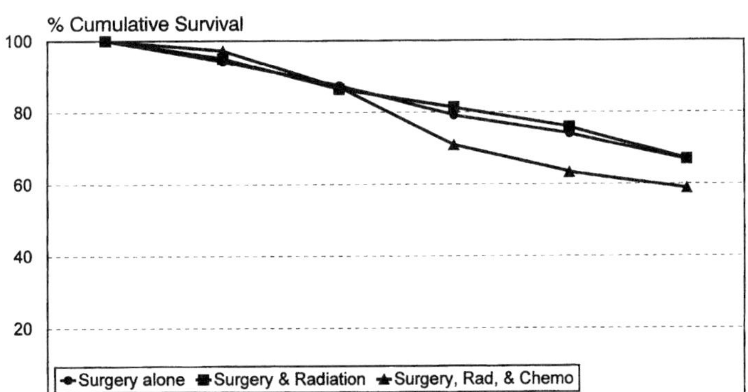

	0	1	2	3	4	5
Surgery alone	100	94.2	87.4	79.1	74	66.6
Surgery & Radiation	100	95	86.4	81.3	75.8	66.9
Surgery, Rad, & Chemo	100	97.2	87	70.9	63.3	58.8

Years Following Diagnosis

FIGURE 4.—Relative survival of American Joint Committee on Cancer stage I patients treated with local excision; cases diagnosed in 1989-1990. *Abbreviations: Rad*, radiation; *chemo*, chemotherapy. (Courtesy of Jessup JM, Stewart AK, Menck HR: The National Cancer Data Base report on patterns of care for adenocarcinoma of the rectum, 1985-1995. *Cancer* 83:2408-2418. Copyright 1998 American Cancer Society. Reprinted by permission of Wiley-Liss, Inc., a subsidiary of John Wiley & Sons, Inc.)

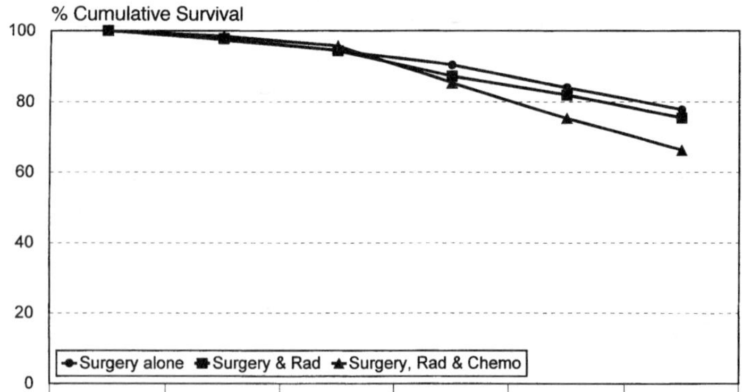

	0	1	2	3	4	5
Surgery alone	100	97.4	94.4	90.4	84	77.8
Surgery & Rad	100	97.8	94.4	87.2	81.9	75.4
Surgery, Rad & Chemo	100	98.5	95.7	85.3	75.3	66.4

Years Following Diagnosis

FIGURE 5.—Relative survival of American Joint Committee on Cancer stage I patients undergoing curative resection, cases diagnosed in 1989-1990. *Abbreviations: Rad*, radiation; *chemo*, chemotherapy. (Courtesy of Jessup JM, Stewart AK, Menck HR: The National Cancer Data Base report on patterns of care for adenocarcinoma of the rectum, 1985-1995. *Cancer* 83:2408-2418. Copyright 1998 American Cancer Society. Reprinted by permission of Wiley-Liss, Inc., a subsidiary of John Wiley & Sons, Inc.)

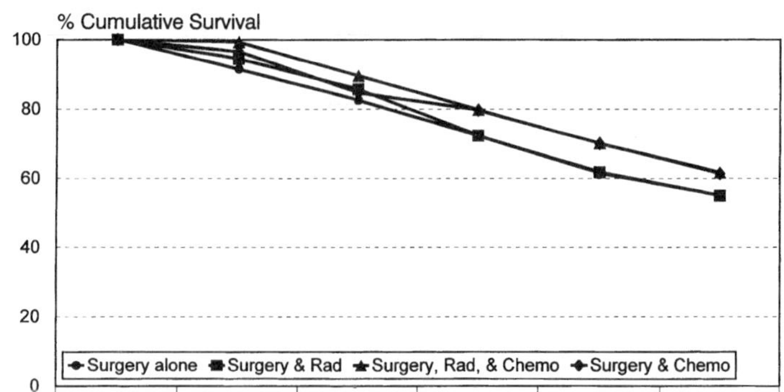

	0	1	2	3	4	5
Surgery alone	100	91.5	82.5	72.3	61.5	55
Surgery & Rad	100	94.5	85.7	72.3	61.8	55
Surgery, Rad, & Chemo	100	99.3	89.6	79.7	70.1	61.6
Surgery & Chemo	100	96.6	84.7	79.6	70.1	61.4

Years Following Diagnosis

FIGURE 6.—Relative survival of American Joint Committee on Cancer stage II patients undergoing curative resection, cases diagnosed in 1989-1990. *Abbreviations: Rad*, radiation; *chemo*, chemotherapy. (Courtesy of Jessup JM, Stewart AK, Menck HR: The National Cancer Data Base report on patterns of care for adenocarcinoma of the rectum, 1985-1995. *Cancer* 83:2408-2418, Copyright 1998 American Cancer Society. Reprinted by permission of Wiley-Liss, Inc., a subsidiary of John Wiley & Sons, Inc.)

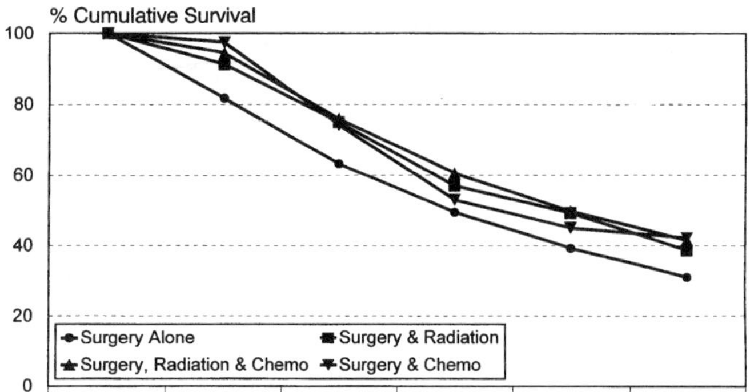

	0	1	2	3	4	5
Surgery Alone	100	81.7	63.2	49.4	39.2	30.9
Surgery & Radiation	100	91.3	75	57	49.2	38.6
Surgery, Radiation & Chemo	100	94.4	75.9	60.5	49.7	41.5
Surgery & Chemo	100	97.4	74.2	52.9	45	42.1

Years Following Diagnosis

FIGURE 7.—Relative survival of American Joint Committee on Cancer stage III patients undergoing curative resection, cases diagnosed in 1989-1990. *Abbreviations: Rad*, radiation; *chemo*, chemotherapy. (Courtesy of Jessup JM, Stewart AK, Menck HR: The National Cancer Data Base report on patterns of care for adenocarcinoma of the rectum, 1985-1995. *Cancer* 83:2408-2418. Copyright 1998 American Cancer Society. Reprinted by permission of Wiley-Liss, Inc., a subsidiary of John Wiley & Sons, Inc.)

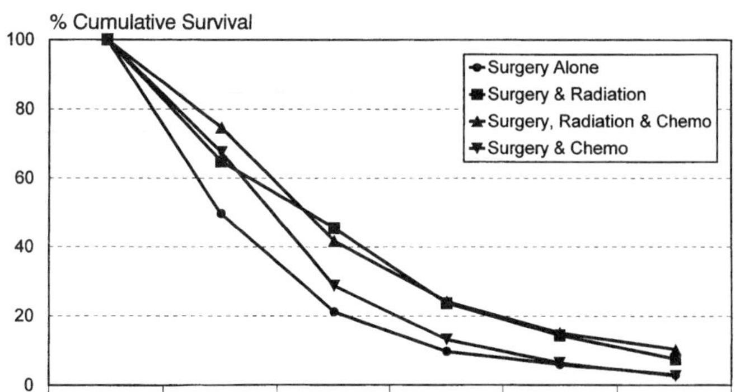

	0	1	2	3	4	5
Surgery Alone	100	49.7	21.2	9.8	6	2.8
Surgery & Radiation	100	64.8	45.5	23.7	14.4	7.5
Surgery, Radiation & Chemo	100	74.6	41.7	24.1	15.1	10.3
Surgery & Chemo	100	67.5	28.7	13.2	6.5	2.6

Years Following Diagnosis

FIGURE 8.—Relative survival of American Joint Committee on Cancer stage IV patients undergoing curative resection, cases diagnosed in 1989-1990. *Abbreviations: Rad*, radiation; *chemo*, chemotherapy. (Courtesy of Jessup JM, Stewart AK, Menck HR: The National Cancer Data Base report on patterns of care for adenocarcinoma of the rectum, 1985-1995. *Cancer* 83:2408-2418. Copyright 1998 American Cancer Society. Reprinted by permission of Wiley-Liss, Inc., a subsidiary of John Wiley & Sons, Inc.)

There was an increase in the frequency of local excisions and anterior/posterior resections and a decrease in the frequency of abdominoperineal resections. Five-year survival data reveal that the survival rate decreases with increasing disease stage (Fig 3). Surgery plus radiation conferred little benefit over surgery alone (Fig 4). Stage I patients treated with surgery alone had improved survival rates when compared with patients treated with surgery plus radiation or with patients treated with radiation plus chemotherapy (Fig 5). Stage II patients treated with surgery or with surgery plus radiation fared worse than patients treated with surgery, radiation, and chemotherapy or with surgery plus chemotherapy (Fig 6). Stage III patients who received multimodality therapy had improved survival compared with patients treated with surgery only (Fig 7). Patients with metastatic disease treated with multimodality therapy fared better than those treated with other regimens (Fig 8). Stage and grade were significant predictors of survival. Patients with stage II, III, or IV disease were 2, 2.8, and 13.6 times more likely to die than were patients with stage I disease.

Conclusion.—Rectal adenocarcinoma is being diagnosed at a later stage. Multimodality therapy is improving survival for patients with stage II to IV disease. Stage and grade are the most important predictors of survival.

▶ This is a very interesting article looking at the National Cancer Data Base supported by the American College of Surgeons Commission on Cancer and the American Cancer Society. These data are maintained in individual hospitals on a voluntary basis and normally require input of data in the medical records department by individuals who are not primary caregivers of the patients. The survival rates listed for the different stages of cancer are a little disappointing for a leading industrial nation. Five-year survival rates of 71.5% for stage I cancers, 52.4% for stage II cancers, 36.9% for stage III cancers, and 3.6% for stage IV cancers are below previously reported survival rates from specific institutions that deal with rectal cancer on a frequent basis (see Fig 3).

The addition of multimodality therapy to each stage of cancer of the rectum has been shown to improve survival only in stage II and III disease, but not significantly. This may indicate the selection bias of physicians who choose multimodality therapy for only the worst, largest, most aggressive cancers as opposed to surgery alone for favorable lesions even in the more advanced stages. These data are not available to us and certainly taint the interpretation of these data (see Figs 4, 5, and 6). The National Cancer Data Base seems to have improved in its data collection but still needs refinement to be able to draw major treatment conclusions. It is interesting that more patients with stage I rectal cancer are being treated with local excision alone. This trend needs to be watched carefully because of the potential for worsening survival in early stage lesions if the local excision is not performed properly.

J.W. Fleshman, Jr., M.D.

Surgical Resection of Locally Recurrent Colorectal Adenocarcinoma

Delpero JR, Pol B, Le Treut YP, et al (Institut J Paoli-I. Calmettes, Marseille, France; Hôpital de la Conception, Marseille, France)

Br J Surg 85:372-376, 1998 5–75

Introduction.—The recurrence rate after curative surgery for colorectal adenocarcinoma is 50%, with 30% of the deaths resulting from locoregional recurrence. Isolated local recurrences are uncommon, so the number of patients who could benefit from further surgery is small. The results of surgery in 120 patients with locoregional recurrence of colorectal adenocarcinoma are reported.

Patients.—Over a 20-year period, 120 patients at 2 centers underwent surgery for locally recurrent colorectal adenocarcinoma. Fifty-six patients had a colonic primary tumor, whereas 64 had a rectal primary tumor. The mean interval between primary surgery and local recurrence was 24 months. According to surgical assessment, 69 resections were curative and 51 were palliative. Extended resection of contiguous viscera was required in 61 cases. Nine patients underwent synchronous hepatic resection. Adjuvant radiation or chemotherapy was used in 56 patients.

Outcomes.—Seven percent of the patients died in the hospital, and 40% experienced immediate postoperative morbidity. Neither mortality nor morbidity was influenced by type of local recurrence. The overall 5-year survival rate was 27%, whereas the recurrence-free survival rate was 22%. The survival rate was 44% for patients undergoing curative resection vs. 0% for those undergoing palliative resection. Forty-four percent of the female patients survived, compared with 11% of the men; the survival rate was 45% for patients operated on for intramural recurrence vs. 19% of those with extramural recurrence. On multivariate analysis, the most important prognostic factor was curative resection.

Conclusions.—This retrospective study suggests that long-term survival is possible for some patients with locally recurrent colorectal adenocarcinoma selected for surgical resection. The results suggest that such resection should be attempted whenever possible. The use of adjuvant therapy may further improve the long-term results.

▶ The authors present a heterogenous group of patients treated surgically for recurrent colorectal cancer. For obvious reasons, the conclusions from this paper must be drawn very carefully. Local recurrence in patients with inadequate operation most certainly should be treated surgically. Palliative operation for small local recurrence is a reasonable recommendation, but attempts to perform radical extended excision for local recurrence should be undertaken only if clear margins can be obtained. The authors do not have a large enough series to make a recommendation on adjuvant therapy. However, the comment in their conclusion that adjuvant chemoradiation should theoretically improve outcome is relevant. Curative resection in females for intraluminal local recurrence was more effective in producing long-term survival. Early detection of asymptomatic recurrence using CEA was not a factor in producing long-term survival.

The issues of postoperative follow-up after treatment of colorectal cancer and the management of a recurrence are controversial. Institutions with large experience which accurately preoperatively stage patients with recurrent cancer seem to achieve the best results. Preoperative PET scan and CT scan would seem to be indicated to avoid inappropriate resection in these individuals with already poor prognosis.

J.W. Fleshman, Jr., M.D.

Outcome After Proctectomy for Rectal Cancer in Department of Veterans Affairs Hospitals: A Report From the National Surgical Quality Improvement Program

Longo WE, Virgo KS, Johnson FE, et al (St Louis Univ; Hines VA Cooperative Studies Program Coordinating Ctr, Ill; Harvard Med School, Boston)

Ann Surg 228:64-70, 1998 5–76

Background.—The National Veterans Affairs Surgical Quality Improvement Program (NSQIP) consists of a prospective registry of more than 287,000 operations, which can be used to construct risk-prediction models with standard statistical techniques. Data from NSQIP were analysed to identify risk factors that predict outcome after proctectomy for rectal cancer in patients of Department of Veterans Affairs Medical Centers.

Study Design.—The study group included all 591 patients from the NSQIP database who had a proctectomy for rectal cancer between 1991 and 1995. A total of 68 presurgical and 12 intraoperative risk factors were examined for their effects on 21 specific adverse outcomes. Stepwise logistic regression analysis was used to construct models predicting 30-day mortality rates.

Findings.—Of the 591 patients, 30% had complications after proctectomy. The most common complications were prolonged ileus, urinary tract infection, pneumonia, and deep wound infection. The 30-day mortality rate was 3.2%. Patients with complications had a significantly higher 30-day mortality rate than patients without complications. For patients with cardiac arrest requiring resuscitation, with deep venous thrombosis or thrombophlebitis, with coma longer than 24 hours, with acute renal failure, with cerebrovascular accident, and with pulmonary embolism, 30-day mortality rates were greater than 50%.

Conclusions.—The mortality rates after proctectomy for rectal cancer in this series of patients were comparable to those reported in other large series. The complication rate after proctectomy was high. Complications were associated with increased 30-day mortality rate. Elevated blood urea nitrogen, impaired sensorium, and low serum albumin before surgery were all predictors of complications and increased risk of 30-day mortality.

▶ A prospective database from Veterans Affairs hospitals across the country is being used to assess the quality of surgery at each of the institutions. This study includes a very large group of patients and evaluates the 30-day morbidity and mortality after treatment of rectal cancer. A complication rate of 30% and a mortality rate of 3.2% were identified. Preoperative factors such as elevated blood urea nitrogen, impaired sensorium, low albumin, and autoanticoagulation were predictors of mortality. Although this study does not evaluate the cancer outcome, it does indicate the baseline early results of rectal cancer management in a Veterans Affairs system. Unfortunately, the results are not stratified by operating surgeon and level of experience, which are quite variable in the Veterans Affairs system.

J.W. Fleshman, Jr., M.D.

Circumferential Margin Involvement After Mesorectal Excision of Rectal Cancer With Curative Intent: Predictor of Survival but Not Local Recurrence?

Hall NR, Finan PJ, Al-Jaberi T, et al (Gen Infirmary at Leeds, England; Univ of Leeds, England)

Dis Colon Rectum 41:979-983, 1998 5–77

Objective.—Total mesorectal excision, which spares autonomic nervous function, reduces the risk of local recurrence for patients with rectal cancer. The finding of tumor at the circumferential resection margin is believed to be an indicator of inadequate surgical excision, and is associated with an increased risk of local pelvic recurrence. However, the studies on which this association is based may not reflect the clinical use of mesorectal excision. A prospective audit was performed to determine the prognostic significance of circumferential margin involvement after potentially curative mesorectal excision for rectal cancer.

Methods.—The 8-year study included 152 patients undergoing mesorectal excision of rectal or rectosigmoid cancer with curative intent. Total mesorectal resection was performed in 44 patients with tumors in the lower third of the rectum and 54 patients with tumors in the middle third. Fifty-four patients with tumors in the upper third underwent mesorectal excision at least 5 cm distal to the primary tumor. Careful histologic examination was performed to assess the presence of circumferential margin involvement. Patients were monitored to detect local and distant recurrences.

Results.—In 13% of patients, tumor was found within 1 mm of the circumferential margin. Median follow-up for survivors was 41 months. The recurrence rate was 24% for patients with a negative circumferential margin vs. 50% for those with a positive margin. Marginal involvement had a significant effect on both disease-free survival and cancer-specific mortality. However, it had no effect on local recurrence rate. The 5-year rate of freedom from local recurrence was 83%. Overall survival was 68%.

Conclusions.—For patients undergoing curative mesorectal excision for rectal cancer, positive circumferential margins are associated with reduced disease-free and overall survival, but are unrelated to local recurrence rate. The results suggest that circumferential margin involvement reflects advanced disease more than it reflects inadequate local surgery. Some patients with positive margins may die of distant metastases before local recurrence appears. More research is needed to define the role of adjuvant therapy for patients undergoing mesorectal excision.

▶ This article once again addresses the issue of complete mesorectal excision in patients with rectal cancer. However, the data are evaluated from a unique point of view. The pathologist, P. Quirke, and the colorectal surgeon, P. Finan, have accumulated a prospective series of patients treated using mesorectal excision. Evaluation of circumferential margins in this group has shown that the presence of positive radial margins has a poor prognosis in terms of long-term survival but not in terms of local recurrence. This finding is in contradiction to that of a previous study by the same authors, which looked at a group of patients treated by a number of surgeons using various techniques. The previous article suggested that positive radial margins increased local recurrence and thereby increased death due to cancer. This article, in fact, suggests that circumferential margin positivity indicates a more aggressive tumor, rather than failure of the surgical technique, when a mesorectal excision is performed. This finding, suggests that preoperative adjuvant radiotherapy or chemoradiation is indicated in patients with local extension of rectal cancer, because of the distant metastatic potential for locally aggressive rectal cancer.

The finding of a local recurrence rate of 11% in this group of patients treated with good surgical technique by a colorectal surgeon suggests that surgical therapy alone is inadequate to ensure excellent outcome for all patients with rectal cancer. As a result, the authors suggest that adjuvant therapy be used selectively in these patients.

J.W. Fleshman, Jr., M.D.

Indication for Using High Ligation of the Inferior Mesenteric Artery in Rectal Cancer Surgery: Examination of Nodal Metastases by the Clearing Method

Hida J, Yasutomi M, Maruyama T, et al (Kinki Univ, Osaka, Japan)
Dis Colon Rectum 41:984-991, 1998 5–78

Background.—There is debate about whether the inferior mesenteric artery (IMA) in patients undergoing surgery for rectal cancer should be ligated at a high or low position: i.e., at its origin or below the origin of the left colic artery. High ligation facilitates en bloc dissection of lymph node metastases, but low ligation is easier and reduces the risk of injury to the hypogastric nerve plexus. This retrospective study examined the indications for high ligation of the IMA during rectal cancer surgery.

Methods.—The review included 198 patients undergoing surgery with high ligation of the IMA over 9 years. The extent of the primary tumor was graded as pT1 in 8 patients, pT2 in 38, pT3 in 128, and pT4 in 24. All patients underwent adequate intestinal resection and nodal dissection, with ligation of the IMA close to the aorta and the inferior mesenteric vein at the inferior border of the pancreas. Lymph node metastases were resected en bloc, according to a previously described clearing method.

Results.—The overall incidence of nodal metastasis was 56.6%, whereas the incidence of metastasis to the IMA root nodes—those surrounding the origin of the IMA—was 8.6%. Patients with more invasive cancer were more likely to have IMA root node metastases. Five-year survival was 38.5% for patients with IMA root node metastases vs. 73.4% for patients without such metastases.

Conclusions.—This study finds nearly a 9% incidence of metastases to the IMA root nodes among patients undergoing surgery for rectal cancer. Survival is significantly reduced in patients with IMA root node metastases. The results suggest that dissection of the IMA root nodes is indicated after high ligation of the IMA in patients with pT3 and pT4 rectal cancer.

► The authors have not convinced me that high ligation of the IMA improves survival in patients with rectal cancer. They have convinced me that a larger lymph node sampling and thereby prognostic indication are possible when high ligation is performed. The presence of lymph nodes with metastases in patients who have a wide mesenteric resection may, in fact, improve survival by providing an indication for adjuvant chemotherapy postoperatively. This possibility has not been shown with this study, but should be the subject of a randomized, prospective trial in the future. The overall survival rate of 78% in patients with no lymph node metastasis is an excellent outcome and indicates that anatomic resection with attention to blood supply and anatomy is of paramount importance in the treatment of rectal cancer.

J.W. Fleshman, Jr., M.D.

Surgeon-Related Factors and Outcome in Rectal Cancer

Porter GA, Soskolne CL, Yakimets WW, et al (Univ of Alberta, Edmonton, Canada)

Ann Surg 227:157-167, 1998 5–79

Introduction.—The outcomes of patients with rectal cancer vary widely among centers and among surgeons. However, there are few data on the prognostic significance of surgeon-related factors. This study examined the prognostic impact of the surgeon's subspecialty training in colorectal surgery and experience with rectal cancer resection.

Methods.—The study included 683 patients undergoing potentially curative low-anterior resection or abdominoperineal resection for primary rectal adenocarcinoma between 1983 and 1990. The operations were

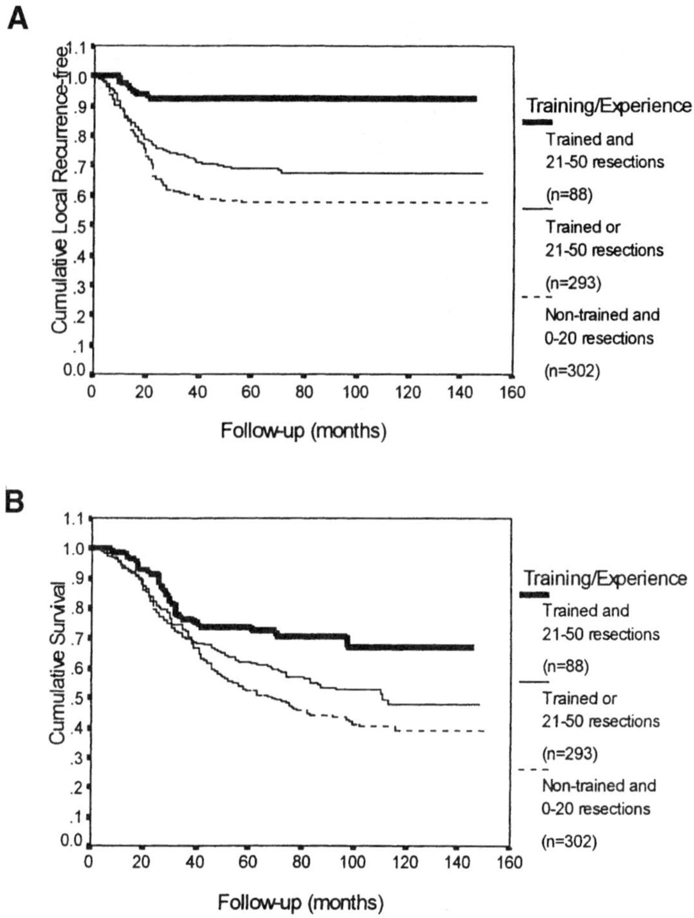

FIGURE 2.—Kaplan-Meier curves for (**A**) local recurrence and (**B**) disease-specific survival, by surgeon group. (Courtesy of Porter GA, Soskolne CL, Yakimets WW, et al: Surgeon-related factors and outcome in rectal cancer. *Ann Surg* 227:157-167, 1998.)

performed by 52 surgeons at 5 Canadian general hospitals. A wide range of preoperative, intraoperative, pathologic, and adjuvant therapy variables were analyzed for their impact on local recurrence (LR) and disease-specific survival (DSS). Cox proportional hazards regression was used to determine survival and to control for confounding and interacting variables.

Results.—Five-year follow-up data were available on 663 patients. Sixteen percent of the operations were performed by 5 surgeons with subspecialty training in colorectal surgery, whereas 47% were performed by surgeons who had a volume of fewer than 21 rectal cancer resections during the study. Patients operated on by surgeons without subspecialty training and by low-volume surgeons were at increased risk of LR, with hazard ratios of 2.5 and 1.8, respectively (Fig 2). Other factors signifi-

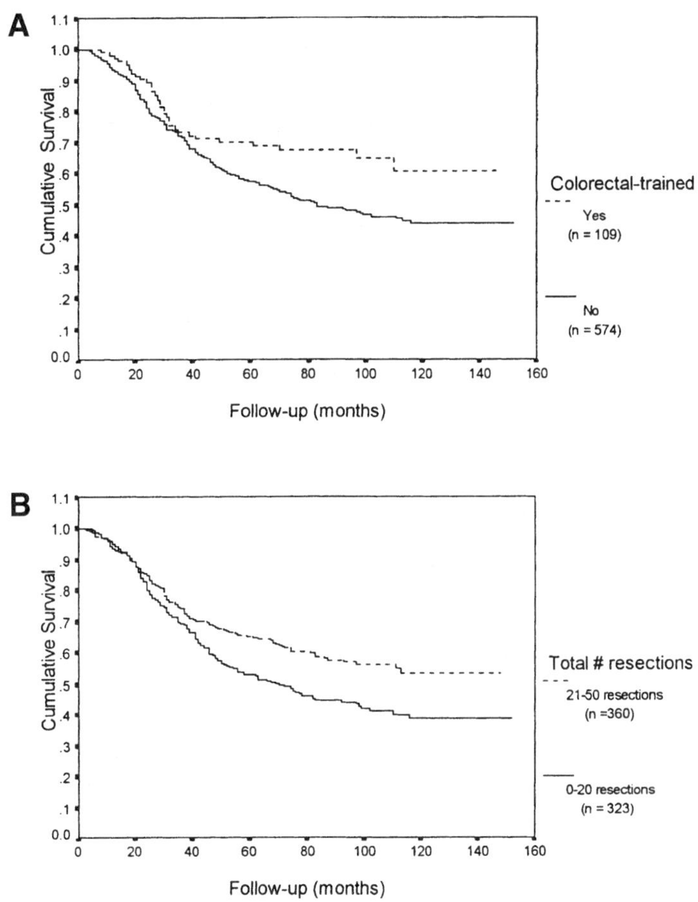

FIGURE 3.—Kaplan-Meier curves for disease-specific survival by (A) presence of colorectal-trained surgeon and (B) by number of rectal cancer resections performed by the surgeon. (Courtesy of Porter GA, Soskolne CL, Yakimets WW, et al: Surgeon-related factors and outcome in rectal cancer. *Ann Surg* 227:157-167, 1998.)

cantly associated with LR on multivariate analysis were disease stage, use of adjuvant therapy, rectal perforation or tumor spill, and vascular/neural invasion. Resection performed by nonsubspecialist or low-volume surgeons was also associated with decreased DSS, with hazard ratios of 1.4 and 1.5, respectively (Fig 3). Other significant prognostic factors for DSS were disease stage and grade, patient age, rectal perforation or tumor spill, and vascular/neural invasion.

Conclusions.—For patients undergoing surgery for rectal cancer, the surgeon's training and experience with rectal cancer surgery have a significant impact on outcomes. Operations should therefore be performed by surgeons with subspecialty training in colorectal cancer or by surgeons performing a higher volume of such procedures. The improved outcomes are likely related to specific operative techniques used by surgeons with more specific training and greater experience.

▶ This article from Edmonton, Alberta, follows the same logic as the article from Uppsala, Sweden (Abstract 5–86), looking at survival and local recurrence after treatment of rectal cancer. These authors were able to identify the factors of colorectal training and frequent management of patients with rectal cancer as independent factors determining outcome after treatment of rectal cancer. The authors conclude that surgical treatment of rectal cancer should be performed exclusively by surgeons with colorectal training and surgeons with a large amount of experience, on an ongoing basis, in the treatment of rectal cancer. This article also indicates that any future trials should include surgeon-related factors as an independent variable in the randomization process.

J.W. Fleshman, Jr., M.D.

Radical and Nerve-Preserving Surgery for Rectal Cancer in The Netherlands: A Prospective Study on Morbidity and Functional Outcome

Maas CP, Moriya Y, Steup WH, et al (Univ Hosp Leiden, The Netherlands; Natl Cancer Ctr Hosp, Tokyo; European Organization for Research and Treatment of Cancer Datacenter, Brussels, Belgium)

Br J Surg 85:92-97, 1998 5–80

Objective.—More radical tumor excision techniques have been proposed in an attempt to improve the results of treatment for primary rectal cancer. Japanese surgeons have reported the use of combined pelvic nerve-sparing and radical tumor resection techniques, with the goals of optimizing local tumor control while minimizing bladder and sexual dysfunction. This technique was prospectively evaluated for morbidity and functional outcomes in a series of Dutch patients with rectal cancer.

Methods.—The study included 47 patients with primary rectal adenocarcinoma. There were 33 men and 14 women (mean age, 63 years) in the study. A sphincter-preserving procedure was performed in 28 patients, abdominoperineal resection in 18, and a Hartmann's procedure in 1. All operations were performed by a noted Japanese surgeon, with a special emphasis on maximal preservation of the superior hypogastric plexus (SHP) and inferior hypogastric plexus (IHP) (Fig 1). Outcomes evaluated were morbidity, death, voiding, and sexual function.

Results.—Mean operating time was 185 minutes. The overall postoperative complication rate was 53%, comparable to the rates reported in previous studies. The only complications that were more frequent than previously reported were prolonged paralytic ileus (11%) and perineal wound dehiscence (28% of patients undergoing abdominoperineal resection). None of the patients died, and none developed urinary incontinence. The postoperative rate of sexual activity was 27% for women and 63% for men. Two men were rendered impotent; this complication was linked to

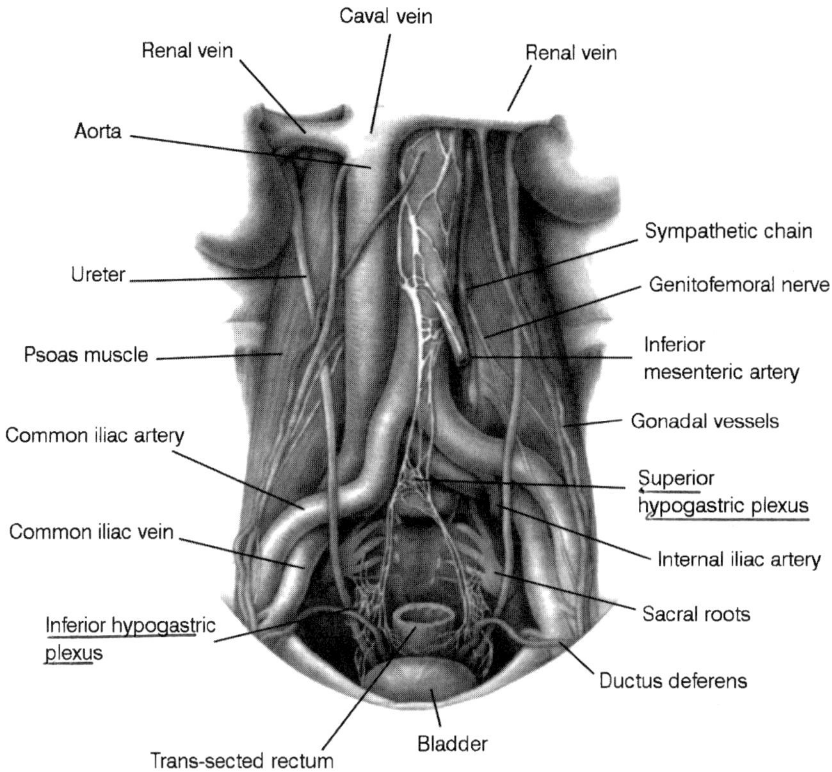

FIGURE 1.—The abdominal and pelvic autonomic nervous system. Reproduced with permission from Steup WH. Colorectal cancer surgery with emphasis on lymphadenectomy. *Thesis*, Leiden, The Netherlands, 1995. (Courtesy of Maas CP, Moriya Y, Steup WH, et al: Radical and nerve-preserving surgery for rectal cancer in the Netherlands: A prospective study on morbidity and functional outcome. *Br J Surg* 85:92-97, 1998, Blackwell Science Ltd.)

sacrifice of the IHP. Preservation of the SHP was essential to ejaculatory function.

Conclusions.—Promising results were observed with a radical, nerve-preserving technique of rectal cancer surgery. Morbidity is acceptable and functional outcomes are good. Nerve-preserving surgery should be considered as the new standard for treatment of primary rectal cancer. Sacrifice of the IHP and sacrifice of the SHP are specifically linked to impotence and ejaculatory dysfunction, respectively.

► This article reinforces the concept of nerve-sparing resection of the rectum as an anatomic dissection for rectal cancer. Clear anatomic dissection and knowledge of the anatomy are required to avoid postoperative sexual dysfunction. This article clearly defines the technique and the positions of the nerve plexes and suggests that identification of the superior hypogastric plexus and the inferior hypogastric plexus is of paramount importance when trying to avoid the outcome of impotence in males after a total mesorectal excision for rectal cancer. Figure 1 is an excellent drawing.

J.W. Fleshman, Jr., M.D.

Surgical Resection of Villous Adenomas of the Rectum

Winburn GB (Med College of Georgia Hosp and Clinics, Augusta)

Am Surg 64:1170-1173, 1998 5–81

Purpose.—Only about 5% of adenomas of the large intestine are villous adenomas. However, these lesions have a 40% incidence of malignancy and therefore require complete resection. Several techniques have been described for resection of villous adenomas of the rectum. The results of 2 sphincter-preserving approaches—low anterior resection and transanal excision—are reported.

Methods.—The retrospective study included 16 patients undergoing resection of villous adenomas of the rectum over 6 years. There were 10 women and 6 men (average age, 61 years) in the study. Fourteen patients underwent transanal excision, and 2 had low anterior resection. The surgical results, patient outcomes, and complications were analyzed.

Results.—The lesions' average size was 5 cm. They were located an average of 9 cm from the anal verge, with one half located within 8 cm of the anal verge. Lesion histology was tubulovillous in 75% of cases and pure villous in 25%. Adenocarcinoma was found in 37% of lesions. Within 6 months after surgery, 31% of patients required treatment for residual disease and 12% for recurrent disease. Urinary retention occurred in 12% of patients. There was also a 12% rate of serious complications: 1 case each of perforation and postoperative hemorrhage.

Conclusions.—The authors report good results with sphincter-preserving surgery for large villous adenomas of the rectum. Morbidity is low and the recurrence rate is acceptable. These patients need close follow-up because of their lifelong risk of recurrence.

▶ Although this is a very small series of patients with rectal villous adenoma, it serves to illustrate several points which should be made. Alternatives to transanal excision and low anterior resection are low anterior resection, mucosectomy, and coloanal anastomosis with J-pouch construction or transanal endoscopic microresection. It is essential to completely remove the lesion with cold dissection, because of cautery artifact, which may distort margins and thereby make it difficult to stage and recommend treatment for patients who have cancer present. This series has a very high incidence of cancer present in the lesions and, therefore, reinforces this concept. The majority of individuals treating superficial low rectal cancers would add adjuvant treatment to any lesion with a depth greater than T_1. This treatment could include chemotherapy and radiation in different combinations. Close follow-up is essential after excision. A word of warning is needed about the use of repeat laser or coagulation ablation of the tumor without complete reexcision. The risk is that deep cells of cancer may be left behind and covered by regrowth of normal epithelium, only to present later as a large, deep, extramural tumor.

J.W. Fleshman, Jr., M.D.

Rectal Cancer: The Basingstoke Experience of Total Mesorectal Excision, 1978-1997

Heald RJ, Moran BJ, Ryall RDH, et al (Univ of British Columbia, Vancouver, Canada; North Hampshire Hosp, Basingstoke, England; Wessex Radiotherapy Centre, Southampton, England)

Arch Surg 133:894-899, 1998 5–82

Introduction.—Standard abdominoperineal or anterior resection approaches to colorectal cancer have yielded disappointing results. At the authors' center, total mesorectal excision (TME) was developed in an attempt to reduce the local recurrence rate of rectal cancer. The good results achieved with TME highlight the importance of meticulous dissection in the management of colorectal cancer. The results of 519 consecutive patients undergoing TME for rectal cancer are reported.

Methods.—The patients were treated with curative or palliative intent over 19 years. Four hundred sixty-five patients underwent anterior resections with low stapled anastomoses, for a total of 407 mesorectal excisions. Thirty-seven patients had abdominoperineal excisions, 10 had Hartmann resections, 10 had local excisions, and 3 had laparotomy only. Forty-nine patients received preoperative radiotherapy. Patient characteristics and histopathologic diagnoses were prospectively recorded. The surgical technique emphasized meticulous development of an avascular plane between the mesorectum and surrounding parietal tissues, all the way to the distal pelvic extremities. The results were assessed in terms of local recurrence and cancer-specific survival.

Results.—Overall cancer-specific survival was 68% at 5 years and 66% at 10 years. Local recurrence rates were 6% and 8%, respectively. For the 405 patients undergoing curative resection, local recurrence rate was 3% at 5 years and 4% at 10 years. Disease-free survival for this group was 80% and 78%, respectively. The only significant histopathologic risk factors for recurrence were Dukes stage, extramural vascular invasion, and tumor differentiation.

Conclusions.—This extensive experience with TME for rectal cancer suggests that surgical excision can be curative for two thirds of patients across stages, and for four fifths of patients undergoing curative resection. Completeness of the mesorectal excision appears to be the major predictor of cure. The TME technique is being adopted throughout Europe; its slow adoption in North America appears to be a result of managed care. Total mesorectal excision should be regarded as the surgical technique of choice in future trials of adjuvant chemotherapy and radiotherapy for rectal cancer.

▶ This article reviews a 20-year experience with the anatomic dissection of total mesorectal excision for patients with rectal cancer. It is a personal series with excellent follow-up, but should not be misconstrued as a randomized prospective trial. As in the articles from Zaheer (Abstract 5–85) and Arenas (Abstract 5–84), the use of clear anatomic dissection yields a low local recurrence rate of less than 10% in patients with rectal cancer. Of note in this article is the change in local recurrence rate in the second decade, when preoperative radiation was introduced as adjuvant therapy for more advanced local disease. In fact, the local recurrence rate after a curative resection reduced to less than 0.5% in those individuals felt to have a curative low anterior resection.

The high rate of diverting stoma and the low rate of resection of the anal sphincters reflect the current trend in the management of rectal cancer across the world. I agree totally with the authors that managed health care has failed to recognize the major issue in the treatment of patients with rectal cancer. This issue is the importance of surgical training in the management of rectal cancer. However, I cannot agree completely with the comment that a multimodality therapy will not be necessary in patients with rectal cancer, since this is not a well-conducted, randomized trial, but rather a large prospective series comparing results to historical data.

It is also interesting that Professor Heald clearly indicates that he no longer advocates total mesorectal excision for patients with upper rectal tumors, but rather a clear dissection of the mesorectum to at least 5 cm below the tumor margin, such that the mesorectum is resected in an intact envelope. The leak rate in these circumstances, as a result, has decreased significantly over the last decade of his experience: the clinical leak rate to 6% and the overall leak rate to 11%.

J.W. Fleshman, Jr., M.D.

Feasibility Study for Use of Brush Cytology as a Complementary Method for Diagnosis of Rectal Cancer

Farouk R, Dodds J, MacDonald AW, et al (Univ of Hull, England; Castle Hill Hosp, Hull, England)

Dis Colon Rectum 40:609-613, 1997 5–83

Background.—Brush cytology is an alternative method for diagnosing colorectal cancer. The accuracy, reliability, and cost associated with brush cytology diagnosis of colorectal cancer were prospectively analyzed.

Study Design.—The study group consisted of 357 patients from 3 centers with a rectal lesion of more than 1 cm in diameter that had been identified by rigid proctoscopy between January 1990 and March 1996. All lesions were brushed and then submitted to biopsy. Results were compared with the final histologic diagnosis. The brushings from 92 patients were independently examined by 4 cytologists and a pathologist to determine interobserver variability.

Results.—Rectal adenocarcinoma was confirmed in 303 patients. Brush cytology accurately diagnosed 278. Biopsy accurately diagnosed 260. Brush cytology accurately identified 53 of 54 adenomas as benign, whereas biopsy accurately identified all 54 as benign. The sensitivity and specificity of brush cytology were 92%. Interobserver agreement was 84%. The cost of brush cytology was $17.00 per patient.

Conclusion.—Brush cytology can safely be used to accurately diagnose rectal cancer with low interobserver variation. The procedure was rapid and well tolerated by patients. Use of brush cytology could reduce the number of reexaminations required to identify malignancy, resulting in cost savings. This method is also a viable alternative when biopsy is contraindicated.

▶ Brush cytology may have a limited role as an adjunct to tissue biopsy in the diagnosis of rectal cancer. It may be appropriate for the small number of patients who are anticoagulated at the time of diagnostic endoscopy. This study fails to clearly show its value for the average patient, however. The authors classify a cytologic interpretation of "suspicious" as being positive, when, presumably, most of the lesions sampled were "suspicious" at endoscopy. Their data are thus biased toward improving the observed sensitivity of brush cytology.

T.E. Read, M.D.

▶ The major question, which is unanswered by this study, is whether a "suspicious" brush cytology is adequate to recommend external beam radiation or surgical treatment of a rectal lesion. In most circumstances, anticoagulation can be reversed or adjusted to obtain a biopsy adequate for a diagnosis.

J.W. Fleshman, Jr., M.D.

Total Mesenteric Excision in the Surgical Treatment of Rectal Cancer: A Prospective Study

Arenas RB, Fichera A, Mhoon D, et al (Univ of Chicago)
Arch Surg 133:608-612, 1998 5–84

Introduction.—A growing number of patients with rectal cancer are being treated with sphincter-sparing procedures with a lower risk of local recurrence; however, cancer-related mortality rates remain unchanged. Optimal surgery for rectal cancer may involve total mesorectal excision (TME) with low anterior or abdominoperineal resection; if the entire rectal mesentery is removed as an intact unit, it increases the chances of obtaining a negative surgical margin. This study evaluated the effectiveness of TME in providing locoregional control of rectal cancer.

Methods.—Seventy three consecutive patients whose rectal cancer was located within 10 cm of the anal verge were studied prospectively. The patients were treated over a 13-year period by a single surgeon. Seven patients underwent transanal cancer resection and 1 had a permanent diverting stoma as the only precedure. Of the remaining 65 patients, 26 underwent sphincter-ablating surgery and 39 had sphincter-sparing surgery; in both of these groups, TME was performed en bloc. Locoregional control was assessed, along with perioperative factors associated with the selection of sphincter-sparing vs. sphincter-ablating surgery. Long-term prognostic factors were identified as well.

Results.—One patient died of postoperative myocardial infarction; the other 64 patients were followed up for a mean of 39 months. The 5-year actuarial survival rate was 88% for patients with stage I or II disease and 65% for those with stage III disease. Six percent of the patients experienced local recurrence, but only 3% of those with potentially curable (stage I to III) disease. Among patients who did not receive adjuvant chemoradiation therapy, the local recurrence rate was 8% overall but 0% for those with potentially curable disease. Significant prognostic factors for survival included tumor stage and the presence of vascular or lymphatic invasion. Factors associated with selection of a sphincter-ablating procedure were the presence of circumferential lesions, gross invasion of contiguous organs, and tumor location less than 5 cm from the anal verge.

Conclusions.—For patients with rectal cancer, TME can reduce the risk of locoregional recurrence. As shown in previous studies, tumor stage and the presence of microinvasion are important prognostic factors. The study also identifies key factors associated with patient selection for sphincter-ablating surgery (i.e., circumferential lesions, distance from the anal verge, and gross invasion of contiguous organs).

▶ The controversy over total mesorectal excision stems from the fact that many colorectal surgeons and general surgeons who have been treating rectal cancer for many years have been doing anatomic dissections and consider total mesorectal excision a nonissue since the appropriate operation has been around for many years. The real advance is the use of an anatomic dissection to maintain the envelope of the mesorectum and the lymph node–bearing tissue within the pelvis as a single unit. This has the advantage of removing all of the lymph node material behind the rectum, which contains 90% of all metastases in most lesions and increases the likelihood that radial margins will be clear after removal of the rectum. The article by Arenas et al. looked at 65 patients prospectively from their database. They were able to show that local recurrence could be reduced to a very low level by means of complete anatomic dissection with either a wide pelvic lymphadenectomy or total mesorectal excision. This is certainly a laudable achievement. They were able to show once again that stage and lymph node metastases predict survival better than any other features.

Unfortunately, the authors have made a claim that total mesorectal excision may negate the need for adjuvant radiation therapy. As those commenting on the article astutely point out, the authors actually treated almost two thirds of their patients with adjuvant chemoradiation therapy and, therefore, really cannot make this statement. In fact, the local recurrence was double for those treated with surgery alone (8% vs. 4%). The selection criteria for those patients receiving adjuvant therapy and surgery alone were probably not the same. The authors also failed to mention the true incidence of local recurrence since they do not give us a number for the patients who suffered local and distant recurrence simultaneously.

In fact, at the end of the response to the commentary, the authors admit that they do not do a true total mesorectal excision for a midrectal cancer. They simply do an anatomic dissection and resect an envelope of the mesorectum well below the tumor level without skimping on their margins. This is rapidly becoming the recommendation for most individuals who deal with rectal cancer.

J.W. Fleshman, Jr., M.D.

Surgical Treatment of Adenocarcinoma of the Rectum

Zaheer S, Pemberton JH, Farouk R, et al (Mayo Clinic and Mayo Found, Rochester, Minn)

Ann Surg 227:800-811, 1998 5–85

Background.—The best operation and the best adjuvant treatment for patients with rectal cancer continue to be debated. Survival and recurrence rates in patients undergoing abdominoperineal resection (APR), coloanal anastomosis (CAA), and anterior resection (AR) without adjuvant therapy were reported.

Methods.—Five hundred fourteen patients undergoing only surgery were reviewed. One hundred sixty-nine had APR, 19 had CAA, 272 had AR, and 54 had other procedures. In 87%, surgery was done with curative intent. In APR and CAA, the envelope of rectal mesentery was excised posteriorly and the supporting tissues were removed laterally from the sacral promontory to the pelvic floor. In AR, an appropriately wide rectal mesentery resection technique was used if the tumor was high. If the tumor was in the middle or lower part of the rectum, all mesentery was resected. A mean distal margin of 3 cm was achieved in AR. Mean follow-up was 5.6 years. Follow-up data were complete for 92% of the patients.

Findings.—Twelve patients died, for a mortality rate of 2%. Five percent had anastomotic leaks after AR, and 15% had a transient urinary retention. Wound infection occurred in 11% of the patients. At 5 years, the rates of local recurrence and disease-free survival were 7% and 78%, respectively, after AR; 6% and 83% after CAA; and 4% and 80% after APR. The disease-free survival rate in patients with stage III disease was 60%.

Conclusions.—In patients with tumors low in the rectum, complete resection of the envelope of supporting tissues during APR, CAA, and AR is associated with low mortality, low morbidity, low local recurrence, and a good 5-year survival rates. Likewise, appropriate tumor-specific mesorectal excision during AR in patients with tumors high in the rectum is consistent with a low rate of local recurrence and good long-term survival. However, the overall failure rate among patients with stage III disease is 40%, independent of operative technique, indicating that surgery alone is not sufficient for improving long-term survival rates.

▶ The Mayo Clinic has the opportunity to review their large database to answer questions or at least stimulate thought on numerous issues. The Colorectal Group has evaluated the use of an anatomic dissection for rectal cancer without adjuvant therapy in 514 patients. Operations performed extended from AR for rectosigmoid tumors to low AR, CAA, and APR for lower lesions. They present an overall local recurrence rate of 7%, and there is no difference in recurrence rate by procedure. The local recurrence rate is influenced by stage, however. The Mayo Clinic group was able to establish a leak rate of 2.4% to 6.9%, depending on the distance of the anastomosis from the dentate line. The lower the anastomosis, the higher the leak rate. They have been able to show that tumor depth of T_3 or T_4 lesions was a predictor of local recurrence and survival, even in a multivariate analysis. In fact, 35% of the T_3 lesions recurred locally, and T_4 lesions were found to recur in 100% of the cases. The presence of three lymph node metastases increased the risk of local recurrence to 60%. These two features and the presence of distant metastases affected survival adversely. Unfortunately, radial margins were not assessed in this group.

Although the authors suggest that an anatomic dissection and good surgical technique reduce local recurrence and improve survival, they certainly cannot make a statement that adjuvant chemoradiation therapy should not be used in T_3 and T_4 lesions. In fact, the current Mayo policy is that all patients with rectal cancer with T_3 N_1 or greater stages should receive chemoradiation either preoperatively or postoperatively. Because they also found a distant failure rate of up to 30%, they continue to recommend chemotherapy in an adjuvant setting as well.

The most important finding in this article is that the anatomic dissection of the rectum with adequate distal mesorectal excision rather than a total mesorectal excision yields the same results as a total mesorectal excision. The anastomotic leak rates are much lower than the literature reports for total mesorectal excision (17%). This anatomic dissection is familiar to all colorectal surgeons and general surgeons who treat rectal cancer frequently and should be the standard of care. The question of chemotherapy and radiation in rectal cancer remains to be answered and should be addressed in a randomized, controlled trial.

J.W. Fleshman, Jr., M.D.

Improved Survival in Patients With Rectal Cancer: A Population-Based Register Study

Dahlberg M, Påhlman L, Bergström R, et al (Univ of Uppsala, Sweden)

Br J Surg 85:515-520, 1998 5–86

Background.—Combined preoperative radiotherapy and total mesorectal excision (TME) was used as the primary treatment of rectal cancer at only one center in Uppsala, Sweden, between 1985 and 1989. The impact of this approach on general outcomes was investigated.

Methods and Findings.—Data on 94,262 patients with colorectal cancer from the total population of Sweden between 1960 and 1989 were obtained for survival analysis. Relative survival rates in the first year of follow-up improved continuously in patients with cancer of the colon and rectum. Improvement also occurred in follow-up years 2 to 5, although it was much more marked between 1985 and 1989 for rectal cancer in Uppsala. This improvement was especially pronounced in follow-up years 3 to 5.

Conclusions.—The introduction of TME with preoperative radiotherapy in Uppsala appears to have improved survival rates in patients with rectal cancer beyond the first year. The current authors believe that it was the combination of interventions that led to this improvement.

► The Swedish have a unique registry in which all patients are entered and must be followed up routinely. Thus, all patients with rectal cancer diagnosed between 1960 and 1989 were studied. The group of authors used the overall Swedish registry and compared it with the registry from the University of Uppsala. Uppsala surgeons began using TME for rectal cancer in 1985. This afforded them the ability to compare a standard operation with an anatomic TME as taught them by R.J. Heald. Their findings suggest that TME reduced the relative risk of dying of cancer by half and increased the rate of survival after treatment for rectal cancer. However, the authors are unable to quantitate the effect that changing their operative technique has had on the outcome because they also added radiation therapy in Uppsala in 1985. The patients were not given adjuvant chemotherapy before 1989 because to that point there had been no studies that showed benefit. This use of a database and a national registry to provide evidence that a particular treatment method affects outcome is a unique approach. It is possible only in countries in which there is compulsory registry. It does show that improvements are possible in the treatment of rectal cancer and can be identified in a population-based study.

J.W. Fleshman, Jr., M.D.

Significance of Local Recurrence of Rectal Cancer as a Local or Disseminated Disease

Maetani S, Onodera H, Nishikawa T, et al (Kyoto Univ, Japan; Shiga Med Centre for Adult Diseases, Moriyama, Japan)

Br J Surg 85:521-525, 1998 5–87

Background.—Questions about the nature of local recurrence in patients with rectal cancer remain. It is unknown whether recurrence represents localized or disseminated disease, what proportion of patients are really cured by surgery, and which patients have prolonged survival with surgery.

Methods.—Fifty-nine patients with locally recurrent rectal cancer who were undergoing extended repeat resections were reviewed. Forty-three patients had sacrectomy and 39 had total pelvic exenteration. Before or at the time of surgery, 12 patients had distant metastases.

Findings.—The overall survival rate at 5 years was 25%. Forty-five patients, including 5 of those surviving for 5 years, had a second recurrence. Thirty-six patients with recurrences had locoregional manifestations and 29 had distant metastases. The most significant prognostic indicator was the postoperative carcinoembryonic antigen doubling time (CEADT), followed by the preoperative CEADT, carcinoembryonic antigen levels, and the occurrence of distant metastases. Late onset of the first recurrence was also a favorable factor. Thus, tumor growth rate had a greater effect on survival than the current extent of tumor progression. After surgery, the CEADT decreased in patients with a second recurrence.

Conclusions.—Locally recurrent rectal cancer is a manifestation of disseminated disease spreading locoregionally, often to distant organs. The probability of long-term cure is low. However, survival varies greatly, depending on tumor growth rate, which is influenced by surgery.

▶ The difficulty with operating on patients with locally advanced or locally recurrent rectal cancer remains the inability to predict those who will benefit from a large, highly morbid procedure. This review of 59 patients from Kyoto University offers some insight into this problem. The doubling time of CEA (CEADT) after the operation can be used as a predictor of tumor progression and is more likely related to biology of the tumor than to anything else. The 25% 5-year survival rate is actually better than that reported from other series. This gives some hope for the future. Even so, the preoperative selection of patients who are amenable to surgical treatment and who will have eventual good outcome is difficult. The use of PET scan to identify patients with localized disease may play a major role in this area. The presence of a rapidly rising CEADT may do more to indicate patients who are more suited to systemic therapy.

J.W. Fleshman, Jr., M.D.

Preoperative Hyperthermia Combined With Radiochemotherapy in Locally Advanced Rectal Cancer: A Phase II Clinical Trial

Rau B, Wust P, Hohenberger P, et al (Humboldt Univ, Berlin)
Ann Surg 227:380-389, 1998 5–88

Objective.—The prognosis is poor for patients with locally advanced rectal cancer. Intensified preoperative therapy in these cases might improve the outcome for these patients. The addition of hyperthermia to preoperative radiotherapy in combination with systemic chemotherapy for primary, locally advanced rectal cancer was evaluated for toxicity, response, surgical treatment, and morbidity in a phase II trial.

Methods.—Combined-modality therapy was administered to 37 patients with locally advanced rectal cancer. Regional hyperthermia was administered weekly with a SIGMA 60 ring applicator at 90 MHz for as long as 1 hour during the 5 weeks of preoperative radiotherapy (4,500 cGy) and chemotherapy (5-fluorouracil and leucovorin) followed by surgery after 4 to 6 weeks. Temperature distributions, depth of infiltration, nodal status, and tumor height above the anal verge were analyzed statistically to determine predictors of response.

Results.—Thirty patients completed the preoperative hyperthermia and radiochemotherapy. Adverse reactions included diarrhea, cramping, proctitis, and erythema and epitheliolysis of the rima ani. Fifteen patients (16%) had grade III toxicities. The primary tumor was resected in 32 of 36 patients (86.5%). One patient refused surgery. Margins were negative in 31 patients. Five patients (14%) had no evidence of residual tumor. Seventeen patients (46%) had a partial response. The overall survival rate was 56% at a median of 21 months. The actuarial survival rate was 86% at 38 months. There were no local recurrences, but distant metastases developed in 5 patients.

Conclusion.—Preoperative hyperthermia combined with radiotherapy in locally advanced rectal cancer is a safe and effective local control modality. A controlled phase III study is needed to demonstrate specific and significant benefits.

▶ Advanced and locally invasive rectal cancer remains a major problem, and resectability rates, while improved after radiochemotherapy, are not complete. The addition of hyperthermia to the regimen may facilitate the resectability and the local control of these lesions. Hyperthermia itself is relatively simple to deliver with radio waves. A core is placed around the patients, and antennas direct the radio waves to focus them and raise the temperature of the specific area of the body that needs to be treated. This, therefore, does not require intraluminal manipulation and can be readily applied to all types of patients.

This particular study is of preoperative hyperthermia in conjunction with radiochemotherapy in tumors that were staged by ultrasound as locally invasive and advanced. The complete response rate of 14% is somewhat higher than the 10% that has been shown in patients with radiation and chemotherapy. This modality deserves a trial, and apparently this is under way in Europe. In the United States, there are also centers that are interested in hyperthermia and will be looking at this. This may be the next step in increasing and improving survival in patients with rectal cancer.

J.W. Fleshman, Jr., M.D.

Preoperative Irradiation Affects Functional Results After Surgery for Rectal Cancer: Results From a Randomized Study

Dahlberg M, Glimelius B, Graf W, et al (Akademiska sjukhuset, Uppsala, Sweden)

Dis Colon Rectum 41:543-551, 1998 5–89

Background.—The Swedish Rectal Cancer Trial has shown that preoperative high-dose radiotherapy decreases local failure rates and improves overall survival in patients with rectal cancer. The effect of preoperative high-dose radiotherapy on long-term bowel function in patients treated with anterior resection was investigated in the current study.

Methods.—Two hundred twenty patients in the Swedish Rectal Cancer Trial who had survived for at least 5 years were asked to complete a questionnaire. After exclusions, 171 questionnaires were analyzed.

Findings.—Median bowel frequencies per week for patients undergoing irradiation and for those having surgery only were 20 and 10, respectively. Incontinence, urgency, and emptying problems were more common after irradiation, although sensory functions did not differ between groups. Thirty percent of the irradiated group and 10% of the surgery-alone group reported that bowel dysfunction impaired their social life.

Conclusions.—High-dose radiotherapy affects long-term bowel function in patients treated for rectal cancer. Predictive factors for local recurrence need to be identified to optimize the use of radiotherapy.

▶ The results of the randomized prospective trial of preoperative radiation for rectal cancer showed an improved survival and an improved controlled local recurrence for rectal cancer. This study focuses on the functional outcome after radiation therapy, using the randomized patients who are available for follow-up. The authors found a decrease in anal sphincter function and an impairment of social life because of incontinence, urgency, and emptying difficulties.

The authors admit in their response to the editorial commentary that the radiation therapy need not have affected the anal canal in a large number of their patients, because they arbitrarily treated the anal sphincter in all of the patients undergoing preop radiation. The authors now recommend sparing the anal sphincter in patients with rectal cancers 6 cm above the dentate line. The study does not address the biologic equivalency of the radiation therapy. Twenty-five hundred cGy delivered in 5 fractions of 500 cGy is a very aggressive dose and may also influence the functional outcome of the patients, since the anal sphincter is included. The American standard for preoperative radiation therapy is 4,500 to 5,000 rads, which is somewhat lower and has less effect. Before completely condemning the use of preoperative radiation, one must also compare the postoperative radiation therapy functional results to the preoperative radiation therapy results.

J.W. Fleshman, Jr., M.D.

Decision-making in Rectal Cancer Surgery: Survey of North American Colorectal Residency Programs

Hool GR, Church JM, Fazio VW (Cleveland Clinic Found, Ohio)

Dis Colon Rectum 41:147-152, 1998 5–90

Background.—Treatments for rectal cancer and outcomes vary greatly in the United States. The degree of variability in the investigation and management of patients with rectal cancer was studied.

Methods.—A questionnaire eliciting information about preoperative assessment, operative technique, and follow-up of primary rectal cancer was mailed to all colorectal surgeons associated with colorectal residency programs in North America. One hundred ten surveys were returned, a response rate of 71%.

Findings.—More than 75% of the respondents agreed about the routine preoperative use of endorectal US and carcinoembryonic antigen and the postoperative use of endorectal US. The respondents also generally agreed about the use of adjuvant therapy and radical resection for a poorly differentiated uT2,NO cancer, the use of total mesorectal excision for mid-rectal cancer, and the use of loop ileostomy if diversion is necessary. Two thirds of the survey respondents used adjuvant therapy and radical resection for a uT3,NO cancer and preferred a follow-up schedule of visits every 3 months for 2 years and visits every 6 months for the next 3 years. There was less agreement about the need for a preoperative liver scan, the approach to a moderately differentiated uT2,NO cancer, the use of rectal irrigation before resection, the timing of colonoscopy in a patient with stenosing rectal cancer, and the frequency of postoperative colonoscopies.

Conclusions.—Colorectal surgeon educators vary markedly in their management of low rectal cancer. Opinion is divided about which procedure is best for each histologic and pathologic stage. Careful analysis of outcomes is needed.

► A survey is a nonscientific method of defining surgical practice. However, in some ways it allows us to see state-of-the art practice. One would expect that surveying the surgeons involved in training programs for colorectal surgery fellows would identify current status and trends for the most up-to-date treatment of colorectal cancer. The authors identified areas of agreement, such as the use of preoperative endorectal ultrasound, ileostomy for diversion, and coloanal anastomosis for low, favorable cancers. One must remember, however, that there is still a large amount of controversy over each of these areas and, even more relevantly, there is lack of data to support some of the practices. This article may be used as a type of practice parameter for the treatment of rectal cancer, in that it identifies certain types of patients and gives consensus for treatment. However, until randomized, prospective trials have been completed, one cannot definitely say that these are standards of care.

J.W. Fleshman, Jr., M.D.

Patterns of Neoplastic Spread in Colorectal Cancer: Implications for Surveillance CT Studies

Giess CS, Schwartz LH, Bach AM, et al (Cornell Univ, New York)

AJR 170:987-991, 1998 5–91

Background.—Routine follow-up for colorectal cancer includes cross-sectional imaging for the presence of locoregional recurrence and distant metastases. Though the value of preoperative CT scanning in such cases is unclear, it is the most commonly used imaging modality in follow-up. The current study investigated patterns of metastatic disease on CT in patients with colorectal cancer and determined the diagnostic yield of routine pelvic CT in follow-up surveillance.

Methods and Findings.—The pathologic records and 3,073 CT studies of 1,119 patients with colorectal cancer were reviewed. Metastatic disease was observed in 34% of all CT studies. Thirty-three percent of these metastases were in the abdomen, and 7% were in the pelvis. Six percent of the studies showed metastases in both the abdomen and the pelvis. Forty-one percent of the patients with abdominal primary colonic tumors had metastatic disease: 40% in the abdomen and 8% in the pelvis. Isolated pelvic metastases were seen in 4 studies from 4 different patients with abdominal primary colon tumors; 3 of these patients had primary tumors of the cecum. Thirty-one percent of the studies demonstrating pelvic primary colonic tumors also showed metastatic disease, 29% in the abdomen and 7% in the pelvis. Isolated pelvic metastases were seen on 29 studies in 26 patients with pelvic primary colonic tumors.

Conclusions.—Pelvic metastases are uncommon and isolated pelvic metastases rare in patients with colorectal tumors arising in the abdomen. The diagnostic yield of routine pelvic CT in the follow-up of such patients is low.

▶ Surveillance and preoperative CT scanning in the management of patients with colorectal cancer is very expensive. The authors have looked at a very large number of patients undergoing CT scans at Memorial Sloan-Kettering. Their finding that colonic primary tumors rarely metastasize to the pelvis is important when we consider the need for including the pelvic CT as an additional study. Only colonic cancers that arise within the pelvis, such as the cecum or the sigmoid colon, develop pelvic disease; and this knowledge should be able to guide the use of pelvic scanning in the preoperative and follow-up evaluation of patients with colorectal cancer. One might question whether abdominal or pelvic CT scanning is necessary in patients with colonic primaries if the patients are undergoing abdominal exploration. Also, routine CT scanning in the follow-up of patients with colorectal cancer is not recommended unless there are symptoms guiding the imaging.

J.W. Fleshman, Jr., M.D.

Anal Cancer

Treatment of Anal Canal Carcinoma With High Dose Radiation Therapy and Concomitant Fluorouracil-Cisplatinum: Long-term Results in 95 Patients

Gerard J-P, Ayzac L, Hun D, et al (Centre Hospitalier Lyon-Sud, France)

Radiother Oncol 46:249-256, 1998 5–92

Background.—Since 1982, the authors' center has used a combination of 5-fluorouracil and cisplatinum (FU-CCDP) for the treatment of anal canal carcinoma (ACC). The long-term results of this combined concomitant radiochemotherapy are presented.

Methods.—The experience included 95 patients (87 women), median age, 63 years. Patients with carcinomas of the anal margin were excluded. Most patients had advanced squamous ACC. They received high-dose external beam radiotherapy, with a total dose of 30 Gy to the perineal field and 18 Gy to the sacral field, with no elective irradiation to the iliac or inguinal nodes. Ten patients with synchronous inguinal nodes underwent irradiation of the involved area 4 weeks after inguinal dissection. Interstitial brachytherapy with a 192-iridium implant was performed a median of 8 weeks after the end of perineal field irradiation, to a median dose of 19.1 Gy. Chemotherapy—consisting of 5-FU, 1 g/m^2/day in a 96-hour continuous infusion on days 1 to 4, and CCDP, 25 mg/m^2 by bolus on days 1 to 4—was given during external bean radiotherapy. The patients were studied for a median of 64 months.

Results.—The complete response rate was 47%, and the locoregional control rate 89%. Three patients with progressive lesions underwent abdominoperineal resection. Fourteen patients had local recurrences. Salvage abdominoperineal resection achieved local control in 6 of these patients, 2 of whom went on to have distant metastases develop. For patients achieving complete response, 5-year overall survival was 92%, disease-specific survival 94%, and colostomy-free survival 86%. Colostomy-free survival was better for patients with primary tumors no larger than 50 mm (83% vs. 60%). However, tumor response was the only significant factor on multivariate analysis; lymph node status had no influence.

Conclusions.—These and previous studies suggest that combined concomitant radiochemotherapy should be the standard treatment of ACC. The authors' approach, using 5-FU-CDDP and high-dose, small-volume irradiation, achieves an overall 5-year survival of 84% and specific survival of 90%. Anal preservation is possible in 82% of patients. The results demonstrate the possibility of long-term survival in patients with stage N2 disease. The authors have replaced the radiation technique of Papillon with a 3- or 4-field technique including the anus and perirectal area.

▶ The group in Lyon, France have completed a long-term follow-up in a very large group of patients with anal canal cancer who were treated with a combined modality therapy using 5 FU and cisplatinum, with high-dose radiation therapy delivered locally and external beam radiation to the pelvis. The Papillon boost technique is able to be replaced, however, with a 3- or a 4-field technique that encompasses the anus and the perirectal area to deliver the high-dose boost to the anal canal. The results of the long-term follow-up in a group of patients with clearly advanced disease (63% of the patients had tumors larger than 4 cm) is excellent. Five-year overall and cancer specific survival were 84% and 90%. The major prognostic factor in this group of patients was the response to chemoradiation. The authors do not include the inguinal lymph node or the iliac node fields. A group of patients had recurrence in these areas. This may be an alternate treatment method for future trials. As seen in the past, salvage abdominal perineal resection has a less than stellar performance, but local regional control was able to be achieved in 93% of patients, using both chemoradiation and boost salvage therapy with combined modality therapy and abdominoperineal resection. Some of these patients developed distant metastases and died of their disease, however.

Clearly, combined modality of chemoradiation therapy for anal canal cancer is state of the art and should be considered in all patients, even those with large tumors. According to this study, N_2 disease does not preclude survival. Abdominoperineal resection and radiation therapy alone should no longer be considered in the treatment of anal canal cancer.

J.W. Fleshman, Jr., M.D.

Diverticular Disease

Primary Anastomosis in the Treatment of Acute Disease of the Unprepared Left Colon

Trillo C, Paris MF, Brennan JT (Hilton Head Clinics, Hilton Head Island, SC)
Am Surg 64:821-825, 1998 5–93

Objective.—The experience of one clinic with primary anastomosis of the unprepared left colon in urgent and emergent situations is described.

Methods.—Between June 1990 and December 1996, 58 patients underwent urgent exploration of the unprepared left colon; 43 (20 women), aged 28 to 88, of these (group I) had primary stapled anastomosis without protective colostomy. Unprotected primary anastomosis was thought to be unsafe in the other 15 patients (group II) (8 women), aged 38 to 86 years, because 3 were taking high-dose steroids, 3 had preoperative or intraoperative shock, 4 had gross fecal contamination of the peritoneal cavity, 4 had large pelvic abscesses, and 1 had ischemic colitis. Of the 15 patients in group II, 14 had resection with end colostomy, and 1 had primary anastomosis with a protective transverse colostomy.

NO POSTAGE NECESSARY IF MAILED IN THE UNITED STATES

BUSINESS REPLY MAIL
FIRST-CLASS MAIL PERMIT NO 135 ST LOUIS MO

POSTAGE WILL BE PAID BY ADDRESSEE

SUBSCRIPTION SERVICES
MOSBY, INC.
11830 WESTLINE INDUSTRIAL DRIVE
ST. LOUIS MO 63146-9988

NO POSTAGE NECESSARY IF MAILED IN THE UNITED STATES

BUSINESS REPLY MAIL
FIRST-CLASS MAIL PERMIT NO 135 ST LOUIS MO

POSTAGE WILL BE PAID BY ADDRESSEE

SUBSCRIPTION SERVICES
MOSBY, INC.
11830 WESTLINE INDUSTRIAL DRIVE
ST. LOUIS MO 63146-9988

Want to speed up the process?

To order a *Year Book* or *Advances*, you also may call 1-800-426-4545

To subscribe to a journal today, call toll-free in the U.S.:
1-800-453-4351
or fax 314-432-1158
Outside the U.S., call: 314-453-4351

Visit us at: *www.mosby.com/periodicals*

Mosby, Inc.
Subscription Services
11830 Westline Industrial Drive
St. Louis, MO 63146 U.S.A.

Mosby

Results.—In group I, 27 patients had peritonitis, which was caused by sigmoid diverticular disease in 26. Six patients had intestinal obstruction as a result of diverticular disease, 9 patients had an obstruction caused by colon cancer, and 1 had an obstruction from sigmoid volvulus. In group II, 13 patients had peritonitis, 10 had diverticular perforation with pelvic abscess (n = 4) or diffuse peritonitis (n = 6), 1 had perforated Crohn's colitis, 1 had perforated sigmoid colon carcinoma, and 1 had perforation secondary to ischemic colitis. Two patients had diverticular disease with pelvic abscesses and small bowel obstruction. In group I complications included atelectasis (n = 9), wound infection (n = 2) prolonged ileus (n = 2), pelvic abscess (n = 1), and anastomotic dehiscence in a patient with non-insulin-dependent diabetes (n = 1). There were no deaths. Operative time averaged 85 minutes for group I and 92 minutes for group II patients. Hospital stays averaged 9.7 days for group I patients and 12.8 days for group II patients.

Conclusion.—Intraluminal fecal matter does not present a major healing problem after primary anastomosis in the unprepared left colon.

▶ The idea of performing a colonic anastomosis in unprepared bowel is foreign to most surgeons. This article demonstrates the change that is being felt within the surgical community regarding the need for bowel preparation and the need for protecting stomas in patients with acute disease of the colon requiring resection. The use of bowel preparation in elective situations, however, should not be abandoned because the anastomotic leak rate can actually be reduced below 2%. Because this is the most morbid complication requiring reoperation and may actually result in permanent colostomy, the complication should be completely avoided, if at all possible. The authors also remind us that there are certain systemic diseases, such as diabetes, renal failure, and steroid-requiring conditions, that mandate a stoma for anastomotic protection if an elective operation is not possible.

J.W. Fleshman, Jr., M.D.

Hartmann's Pouch: Radiographic Evaluation of Postoperative Findings

Cherukuri R, Levine MS, Maki DD, et al (Hosp of the Univ of Pennsylvania, Philadelpiha)

AJR 171:1577-1582, 1998 5–94

Objective.—Leakage or blowout of Hartmann's pouch can create a life-threatening situation. The usefulness of contrast-enhanced radiography of the pouch for evaluating postoperative abnormalities was retrospectively assessed.

Methods.—Contrast-enhanced radiography (single-contrast barium studies in 64, water-soluble contrast medium in 17, and both in 3) was performed on 84 patients (26 females), aged 15 to 85 years, between 1990 and 1997. Time from the creation of the pouch to the takedown of the colostomy averaged 8 months. The time between creation of the pouch and contrast-enhanced radiography averaged 10 months.

Results.—Contrast-enhanced radiography detected abnormalities in 16 patients (19%). In 70 patients who had routine contrast-enhanced radiography before takedown, 3 had diversion colitis, 2 had leaks, 2 had adhesions, 2 had recurrent carcinoma, 1 had ulcerative colitis of the pouch, and 1 had stricture. Of the remaining 14 patients who underwent contrast-enhanced radiography because of suspected abnormalities, 2 had leaks, 2 had fistulas, and 1 had recurrent carcinoma.

Conclusion.—Contrast-enhanced radiography revealed postoperative abnormalities in 19% of the patients, including 2 who had silent leaks. To avoid extravasation of barium into the peritoneal spaces, it is advisable to perform these studies with the use of a water-soluble contrast medium.

► The majority of patients undergoing Hartmann resection of the rectosigmoid do so because of diverticular disease. The possibility of closing a colostomy is very high (close to 75%) in these patients. Before closure of the colostomy, a water soluble contrast injection of the rectal pouch is usually performed. This study has shown that 20% of the patients will have an abnormality and that a large percentage of those are asymptomatic. This study also reveals the findings in diversion colitis and perforation of the rectal stump into the sacrum. Hypaque enema of the rectal pouch is usually a good idea in these patients before the colostomy takedown is planned.

J.W. Fleshman, Jr., M.D.

Natural History of Diverticular Disease: When to Operate?

Mäkelä J, Vuolio S, Kiviniemi H, et al (Oulu Univ Hosp, Finland)

Dis Colon Rectum 41:1523-1528, 1998 5–95

Background.—Diverticulosis of the colon is not uncommon among elderly patients, but it can occur among younger patients as well. A large series of patients with diverticulosis of the colon was reviewed to determine optimal treatment for patients of different ages.

Methods.—The study group consisted of 366 patients, aged 29 to 93 years, admitted to the Oulu University Hospital for acute diverticular disease from 1981 to 1990. Patient records were reviewed and data on characteristics, operative procedures, morbidity and mortality, and complications were obtained. Of the 366 patients, 247 were first admissions. There were 74 patients less than 50 years of age. Patients were followed for an average of 10 years.

Results.—There were significantly more men than women among those less than 50 years of age. Young male patients had surgical treatment during the first treatment period more often than did other patients. Recurrences of diverticular disease developed in 22% of those in the study group and were significantly more common among younger patients.

Younger male patients (under 50 years) had significantly more complications.

Conclusion.—Younger male patients with diverticular disease undergo more primary operations, have more recurrences, and are more prone to complications than older patients. Guidelines for the management of diverticular disease state that all patients should be considered for surgical management after 2 attacks of diverticulitis to reduce the risk of the development of complications.

▶ This is a longitudinal study of patients from Finland with diverticular disease. The article is very interesting in that it gives longer than 5-year follow-up on patients who were admitted to the hospital with diverticulitis. The most interesting group is the patients with mild disease who were not operated on after the first admission. The complication and recurrence rate in this group is moderate. The article seems to justify early operation in the group of patients with more severe disease. Following these patients for 5 years reveals that complications occurred in the younger age group more frequently than in the older age group and, thus, possibly even indicates that patients in the younger age group should be operated on after the first episode. Further studies will need to be done to delineate the role of early operation in young patients with diverticulitis.

The use of the Hartmann procedure for diverticulitis is becoming less necessary as primary resection with anastomosis becomes more feasible with low morbidity and low mortality. Only in the elderly, debilitated, medically unstable patient with the most severe disease is a Hartmann operation with colostomy indicated. The closure rate of the colostomy decreases as the patient ages, and, thus, every effort should be made to perform a primary anastomosis if at all possible.

J.W. Fleshman, Jr., M.D.

The Utility of the Hartmann Procedure

Desai DC, Brennan EJ Jr, Reilly JF, et al (Lankenau Hosp, Wynnewood, Pa)

Am J Surg 175:152-154, 1998 5–96

Introduction.—The Hartmann procedure was originally proposed as a less-extensive alternative to abdominoperineal resection for high-risk patients with rectosigmoid cancer. It has come to be applied to a number of different indications, including complicated diverticulitis, ischemic bowel, volvulus, iatrogenic perforations, colitis, and anastomotic dehiscence. A 15-year experience with the Hartmann procedure for various indications is reviewed, focusing on morbidity and mortality and the second stage of the procedure.

Patients.—The authors' hospital performed a total of 185 Hartmann procedures from 1981 to 1995. The patients' average age was 66 years. One hundred eight patients had complicated diverticulitis, e.g., perforation, obstruction, and abscesses; 31 patients had rectosigmoid cancer; and 46 patients had other indications.

Outcomes.—In-hospital mortality was 15%, with most of the deaths resulting from perforated diverticulitis, perforated cancer, or ischemic bowel and subsequent sepsis. The most frequent complications in survivors were pulmonary (8%), wound infection (7%), and ileus (6%). Fifty-seven percent of the surviving patients eventually proceeded to the second stage of the Hartmann procedure to restore bowel continuity. The reanastomosis was performed an average of 149 days after the initial resection. Complications were less frequent after second-stage surgery, the most frequent being wound infection and incisional hernia (4% each). There were no deaths related to second-stage surgery. Bowel continuity was restored in 70% of patients operated on for complicated diverticulitis vs. 13% of those operated on for cancer.

Conclusions.—This large experience with the Hartmann procedure demonstrates low morbidity, and lower mortality than previously reported. For properly selected patients, second-stage surgery to restore bowel continuity can be carried out with low morbidity and no mortality. The Hartmann procedure provides a safe and effective operative approach for patients with complex disease states of the rectosigmoid area, and removes a dangerous source of sepsis in debilitated patients.

► This article reminds us that there are several options for treatment of acute emergencies within the abdominal cavity. The authors provide an updated review of their experience with the Hartmann procedure and reveal some interesting changes in outcome. Even though the mortality rate for a Hartmann operation is 14.6%, the mortality for the Hartmann closure is 0, suggesting that this is a safe procedure. As reported in past publications, the colostomy closure rate is only 57% for the entire group, but is fairly high (70%) for the diverticulitis group. The reversal rate is very low for patients with cancer, probably because of age, advanced state disease of disease initially, and inability to reverse a very low stump.

Much has been written about the possibility for intraoperative lavage, 1-stage operations, etc. However, the Hartmann procedure is still a viable alternative once the disease has been resected to allow the patient to recover from massive sepsis and peritonitis. The reason that closure can be done safely in the majority of patients is probably improved postanesthesia care and the use of antibiotics. I must agree with the authors that there are certainly patients who are much better served by the continued presence of an end colostomy than by conversion to a perineal colostomy. All efforts should be made to document anal sphincter function prior to closure of the Hartmann stump in elderly patients.

J.W. Fleshman, Jr., M.D.

Constipation and Incontinence

Should Patients With Combined Colonic Inertia and Nonrelaxing Pelvic Floor Undergo Subtotal Colectomy?

Bernini A, Madoff RD, Lowry AC, et al (Univ of Minnesota, Minneapolis)
Dis Colon Rectum 41:1363-1366, 1998 5–97

Objective.—The optimum treatment for chronic constipation is controversial. For patients with colonic inertia and nonrelaxation of the pelvic floor, neither biofeedback nor colectomy alone has proven successful. The outcome of preoperative biofeedback and subtotal colectomy was evaluated in patients with combined slow transit constipation and functional outlet obstruction.

Methods.—A questionnaire was given to 134 patients (5 men), with chronic constipation, who underwent subtotal colectomy between 1982 and 1995. Sixteen female patients with combined colonic inertia and nonrelaxation of the pelvic floor (NRPF) also underwent electromyographic relaxation of pelvic floor muscles. The questionnaire requested postoperative information about bowel function, symptoms of abdominal pain and bloating, and degree of satisfaction after surgery.

Results.—There were 106 responders (2 men), aged 23 to 68 years. Responders had been followed up for an average of 78 months. After treatment, 4% of the patients with a normal pelvic floor (NPF) and 38% of patients with NRPF had difficult evacuations, 21% and 12% were incontinent, 44% and 37% had abdominal pain, 45% and 43% had bloating, 14% and 18% had diarrhea, 33% and 31% were free of symptoms, and 78% and 56% were satisfied or highly satisfied with the results and would have the surgery again. The daily stool frequency was 2.8 for NPF patients and 2.1 for NRPF patients.

Conclusion.—Whereas subtotal colectomy provides symptomatic relief for patients with chronic severe constipation, many experience difficult evacuation or incontinence. Almost half of the patients with NRPF were dissatisfied with the results of their treatment.

▶ Operation for colonic inertia is an excellent alternative in patients with pure colonic inertia. This article confirms the findings of other authors that nonrelaxing puborectalis or pelvic floor outlet obstruction is a contraindication to subtotal colectomy in patients with colonic inertia unless the nonrelaxing puborectalis muscle and outlet obstruction can be treated preoperatively. The resolution of the outlet obstruction should make possible an excellent outcome from a subtotal colectomy, thereby resolving the problem. Patients with colonic inertia and nonrelaxing puborectalis muscle make up approximately 10% of the constipation population. The treatment consists of simple biofeedback with electromyography and balloon expulsion.

J.W. Fleshman, Jr., M.D.

Effects of Regular Exercise in Management of Chronic Idiopathic Constipation

Meshkinpour H, Selod S, Movahedi H, et al (Univ of California, Irvine)
Dig Dis Sci 43:2379-2383, 1998 5–98

Objective.—Whereas regular exercise is thought to benefit patients with chronic idiopathic constipation by shortening transit time through the gastrointestinal tract, there have been no controlled studies to test its effectiveness. The influence of regular physical exercise in the management of chronic idiopathic constipation was assessed.

Methods.—Eight patients (1 man), aged 31 to 65 years, with chronic idiopathic constipation participated in 4 weeks of exercise after a 2-week rest period during which they monitored their physical activity level. Patients took an exercise test before and after the study to determine their rate of perceived exertion (RPE). A constipation index that included frequency and consistency of bowel movements and the severity of straining on defecation was prepared.

Results.—There was a significant difference between the mean weekly distance walked during the rest period and during the study period (1.9 vs. 3.2 miles). Whereas the mean maximum time before and after exercise differed significantly (14.3 vs. 15.53 minutes), the mean RPE and the constipation index did not change significantly. There was no correlation between constipation index and physical activity scores.

Conclusion.—The use of physical activity to manage chronic idiopathic constipation is problematic.

► Activity has long been recommended as a potential conservative means for correction of chronic constipation. This is the first study looking at moderate low-impact exercise on constipation. The finding that exercise at a walking level of approximately 3 miles per day does not improve chronic constipation is a surprise in my opinion. Unfortunately, the study does not control for fluid intake, dietary fiber, or eating habits related to the exercise. It is still possible that more aggressive exercise may improve colonic transit in these patients and improve constipation.

J.W. Fleshman, Jr., M.D.

Physiological Modulation of Jejunal Sensitivity in Health and in Irritable Bowel Syndrome

Evans PR, Kellow JE (Univ of Sydney, Australia)
Am J Gastroenterol 93:2191-2196, 1998 5–99

Objective.—Patients with irritable bowel syndrome (IBS) demonstrate enhanced jejunal sensitivity. The effects on intensity of jejunal perception and compliance of feeding, nonperceived distension of the rectum simulating the presence of stool, and a combination of both were evaluated in patients with IBS and in normal controls.

Methods.—Eleven women, average age 49 years, with IBS (5 with diarrhea [IBS-D] and 6 with constipation [IBS-C]) and 7 healthy women participated in the study. Jejunal distension was produced by inflation of a high-compliance latex balloon during fasting, 30 minutes after a 400-kcal meal, and during simultaneous nonperceived rectal stimulation.

Results.—Compared with the control group, jejunal sensitivity after feeding was significantly higher in the IBS-C group but not in the IBS-D group. Jejunal sensitivity was significantly reduced during rectal stimulation in all patients with IBS but not in controls. Jejunal sensitivity was unchanged during simultaneous feeding and rectal stimulation for all patients with IBS and for controls. Jejunal compliance was similar for all patients with IBS and for controls.

Conclusion.—Stimuli applied in different parts of the gut can alter jejunal sensitivity. Differences in responses to these stimuli by patients with IBS strengthen the hypothesis that afferent nerve misinformation or mistransmission is responsible for IBS.

► IBS remains an enigma to physicians. The etiology and true source of the IBS is still unknown. The article from Sydney attempts to identify aberrant responses to different stimuli within the jejunum and other portions of the bowel as the source of IBS. This would then lead to the theory that afferent nerve misinformation or mistransmission is the probable source. There is a large expenditure of resources for patients with IBS, and work is needed to fully define and potentially categorize patients with IBS to allow better management.

J.W. Fleshman, Jr., M.D.

Segmental Colectomy in the Management of Colonic Inertia

You Y-T, Wang J-Y, Changchien C-R, et al (Chang Gung Mem Hosp, Taipei, Taiwan, China)

Am Surg 64:775-777, 1998 5–100

Objective.—Whereas subtotal colectomy and ileorectal anastomosis can relieve symptoms of idiopathic severe chronic constipation, one third of the patients experience intractable diarrhea. This condition can be prevented by resection of the precise colon inertia segment. Patients were assessed preoperatively to determine the best type of colectomy for managing constipation of the colon inertia type.

Methods.—Forty patients (8 men), aged 20 to 70 years (two thirds between 20 and 40), with chronic constipation, underwent a series of colon motility tests and anorectal function examinations to determine right-sided and left-sided transit time. If right colon transit time was prolonged, a right hemicolectomy with ileotransversostomy was performed. If left transit time was prolonged, a left hemicolectomy with transversosigmoidostomy was performed. If both transit times were prolonged, a subtotal colectomy with ileosigmoidostomy was performed.

Patients were followed up at 1 week and every 3 months for at least 2 years.

Results.—Four patients had prolonged right colon transit time, 24 had prolonged left colon transit times, and 12 had both. There were no deaths. One patient had a wound infection, and 2 had intestinal obstructions 1 week after surgery. At 3 months, 28 patients (70%) had firm stools, and 12 (30%) had soft stools. All patients had transit times of 24 hours or less. No patient had diarrhea. Symptoms of constipation disappeared in all patients a week after surgery.

Conclusion.—Segmental colectomy of the exact segment of colon demonstrating inertia significantly improved the ease and frequency of bowel movements without causing diarrhea.

▶ Although this article resurrects the issue of segmental colectomy for constipation, one must remember that selection of these patients is very difficult. In fact, in three of the patients who had segmental resection, total colonic inertia was probably misdiagnosed as segmental inertia. The issue of intractable diarrhea after subtotal colectomy has been long argued as a contraindication to a total abdominal colectomy for constipation, especially in elderly patients. This argument does not hold much credence when you see that the majority of patients are between 20 and 40 years old. Perhaps segmental resection should be reserved for patients who have presumed segmental delay in whom diarrhea may be a problem. Other groups have recently confirmed the need for subtotal colectomy in cases of colonic inertia, especially after the diagnosis and treatment of nonrelaxing puborectalis muscle. As surgeons, we must be careful to select the procedure for the patient based on particular indications with available testing. This is an excellent example of such a need for expertise in the diagnosis and management of a benign disease that is sometimes underrated in its complexity.

J.W. Fleshman, Jr., M.D.

Long-term Clinical Outcome of Surgery for Solitary Rectal Ulcer Syndrome

Sitzler PJ, Kamm MA, Nicholls RJ, et al (St Mark's Hosp, Harrow, England; Royal Infirmary, Glasgow, Scotland)

Br J Surg 85:1246-1250, 1998 5–101

Objective.—Solitary rectal ulcer syndrome is a condition that is difficult to treat. Whereas surgery is required for patients with severe symptoms, little is known about the reoperation rate or the overall failure rate. The effectiveness of procedures used and the ultimate failure rate judged by stoma formation were retrospectively reviewed.

Methods.—Between 1984 and 1993, 81 patients were operated on for solitary rectal ulcer. Two died, 2 were lost to follow-up, and 11 were followed up for less than 12 months. The remaining 66 patients (13 males), aged 15 to 77 years, underwent rectopexy (n = 49), Delorme's operation (n = 9), anterior resection (n = 2), or creation of a stoma (n = 4). Success was defined as complete or substantial abatement of symptoms. Failure was defined as worsening of symptoms or no change.

Results.—Rectopexy failed in 22 patients, 19 of whom had additional surgery. In 4 patients rectal resection with coloanal anastomosis was performed; 3 of these failed. In 11 patients colostomies were perforned. Rectopexy resulted in relief or substantial symptomatic improvement in 29 patients and failure in 20. Fourteen patients ultimately required a stoma. Delorme's operation failed in 4 patients, 3 of whom underwent further surgery. One patient underwent a rectopexy and 1 had a coloanal anastomosis, both of which failed. One patient had an ileostomy. Two ultimately required a stoma, and 5 had a successful outcome. Anterior resection was successful in both patients and was used after unsuccessful rectopexy in 4 patients and after an unsuccessful Delorme's operation in 1. Stomas were created in 4 patients, and stoma creation was used as secondary procedure in 16, for an overall rate of 30%.

Conclusion.—Rectopexy was successful in about 55% of the patients with solitary rectal ulcer. Preoperative incontinence or inability to defecate completely predicted a poor outcome. Anterior resection had a high failure rate.

▶ Solitary rectal ulcer syndrome has been a dilemma in the past. This large series of patients from St. Mark's Hospital in England has long-term follow-up and statistical analysis to make it a worthwhile study. The interesting finding that incontinence before surgery for the solitary rectal ulcer predicts poor outcome after an operation is also contradictory to findings from previous series. In the past, incontinence has been the best indication for operation in cases of solitary rectal ulcer. This series does not define whether the incontinence is due to the condition or whether this is an associated condition. In fact, it does not give any pathophysiologic data to suggest whether there is a primary sphincter mechanism responsible for the incontinence.

The finding that inadequate defecation on proctography indicates a poor prognosis is very important. The lack of prolapse is very important also. This indicates that the solitary rectal ulcer may be somewhat different etiologically in these patients who have no prolapse. Patient selection is very important and is needed to identify the group of individuals who will respond. Although solitary rectal ulcer remains a rare indication for surgery and presents a difficult diagnostic dilemma in some instances, a number of patients will continue to come to surgery for treatment of this problem. It is helpful to know that defecography and preoperative symptomats may aid in the identification of patients who will respond.

The authors suggest that low anterior resection and coloanal anastomosis is not a good operation for this condition. However, their experience is based on only those patients in whom other attempts at operative management failed. A prospective trial of low anterior resection and coloanal anastomosis should be tried before clear statements may be made along these lines.

J.W. Fleshman, Jr., M.D.

Accuracy and Reliability of Transanal Ultrasound for Anterior Anal Sphincter Injury

Sentovich SM, Wong WD, Blatchford GJ (Beth Israel Deaconess Med Ctr, Boston; Univ of Minnesota, Minneapolis; Creighton Univ, Omaha, Neb)

Dis Colon Rectum 41:1000-1004, 1998 5–102

Objective.—Transanal ultrasound (TAUS) has quickly become the gold standard for evaluation of the anal sphincter muscles, but some aspects of the technique had yet to be evaluated. A study was undertaken to determine the accuracy and reliability of TAUS for identification of anterior (obstetric-related) anal sphincter muscle injury.

Methods.—TAUS was performed by means of a 7-MHz transducer with a plastic anal cap and type 1850 anal probe in 20 symptom-free, parous women; 20 symptom-free nulliparous women (controls); and 22 incontinent women with probable anal sphincter injury. Images were obtained at 0.5-cm intervals from the anal verge to the anal canal and were interpreted by 2 colorectal surgeons. Interobserver reliability was assessed with use of the kappa coefficient.

Results.—Sphincter injury was identified individually by the 2 surgeons from static images in 55% and 75% of the nulliparous women (25% to 45% accuracy), 70% and 80% of the parous women, and 100 and 100 of the incontinent women (100% accuracy). With use of the video recording of the TAUS, sphincter injury was identified by the 2 surgeons in 40% and 60% of the nulliparous women (40% to 60% accuracy), 65% and 80% of the parous women, and 100% and 91% of incontinent women (100% accuracy). With the hard copy limited to the distal 1.5 cm of the anal canal, sphincter injury was identified in 5% and 25% of the nulliparous women (85% accuracy), 20% and 30% of the parous women, and 100 and 100 of the incontinent women (100% accuracy). Intact anal sphincters in the nulliparous women were more easily identified than intact external sphincters. Interobserver reliability was 68% ($\kappa=0.26$). Interobserver reliability was 78% in the distal anal canal and 48% in the proximal anal canal. Overall agreement was 81%, but it was higher for the internal sphincter (74%) than for the external anal sphincter (61%).

Conclusion.—TAUS can accurately identify anterior anal sphincter injury, but it has a false positive rate that varies between 5% and 25% for normal sphincters. Overall interobserver reliability was only 68% but improved to 78% when interpretation was limited to the distal 1.5 cm of the anal canal.

▶ The upper portion of the anal sphincter mechanism is composed of the puborectalis, a posteriorly based, U-shaped skeletal muscle that is open in the anterior quadrants. The puborectalis continues down to the external sphincter, which is a circular skeletal muscle in the lower anal canal. The internal sphincter is a circular smooth muscle and is a continuation of the rectal musculature. It is readily identifiable with endoanal ultrasonographic techniques and appears as a hypoechoic ring throughout the anal canal.

TAUS, anal manometry, and electromyography are three common tests used for evaluating the anal sphincter and diagnosing anal sphincter injuries. Although many believe that TAUS is the test of choice, most think that there is a learning curve for the performance and interpretation of these studies and some question the accuracy and reliability of this technique.

The authors have gone to great lengths to eliminate some of these variables in the design of the study. Using the services of two very experienced ultrasonographers, the authors have shown that accuracy in women with known anal sphincter injury is 100%. Of more interest, and some concern, is the issue of accuracy in women with intact anal sphincters. The ultrasonographers falsely identified sphincter injuries in 5% to 25% of the normal anal sphincters. In addition, there was only fair agreement between the experienced ultrasonographers, which improved if the examination was limited to the distal 1.5 cm of the anal canal. It is quite understandable that the authors found it difficult to interpret the upper portion of the anal canal because of the configuration of the puborectalis and external sphincter. Thus, as pointed out by the authors, the technique of endoanal ultrasonography has its limitations. Their recommendation that the results be interpreted together with the results of functional studies before surgical repair is undertaken should be heeded.

E.H. Birnbaum, M.D.

Anorectal Reconstruction After Abdominoperineal Resection: Experience With Double-wrap Graciloplasty Supported by Low-frequency Electrostimulation

Cavina E, Seccia M, Banti P, et al (Univ of Pisa, Italy)

Dis Colon Rectum 41:1010-1016, 1998 5–103

Objective.—A minority of patients with rectal cancer require an abdominoperineal resection (APR). Sphincter reconstruction usually involves transposition of the gracilis muscles, followed by electrostimulation. The safety and efficacy of this procedure and preliminary results of a new technique for electrode implantation are discussed.

Methods.—Between October 1991 and June 1997, 31 patients (17 men), aged 32 to 79 years, underwent total anorectal reconstruction and APR.

Technique.—During the APR the gracilis muscles are mobilized by a second operating team that frees the muscles through 3 small incisions at the proximal, middle, and distal thirds of the thigh. A 4- to 5-cm segment of the colon is delivered through the perineal wound, a double-wrap gracilis transposition is performed, and a new sling is formed in the retrocolic position. Both muscles are sutured to the residual insertions of the levators to restore the perineal floor. The colonic stump is left closed and protected by a catheter. Low-frequency electrostimulation with platinum-iridium electrodes and fully implantable stimulators was started during the first 2 weeks; cyclic stimulation was used to obtain type II fiber conversion during the training period (average duration, 9.8 months). During the follow-up period, the lowest stimulation rate was programmed to reach the best continent contraction at the lowest values.

Results.—Three patients died of their disease at 38, 44, and 58 months after surgery, 1 patient required conversion to an abdominal stoma, and 1 is awaiting closure of a stoma. Thirty-three pulse generators were implanted in 31 patients, and 26 patients were followed up for an average of 37.8 months. Good continence was achieved in 22 patients. No patients required antidiarrheal drugs or dietary restrictions. Local infections occurred in 22% of the patients. Ten patients had a stricture of the colocutaneous anastomosis, most of which developed during the sixteenth postoperative month. Skin erosions developed at the site of leads tunnel in 4 patients. These were treated by removing the stimulators and then reimplanting them with new electrodes.

Conclusion.—Preliminary results of the double-wrap graciloplasty technique with low-frequency electrostimulation demonstrate safety and efficacy.

▶ The treatment of rectal cancer located within the lower third of the rectum frequently requires an APR and a permanent colostomy for management. Many patients accept a permanent colostomy as a not-so-pleasant but necessary byproduct of this cancer operation. Given a choice, many patients may opt for a procedure to restore continence. It is imperative that the principles of cancer surgery not be compromised in an effort to restore continence in these patients. Graciloplasty without electrostimulation has not had good long-term results because it results in a static encirclement of the anal canal. The electrostimulated graciloplasty has been used for fecal incontinence with better results. The authors used an electrostimulated double wrap graciloplasty to restore continence in patients undergoing APR for carcinoma of the rectum. This procedure is often performed as a last resort in an effort to avoid a permanent stoma, but it is not without functional problems, particularly in the realm of difficult evacuation. Prior studies have discussed the need for an irrigating stoma to assist patients with evacuation. It appears from this study that irrigating stomas are not necessary in this select group of patients, but these patients still have evacuating difficulties. The majority of patients required water enemas to evacuate, which eliminates the irrigating stoma but requires the patient to continuously irrigate the neorectum. It is certainly interesting to note that the mean defecation frequency appears to be significantly less than would be expected for patients with coloanal anastomoses, something that is certainly desirable for the patient.

As stated by the authors, however, the procedure is not without complications. Infectious complications are the most common complication after this operation (22%). A diverting stoma was necessary in almost one third of the patients in the postoperative period. Strictures and problems relating to the electrostimulation device make up a significant late complication rate. This procedure and the required technology remain quite expensive, and the potential for significant morbidity remains. The authors' conclusion that this study has shown that a staged operation may not be necessary and early stimulation does not appear to have any detrimental effects on long-term outcome may be a bit premature.

E.H. Birnbaum, M.D.

Simultaneous Endoluminal Sonography and Manometry to Assess Anal Sphincter Complex in Normal Subjects

Wong RF, Bonapace ES Jr, Chung CY, et al (Temple Univ, Philadelphia; Thomas Jeffereson Univ Hosp, Philadelphia)

Dig Dis Sci 43:2363-2372, 1998 5–104

Introduction.—Manometric and US evaluation of the anal sphincter complex provides valuable information in patients with incontinence, constipation, and other anorectal disorders. However, the expected correlation between anal pressure and muscle thickness of the anal sphincters is not always borne out by studies. High-frequency, catheter-based endoluminal US (EUS) permits more accurate localization and measurement of the anal sphincters. The correlation between resting anal pressure and sphincter thickness was assessed using high-frequency EUS.

Methods.—Simultaneous anal EUS and manometry were performed in 11 normal volunteers (mean age, 27 years). The studies were performed using specialized catheters that included both pressure ports and US transducers. The correlation between sphincter thickness, measured as cross-sectional area (CSA), and resting anal pressure was assessed. The relationship was clarified using 3-dimensional reconstructions of pressure and EUS images.

Results.—EUS measured the length of the internal anal sphincter as 27 mm, whereas the length of the high-pressure zone on manometry was 44 mm. The maximal CSA of the internal anal sphincter was found to be a mean of 10 mm proximal to the peak resting pressure. Resting anal pressure was significantly correlated with the CSA of the external anal sphincter, but not with the CSA of the internal anal sphincter. The external anal sphincter plus the internal anal sphincter CSA was significantly correlated with resting anal pressure.

Conclusion.—In normal young volunteers, the ultrasonographically measured internal anal sphincter is shorter than the manometrically measured high-pressure zone. These subjects show a significant distance between the maximum CSA of the internal anal sphincter and the peak resting anal pressure. Together, the CSA of the internal anal sphincter and the external anal sphincter are significantly correlated with resting pressure, though the CSA of the internal anal sphincter is not. The findings indicate that the external anal sphincter makes a significant contribution to resting anal pressure. Simultaneous anal manometry and EUS may aid in physiologic and clinical evaluation of the anal sphincter complex.

▶ The anal sphincter is a complex group of muscles and is composed of both smooth and striated muscles that work in conjunction for maintenance of continence and normal defecation. The anal sphincter has been studied extensively using various manometric techniques and, more recently, using EUS. It has been presumed that the internal anal sphincter contributes the largest component to the resting anal pressure. It is well known, however, that after a lateral anal sphincterotomy, continence is maintained despite a reduction in rest pressures.

The authors have elegantly demonstrated that the external anal sphincter may contribute a larger component to the resting pressure than previously believed. Radial asymmetry of the anal canal pressures has been demonstrated using various techniques. The authors have demonstrated that not only does this exist but it is the result of the configuration and thickness of both the internal and external anal sphincters.

The authors have provided us with a visual explanation of why and how the inconsistencies with manometry and US may occur. They have confirmed what many prior authors have believed and have shown us that the internal and external sphincters, although considered separate entities, should be evaluated together.

E.H. Birnbaum, M.D.

Cost-effectiveness of Dynamic Graciloplasty in Patients With Fecal Incontinence

Adang EMM, Engel GL, Rutten FFH, et al (Univ of Maastricht, The Netherlands; Erasmus Univ Rotterdam, The Netherlands)

Dis Colon Rectum 41:725-734, 1998 5–105

Objective.—Dynamic graciloplasty (DGP), in which a new sphincter is created using neurostimulated graciloplasty, has emerged as a new treatment alternative for the common problem of fecal incontinence. It may be useful for patients in whom anal or postanal surgical repair has been unsuccessful. The cost effectiveness of DGP as a treatment for intractable fecal incontinence was evaluated.

Methods.—The prospective study included 43 consecutive patients with fecal incontinence who had not responded to previous surgeries. The patients were 32 women and 11 men (median age, 48 years). The most common initial cause of fecal incontinence was perineal trauma. All patients underwent DGP, with quality of life assessments performed before and after the procedure. Cost analysis was performed using data from the hospital information system and from patient questionnaires. A randomized trial was considered unethical. Data on the costs of colostomy were based on 7 patients who had had a stoma in place for incontinence for several years. The cost comparison of these 2 approaches included sensitivity analyses.

Results.—Total direct, lifelong costs for the 2 approaches were calculated at approximately $32,000 for DGP vs. $72,000 for colostomy, including stoma care. The baseline analysis assumed a clinical success rate of 74% with DGP. Quality of life was significantly improved after DGP, compared with conventional treatment.

Conclusion.—Although DGP is a more expensive treatment option for intractable fecal incontinence than conventional therapy, it produces a better quality of life. Both cost and outcome considerations suggest that stoma care is the least attractive treatment option. As a result of this study, reimbursement for DGP was recommended to the Dutch national health insurance programs. The DGP option should become more cost effective over time, as experience with the procedure grows and the cost of a neurostimulator (for patients with failed DGP) decreases.

▶ Much has been written in the medical and lay press regarding cost effectiveness of various procedures and disease treatments. Much of the discussion centers around how to establish the cost of procedures, the cost of life, the cost of morbidity, and the loss of income. Although these are very real costs, they are very difficult to tabulate. Although the up-front cost of technology may be expensive, the long-term benefit in terms of dollars saved may outweigh the initial outlay. It is very difficult in this day and age to make this case and even more difficult to change insurance and governmental policies. The authors must be commended for their efforts because as the result of this paper, the Dutch Health Insurance Executive Board recommended reimbursement for a novel and initially expensive procedure.

Fecal incontinence affects a significant number of men and women, and the costs are both monetary and emotional. Standard treatments for fecal incontinence are not without complications and the failure rate is not inconsequential. Surgical repairs have a high success rate and should be used before utilization of expensive technology. Patients may undergo multiple sphincter repairs, but the success rate of subsequent repairs is lower with each attempt. Thus, a small, select group of patients might be candidates who would benefit from this advanced technology.

Neurostimulated graciloplasty is being evaluated and used for the treatment of fecal incontinence in patients who have failed conventional treatment. This study looked at the costs of this technology vs. the lifelong cost of maintaining a colostomy or purchasing adult diapers. As pointed out in the invited editorial, this study is not without flaws. For example, the calculated lifelong costs of a colostomy appear to be quite high. One might question the authors' conclusion that DGP is more cost effective than a well-made colostomy. The important issues are not just economic ones but also include the psychological toll that patients with fecal incontinence incur. The authors bring this to light in their paper and have been successful in changing medical policy to allow reimbursement for a new technology.

E.H. Birnbaum, M.D.

Glutaraldehyde Cross-linked Collagen in the Treatment of Faecal Incontinence

Kumar D, Benson MJ, Bland JE (St George's Hosp, London)

Br J Surg 85:978-979, 1998 5–106

Background.—There are many causes of fecal incontinence. If surgical repair is not successful or possible, there are few other options available. The use of a bulk-enhancing agent in the anal canal in patients with fecal incontinence has not been evaluated. The usefulness of anal glutaraldehyde cross-linked collagen injections for the treatment of fecal incontinence for patients with a surgically uncorrectable problem and for whom conservative treatment has been unsuccessful was examined.

Methods.—The study group consisted of 5 men and 12 women, aged 42 to 76 years, with grade 2 or 3 fecal incontinence, who had a surgically uncorrectable problem and for whom conservative treatment was unsuccessful. Of the 17 patients, 9 had idiopathic fecal incontinence, 6 had incontinence after surgical procedures, and 2 had an internal sphincter defect after obstetric injury. All patients had anorectal physiology and endoanal US before injections. Clinical outcome was assessed at 1 and 6 month follow-up.

Results.—Anal collagen injection was well tolerated, without complications. After glutaraldehyde cross-linked collagen injection, 11 of 17 patients had significant symptomatic improvement. One patient who did not have improvement initially responded to repeat injections.

Conclusion.—These initial results suggest that injection of glutaraldehyde cross-linked collagen into the anal canal is a simple, well-tolerated out-patient method for treating fecal incontinence caused by internal sphincter dysfunction.

▶ Incontinence to flatus and stool is a small but very real risk after minor anorectal procedures. Most physicians try to avoid aggressive surgical repair and initially attempt conservative medical management. The authors used a technique that has been successfully used for patients with urinary incontinence. Glutaraldehyde cross-linked collagen was injected into the anal canal of patients with fecal incontinence in an attempt to improve control. It is conceivable that patients with minor keyhole deformities and internal sphincter defects from lateral sphincterotomies would be the group to benefit from bulk-forming agents. Although this study was small (17 patients) and there were multiple etiologic factors causing the fecal incontinence, the authors have shown that glutaraldehyde cross-linked collagen may be effective in treating some patients with minor incontinence. Future studies with larger subgroups might better identify those who would be improved with collagen injections.

E.H. Birnbaum, M.D.

The Malone Antegrade Continence Enema Procedure in the Management of Patients With Spina Bifida

Hensle TW, Reiley EA, Chang DT (Columbia Univ, New York; Babies' and Children's Hosp of New York; St Joseph's Hosp Med Ctr, Paterson, NJ)

J Am Coll Surg 186:669-674, 1998 5–107

Background.—Bowel and bladder dysfunction are common among patients with spina bifida and cause both medical and emotional problems. Although urinary incontinence has become easier to manage, traditional bowel management has not been successful for most patients with spina bifida. These authors describe successful management of bowel incontinence in patients with spina bifida with the Malone antegrade continence enema (ACE).

Methods.—The study group consisted of 17 male and 10 female patients with spina bifida, aged 10 to 31 years, who underwent Malone ACE procedures from 1994 to 1997. Of the 27 participants, 22 were bed or wheelchair bound. Many had undergone previous major surgical procedures. All patients had preoperative mechanical bowel cleanout. The appendix was used as a catheter channel in the majority of patients, but some had a neoappendix created using a small-bowel tube. Antegrade irrigation was initiated in patients beginning on postoperative days 5 to 7. The amount of saline used for irrigation ranged from 60 to 2000 mL, with a transit time of 10 to 120 minutes.

Results.—Patients were followed for 9 to 30 months. Of the 27 patients, 18 performed the catheterization and irrigation independently and 9 required assistance. All of those requiring assistance were bed or wheelchair bound and 3 were intellectually impaired. Nineteen of the 27 patients had predictable bowel control using the ACE, whereas 6 had occasional soiling. Two patients, both teenaged girls, had a successful procedure but refused to use the ACE stoma. No stoma leakage was reported. Complications included stomal stenosis in 5 patients, cecal flap necrosis in 1, false passage of a cecal flap in 1, and stomal granulations in 3. Of the 27 patients who underwent Malone ACE procedures, 25 reported significant quality-of-life improvement because of decreased concerns about soiling accidents.

Conclusion.—The results of this small study of bowel continence in 27 patients with spina bifida suggest that the Malone antegrade continence enema procedure provides reliable colonic emptying without fecal soiling in the majority of patients. Most patients found that it significantly enhanced their quality of life.

▶ Spina bifida affects young individuals in whom a myriad of bowel and bladder dysfunctions develop. It has been recognized that significant emotional trauma and lack of independence resulting from the problems associated with the management of this dysfunction affect these patients throughout their lives. Creation of intestinal stomas would eliminate the need for enemas, disimpaction, and other bowel maintenance routines that these patients endure. Colostomies can be irrigated, which allows patients to control their bowel function to some degree. There is some emotional stigma felt on the part of patients and their physicians when discussing intestinal stomas, particularly for benign diseases.

The authors have outlined 1 method of management for bowel dysfunction which, if successful, could allow these patients more independence from their caregivers and permit them to eliminate stool the "natural" way. The technique, outlined nicely in the paper, provides a small stoma through which an antegrade colonic washout can be performed. Although the complication rate can be quite high (30%), 25 of 27 patients reported improvement in their quality of life, 19 attaining complete and predictable bowel control. Although, clearly, this procedure does not completely liberate these patients, it is a useful technique for highly motivated patients to gain some independence.

E.H. Birnbaum, M.D.

Restoration of Anal Sphincter Function by Single-Stage Dynamic Graciloplasty With a Modified (Split Sling) Technique

Rosen HR, Novi G, Zoech G, et al (Danube Hosp, Vienna)

Am J Surg 175:187-193, 1998 — 5–108

Introduction.—"Dynamic graciloplasty" uses electrostimulation to transform fast-twitching type II muscle fibers into slow-twitching type I fibers, thus providing skeletal muscles with the capacity for tetanic contraction. This technique has given promising results in the treatment of patients with fecal incontinence or those who have undergone excision of the anal sphincter. The results of dynamic graciloplasty in 28 patients are presented.

Methods.—The 5-year experience included 16 men and 12 women, median age 53.5 years, who had fecal incontinence or had undergone abdominoperineal resection (APR) of the anal sphincter. Twelve patients underwent APR with synchronous graciloplasty to restore the excised sphincter. Six underwent total anorectal reconstruction after previous APR. Four patients had acquired fecal incontinence and 6 had congenital atresia. In a 1-stage procedure, the muscle was transposed and the stimulation electrodes and pulse generator implanted. The neosphincter was wrapped using a modified split-sling technique. This was followed by controlled neuromuscular stimulation to transform the muscle, performed over 8 weeks in the early part of the experience and 4 weeks in the latter part.

Results.—There were no postoperative deaths. Early in the experience, 4 patients had rectal injury, most often resulting from overstimulation causing excessive tension of the muscle sling. Median resting pressure increased from 27.5 mm Hg preoperatively to 42.8 mm Hg after graciloplasty, with no further change after muscle transformation. Median squeeze pressure increased from 39.2 to 89.3 mm Hg. Ninety percent of patients with congenital or acquired incontinence achieved a continence for solids and liquids or solids alone. In contrast, only 55.5% of APR patients had satisfactory outcomes, defined as continence for solids or liquids, solids alone, or with occasional episodes for liquids. Defecation disorders were the major functional problem for patients who had undergone APR and who required enemas for treatment.

Conclusions.—By the 1-stage technique used in this study, dynamic graciloplasty can achieve continence within 7 weeks in patients with an insufficient or excised anal sphincter. The muscle wrap must be placed under correct tension to avoid direct injury to the rectum. The authors have created a modified intraoperative anal manometry device to provide objective data on the pressures created by the neosphincter. To achieve satisfactory results with dynamic graciloplasty, patients must be carefully selected and informed about potential postoperative problems with this last-resort technique.

▶ The authors present a very detailed and honest review of their experience with a small group of patients undergoing stimulated graciloplasty to correct anal incontinence. Once again, the most appropriate group seems to be those with acquired anal incontinence, because sensation is intact, and such patients have the best results. However, there is some promise in the reconstruction of the anorectal area for patients with abdominoperineal or total proctocolectomy who wish restoration. One must be aware of the potential severe complications that accompany this procedure: severe sepsis, obstipation and erosion, etc. In fact, up to one third of patients simply have a perineal colostomy and have no control whatsoever. Another one third will require neoanal irrigations to stimulate bowel movement. One's enthusiasm must be tempered by these early results. This is a very large operation and affects the patient's ambulation. With those negative comments aside, the potential for helping individuals is unlimited with this technique, should it become more refined and user-friendly. The reader should remember that there is also an artificial bowel sphincter being developed, which may be more appropriate for patients with in situ anal sphincter mechanisms, thus limiting the stimulated graciloplasty to patients with no sphincter mechanism after extirpative surgery.

J.W. Fleshman, Jr., M.D.

Vaginal Endosonography of the Anal Sphincter Complex Is Important in the Assessment of Faecal Incontinence and Perianal Sepsis

Poen AC, Felt-Bersma RJF, Cuesta MA, et al (Vrije Universiteit, Amsterdam)

Br J Surg 85:359-363, 1998 5–109

Objective.—Anorectal endosonography has become a standard technique for the staging of rectal cancer and other anorectal diseases. The technique is usually well tolerated and easily performed; however, it may have difficulty in providing visualization of the anterior portion of the sphincter complex, and it may be impossible in patients with anal canal stenosis or pain. Vaginal endosonography may offer an alternative. Vaginal endosonography was examined for use in patients with fecal incontinence and perianal sepsis.

Methods.—The study included 56 women undergoing anal and vaginal endosonography in a single session. There were 36 patients with fecal incontinence (mean age, 50 years) and 20 patients with perianal sepsis (mean age, 39 years). The pelvic floor anatomy was described, and anal sphincter measurements were performed by both techniques. The diagnostic value of vaginal endosonography, added to that of anal endosonography, was assessed.

Results.—Vaginal endosonography provided clear visualization of the pelvic floor. The anal sphincter could not be visualized in 13 of the 56 patients; in the latter half of the experience, this number dropped to 3 of 28. External anal sphincter thickness measurements were smaller with vaginal endosonography; all other anal canal measurements were greater with vaginal endosonography. Vaginal endosonography added significant information to that provided by anal endosonography in 25% of patients.

Conclusions.—Vaginal endosonography of the anal sphincter complex is a useful technique in the diagnosis of fecal incontinence and perianal sepsis. It offers reliable and undistorted images of the anal sphincters, providing additional diagnostic information in many patients. Endosonographers should be familiar with this technique, though its use may be limited to cases in which there is doubt about the presence of obstetric injury or in which fistulous tracts in the anovaginal septum are suspected.

▶ Endorectal ultrasound or anal ultrasonography has become an essential part of the evaluation of the anorectal area and the sphincter mechanism. Surgeons who routinely perform anal sphincter reconstruction use transrectal ultrasound to image the sphincters and identify sphincter defects in patients with borderline physical findings and mild anal incontinence. The ultrasound has become an essential tool in planning procedures and following patients in whom results are less than perfect. The authors of this article suggest that vaginal ultrasonography should also be considered an essential part of the evaluation of the anal sphincter mechanism for both incontinence and perianal sepsis. Although this may give an added piece of information, it is difficult to see that it is essential from their data. The information provided by the vaginal ultrasound was more confirmatory than it was new. The vaginal scan in perianal sepsis may actually have a more important role because the intrarectal probe distorts the sphincter mechanism, hides the internal opening of a fistula tract, and has limited use in the setting of anal pain. Vaginal ultrasound may, therefore, improve diagnostic findings and help the patient. I agree with the author's conclusion that individuals familiar with endorectal ultrasound should also be able to perform vaginal ultrasonography to have an alternative for viewing the anal sphincter mechanism. This is also a viable approach for patients undergoing follow-up after abdominoperineal resection for either anal or rectal cancer.

J.W. Fleshman, Jr., M.D.

Hemorrhoids and Anal Fissure

Anal Endosonography in Patients With Anorectal Symptoms After Haemorrhoidectomy

Abbasakoor F, Nelson M, Beynon J, et al (Singleton Hosp, Swansea, Wales)
Br J Surg 85:1522-1524, 1998 5–110

Objective.—Whereas complications after hemorrhoidectomy are rare, they can lead to anal incontinence. Evaluation of these patients can be difficult. The prevalence of endosonography anal abnormalities in patients with anorectal symptoms after hemorrhoidectomy is assessed.

Methods.—Anal endosonography was performed on 16 patients (6 women), aged 35 to 77 years, with anorectal incontinence (n = 10), pain (n = 4), and obstructive defecation (n = 2) after hemorrhoidectomy and compared with results in a control group of 16 patients, aged 40 to 80 years, who were free of symptoms after hemorrhoidectomy.

Results.—Lesions were found in 12 patients with symptoms. Ten patients with anorectal incontinence had disruption of the internal anal sphincter (IAS) (n = 5) or of both sphincters (n = 2) at the site of hemorrhoidectomy. Four patients with anal pain had IAS injury (n = 1), extrinsic mass (n = 1), intersphincter mass (n = 1), and normal appearance (n = 1). One of 2 patients with obstructive defecation had an isolated external anal sphincter (EAS), and 1 was normal. The endosonographic findings were normal in all control patients.

Conclusion.—Preliminary results of anal endosonography are promising and warrant further evaluation.

▶ The rate of excisional hemorrhoidectomy has diminished since more conservative treatments, such as elastic ligation, have become widely accepted. However, excisional hemorrhoidectomy is still frequently performed and, although presumed to be a minor surgical procedure, it is not without postoperative complications. Pain, infection, and minor and occasional major incontinence can be significant problems for patients. Endoanal ultrasonography is becoming a widely accepted technique for evaluating both the internal and external sphincters. Anal sphincter defects, particularly in the internal anal sphincter, can be clearly identified. The authors used this technology in evaluating a group of patients who had symptomatic fecal incontinence, persistent anal pain, and obstructed defecation after hemorrhoidectomy. The findings were then compared with those in a matched group of symptom-free patients after hemorrhoidectomy. The authors do show that anal endosonography can identify sphincter defects as well as extrinsic masses and even an intersphincteric abscess. Missing from this paper is any clinical evaluation of these patients. It is left for the reader to wonder whether these abnormalities could have been identified by a good clinical examination. Studies have shown that endoanal ultrasonograms can identify occult sphincter injuries, even in patients who have no symptoms. Many of these studies, however, lack longitudinal evaluation to discover whether these occult injuries become symptomatic as the patient population ages. However, as the authors point out, endoanal ultrasonography is a valuable tool for evaluating patients with symptoms in the postoperative period. It is not recommended that endoanal US be used before and after routine hemorrhoidectomy, but it should be considered in patients who have symptomatic incontinence before surgical hemorrhoidectomy is undertaken.

E.H. Birnbaum, M.D.

Surgical Treatment of Piles: Prospective, Randomized Study of Parks vs. Milligan-Morgan Hemorrhoidectomy

Hosch SB, Knoefel WT, Pichlmeier U, et al (Univ of Hamburg, Germany)

Dis Colon Rectum 41:159-164, 1998 5–111

Background.—Over the years, many different treatments have been proposed for hemorrhoids. Hemorrhoidectomy is the most popular treatment for third- and fourth-degree hemorrhoids. The Milligan procedure for eliminating the vascular cushions was originally described in 1937 and often modified since. The Parks technique reconstructs the anal canal, and thus is believed to better preserve sensorial continence and reduce postoperative pain. This randomized trial compared hospital stay, time off work, symptom relief, morbidity, and convenience associated with these 2 techniques.

Methods.—Thirty-four consecutive patients with third- or fourth-degree internal hemorrhoids were randomized to undergo either Parks or Milligan-Morgan hemorrhoidectomy. There were 25 men and 9 women (mean age, 50 years). Preoperative information was collected by a standard questionnaire and rectal examination. The patients were re-examined at 1, 2, 4, 8, and 12 weeks postoperatively.

Results.—Neither group had any serious complications. The Parks procedure group had a significantly shorter hospital stay, 3.2 vs. 4.6 days. This procedure was also associated with a shorter duration of work incapacity, 12.3 vs. 20.2 days. Pain was greater for patients undergoing the Milligan-Morgan procedure, until 2 weeks postoperatively. All patients in both groups were free of symptoms at the 8- and 12-week examinations. All wounds had healed, and all patients were satisfied with their results.

Conclusions.—The Milligan-Morgan and Parks hemorrhoidectomy procedures are both safe, simple, and effective. The Parks procedure is associated with reduced postoperative discomfort, reduced hospital stay, and reduced time off work. Because it reduces pain and is more economical, the Parks procedure is the preferred hemorrhoidectomy technique.

► Randomized, controlled trials in the treatment of hemorrhoids are rare. The authors should be congratulated for having achieved something that is very difficult because of biases held by surgeons and patients alike. Unfortunately, the majority of American surgeons would suggest that the treatment of choice for third-degree hemorrhoids is internal elastic ligation or some other nonoperative approach. Excisional hemorrhoidectomy is most often performed using a closed or Ferguson technique, which also results in an outpatient or at most 23-hour observation stay in the hospital. There are currently attempts to change the treatment of second and third-degree internal hemorrhoids to a stapled technique that may be more expensive and unnecessary. Internal elastic ligation and sclerotherapy continue to be the gold standard, safe and effective. Fourth-degree hemorrhoids are relatively unusual and, when they do require operation, generally respond well to a closed hemorrhoidectomy technique.

J.W. Fleshman, Jr., M.D.

Botulinum Toxin Injections in the Internal Anal Sphincter for the Treatment of Chronic Anal Fissure: Long-term Results After Two Different Dosage Regimens

Maria G, Brisinda G, Bentivoglio AR, et al (Catholic Univ of Rome, Italy)
Ann Surg 228:664-669, 1998 5–112

Objective.—Although most acute anal fissures heal spontaneously, some lead to a chronic ulcer. Anal fissures are managed by dilatation of the internal anal sphincter (IAS). Whereas conservative treatment can be protracted and sphincterotomy weakens the sphincter, chemical denervation with botulinum toxin (BTX) weakens striated muscle. The effects of 2 different dosage regimens of BTX to induce healing in patients with idiopathic anal fissure, as well as complications and long-term results, were evaluated.

Methods.—BTX was administered to 57 consecutive outpatients with chronic idiopathic anal fissure. Group A patients (n = 23, 10 men), aged 20 to 82 years, were treated with 15 units and re-treated with 20 units. Group B patients (n = 34, 18 men), aged 19 to 64, were treated with 20 units and re-treated with 25 units. Scar healing at 1 and 2 months was compared with baseline evaluation.

Results.—At 2 months, 10 group A patients (43.5%) and 23 group B patients (67.6%) had healing scars. Pain disappeared in 24 patients and was reduced in 4 patients. Resting anal pressure was significantly reduced. Thirteen patients in group A and 24 patients in group B had healing scars or symptomatic improvement. Resting anal pressure and maximum voluntary squeeze pressure decreased significantly with treatment, but maximum voluntary pressure was unchanged. Among patients who had complete treatment, 13 of 15 group A patients (86.7%) and 30 of 30 group B patients had fissure healing.

Conclusion.—BTX treatment for chronic anal fissure promotes scarring and provides symptomatic relief. Higher doses are safe and more effective than lower doses.

► It is expected that two thirds of patients with acute anal fissures will heal with medical therapy. Chronic fissures are those that persist for more than

1 to 2 months and are much more difficult to treat medically. Many patients with chronic fissures who have been treated unsuccessfully with other nonaggressive treatment regimens come to be evaluated for surgery. The surgical therapy for anal fissure is a lateral sphincterotomy. This outpatient procedure is simple to perform and has a high success rate but is not without complications, as the authors point out in their discussion. The risk of impaired incontinence after lateral sphincterotomy or anal dilatation is very real. Many efforts, including the use of 0.3% nitropaste, have centered around treating the patients' symptoms and preserving fecal continence. Topical nitroglycerin ointment yields a transient headache as a common side effect. Since this is a short-acting agent, it needs to be applied on a frequent basis until healing of the fissure has been obtained. BTX has been used to weaken striated muscle and has been used in the treatment of disorders in which spasms of these muscles are a problem. Its use for smooth-muscle spasm is less well studied. Use of BTX for the treatment of anal fissures has two desirable features. One is relaxation of the internal sphincter and thus lowering of the anal rest pressures. The second feature is its apparent impermanence, which would allow the sphincter to return to baseline function after the fissure has healed. Small uncontrolled trials using BTX to treat anal fissures have had some positive results. Although long-term follow-up is not available, permanent complications do not seem to be significant. The authors evaluated two treatment doses of BTX and found that the group that was treated with the higher dosage had a higher rate of improvement and had no significant complications or side effects. Once healed, there appeared to be no relapses.

The initial injury leading to an anal fissure is straining at defecation. This then leads to anal spasm and chronically elevated resting pressures caused by continuous spasm of the internal sphincter. Whether this leads to hypoxia, which further contributes to the nonhealing fissure, is currently being debated. Reduction of the resting anal pressures is believed to contribute to improvement in the healing of these fissures. The authors nicely demonstrate that injection of BTX into the anal sphincter causes a reduction in resting pressures and does not alter the voluntary squeeze pressures. Although long-term studies should be forthcoming, the use of BTX appears to be an effective way of treating this vexing problem.

E.H. Birnbaum, M.D.

Clostridium difficile Colitis

Timing of Surgery for Fulminating Pseudomembranous Colitis

Synnott K, Mealy K, Merry C, et al (Trinity College, Dublin; St James's Hosp, Dublin)

Br J Surg 85:229-231, 1998 5–113

Background.—As the use of antibiotics increases, *Clostridium difficile* colitis becomes more common. Because specific anticlostridial chemotherapy is usually effective, surgery for fulminating *C. difficile* colitis is rarely performed. The surgical outcomes of 5 patients with fulminating *C. difficile* colitis were reported.

Methods.—The 5 patients undergoing surgery were unresponsive to medical treatment. All had received antibiotics previously. Surgery was indicated by systemic toxicity with a pyrexia, marked leukocytosis, and abdominal signs resulting in progressive organ failure.

Findings.—At surgery, all patients had a markedly edematous colon with normal serosa but with acute mucosal colitis. Subtotal abdominal colectomy and ileostomy were performed in all patients. Progressive organ failure persisted in 4 patients, who subsequently died. The mortality rate in the unoperated group was 3.8%.

Conclusion.—This increasingly common disease is life threatening in patients who eventually need surgery. Earlier surgical consultation may be indicated to improve the survival of patients with fulminating *C. difficile* colitis unresponsive to antibiotic treatment.

▶ This short article reports on 5 patients who were operated on for fulminant *C. difficile* colitis during a 6-month period in Dublin. The authors suggest that systemic signs of sepsis and peritonitis are indicators for early operation and total abdominal colectomy. However, patients had not received vancomycin enemas nor IV metronidazole therapy before operative therapy. Total abdominal colectomy is rarely necessary in this disease, and, most commonly, patients will respond to maximal medical therapy. Elderly, immune-compromised patients may be the group that responds well to early operative therapy, but there are no data to justify this tactic as 4 of the 5 patients operated on in this series eventually died.

J.W. Fleshman, Jr., M.D.

Recent Trends in Diagnosis and Treatment of *Clostridium difficile* in a Tertiary Care Facility

Butterworth SA, Koppert E, Clarke A, et al (Univ of British Columbia, Vancouver, Canada; St. Paul's Hosp, Vancouver, BC, Canada)

Am J Surg 175:403-407, 1998 5–114

Background.—Given the prevalence of antibiotic use, the diagnosis and management of *Clostridium difficile* disease should be evaluated. Recent trends in the diagnosis and treatment of *C. difficile* in a tertiary care facility were investigated.

Methods and Findings.—One hundred one patients with a culture or toxin positive for *C. difficile* during 1 year were identified. Ninety-six were available for assessment. Forty-five percent of the patients tested for both toxin and culture tested positive for both. Sixty-two patients were treated with antibiotic agents. Metronidazole was used in 90%. Ten antibiotic treatments were changed at a mean of 3 days.

Conclusion.—Either culture or toxin testing produced negative results in 55% of the patients testing positive for *C. difficile*. Metronidazole, which is less expensive than vancomycin, is the drug of choice. Changes in antibiotic regimens in this study were typically made before the 6 days recommended in the literature.

► Antibiotic-associated diarrhea is a frequent problem in major tertiary care facilities. This article evaluates the treatment and diagnosis of *Clostridium difficile* diarrhea in patients in Vancouver, British Columbia. Interestingly, only 18% of all the patients in the hospital with *C. difficile* colitis were surgical patients. The article emphasizes the use of both a culture and a toxin for diagnosis. This may be the recommended method of diagnosis according to world literature and carries a very high sensitivity and specificity when the 2 techniques are combined, but it is not cost effective. A more practical approach is to use the toxin test singly and to only order a culture if the toxin result is negative.

There were no colectomies for *C. difficile* pseudomembranous colitis in this series, although the authors admit that there may have been some that were performed before the culture or toxin was obtained. The treatment of choice is now metronidazole, 1.5 gm/day orally. Oral vancomycin is very expensive and in the setting of vancomycin-resistant enterococcus should be reserved only for metronidazole-resistant *C. difficile*. The medication should not be switched until the patient has had 6 days of therapy, as that is required for response. One interesting finding was that culture positive–toxin negative *C. difficile* colitis is more likely to respond to withdrawal of antibiotics alone. This is important because, occasionally, the patient will contact the physician complaining of diarrhea, the antibiotics will be stopped, culture and toxin will be obtained, and the diarrhea stops. At this point, if the culture is positive and the toxin is negative, it might be reasonable not to begin metronidazole in these patients.

Another point from the article that should be emphasized is that cephalosporins given perioperatively are some of the most likely antibiotics to result in *C. difficile*–associated diarrhea. Their use should be limited to necessary cases only.

J.W. Fleshman, Jr., M.D.

Techniques

New Technique for Mesh Repair of Paracolostomy Hernias

Hofstetter WL, Vukasin P, Ortega AE, et al (Univ of Southern California, Los Angeles; Los Angeles County Med Ctr)
Dis Colon Rectum 41:1054-1055, 1998 5–115

Background.—When they are symptomatic, paracolostomy hernias require treatment. A new technique for repairing paracolostomy hernias and its use in 13 patients were described.

Technique.—The surgeon performs primary repair, leaving a fascial defect around the bowel admitting about 2 fingers. The repair is reinforced with 1-mm polytetrafluoroethylene mesh, which is fashioned by cutting it about three fourths of the way across at its midpoint. The surgeon makes a perpendicular incision, 1.5 cm in each direction, 1.5 cm in from the end of the initial incision. At this 4-corner junction, each corner is divided a distance of 1.5 cm, creating an 8-pointed, star-shaped incision 3 cm in diameter. The surgeon places the mesh around the stoma from the inside against the peritoneum, dorsal to the rectus sheath, to cover the previously sutured defect. The "fingers" of the star are then splayed over the bowel, pointing away from the fascia, and the slit is closed to the bowel with 3-0 silk sutures. The mesh is then stretched to its full size and fixed to the posterior rectus sheath with staples or sutures. The surgeon closes the abdomen in a standard fashion. Postoperatively, the patient is managed with standard laparotomy orders.

Patients and Outcomes.—No parastomal hernias recurred in 13 patients treated by this technique during 8 years. In 2 patients, the mesh appeared to migrate over time, resulting in stomal angulation, which may cause problems in the future. No infections, fistulas, or other complications occurred. In 2 patients undergoing reexploration for unrelated reasons, the mesh was found to be incorporated well to the fascia and bowel by fibrous tissue.

Conclusion.—A new technique using polytetrafluoroethylene mesh in the repair of paracolostomy hernias was presented. This technqiue is safe and simple to perform, allows stomal site preservation, and is associated with a lack of recurrences.

▶ Paracolostomy hernias are a major problem for colorectal and general surgeons. This technique of using soft polytetrafluoroethylene mesh to repair the inner aspect of the abdominal wall around the colostomy is an excellent idea and may replace some of the paracolostomy hernia repairs using an approach around the stoma through the skin. The advantage of leaving the mucocutaneous junction intact is obvious in that it reduces the risk of infection and preserves the existing stoma site. Long-term follow-up, of course, is needed before the technique can be confirmed as a standard treatment. However, the technique offers potential and should be considered in the approach to paracolostomy hernias and even prolapsing hernias. One caveat to consider when using this technique: Cover the underlying bowel with some form of adhesion barrier, as even the soft mesh can cause adhesions and fistulization.

J.W. Fleshman, Jr., M.D.

Long-term Functional Evaluation of Straight Coloanal Anastomosis and Colonic J-Pouch: Is the Functional Superiority of Colonic J-Pouch Sustained?

Joo JS, Latulippe JF, Alabaz O, et al (Cleveland Clinic Florida, Fort Lauderdale)

Dis Colon Rectum 41:740-746, 1998 5–116

Background.—Although the colonic J-pouch has been shown to have functional advantages over a straight coloanal anastomosis, the longevity of this functional superiority has not been proved. The functional and clinical outcomes of straight coloanal anastomosis compared with colonic J-pouch performed after low anterior resection were investigated.

Methods.—Thirty-nine patients undergoing "straight" coloanal anastomosis and 44 undergoing colonic J-pouch between 1989 and 1996 were studied. In all patients, low anterior resection with anastomosis was done less than 4 cm from the dentate line. Daily bowel movements, tenesmus, urgency, incontinence score, and anorectal manometric findings were assessed before and 6 months, 1 year, and 2 years after surgery.

Findings.—The 2 groups did not differ significantly in age, sex, diagnosis, preoperative incontinence score, bowel movements, level of anastomosis, history of perioperative radiation therapy, or manometric findings. The postoperative mortality rate was 5.1% in the coloanal anastomosis group and 2.3% in the colonic J-pouch group, a nonsignificant difference. Anastomotic complications occurred in 17.9% and 4.5%, respectively; strictures, 10.3% and 0%; leaks, 5.1% and 2.3%; bleeding, 2.6% and 0%; and rectovaginal fistula, 0% and 2.3%. Pouchitis developed in 2 patients in the colonic J-pouch group, and another patient had evacuation problems 1 year after surgery. Function was significantly better for up to 1 year after surgery, as judged by less frequent bowel movements, urgency, and incontinence scores. In the coloanal anstomosis group, functional results at 2 years were not significantly better than those at 1 year after surgery. At 1 year after this procedure, rectal compliance of the colonic J-pouch was significantly increased, although the difference was less pronounced after 2 years.

Conclusion.—In this series, the functional superiority of the colonic J-pouch was greatest 1 year after surgery. By 2 years, functional results were similar to those of coloanal anastomosis. However, the reduction in anastomotic complications in patients undergoing colonic J-pouch procedure was nearly fourfold, indicating another potential advantage of this technique.

► Colonic J-pouch has become a standard technique for patients undergoing low rectal cancer resection. The debate regarding the use of a colonic J-pouch, however, is not concluded in that the colonic J-pouch normally requires the use of a diverting ileostomy in most institutions. A straight coloanal anastomosis using a staple/double-staple technique may be safely used for reconstruction in sphincter-sparing procedures and does not always require loop ileostomy. It has been shown in several series that anastomotic leak occurs at a higher frequency (up to 15%) in anastomoses within 5 cm of the dentate line. There has been no randomized, prospective trial to identify the rate of coloanal anastomotic leak when straight coloanal anastomosis or J-pouch coloanal anastomosis is used.

This article suggests that colonic J-pouch may improve the anastomotic leak rate because of a theoretical improvement in the blood supply of the bowel at the level of the anastomosis in the J-pouch. The authors cannot confirm this with either blood flow or oxygenation analysis. The functional outcome is exactly the same for the straight coloanal anastomosis as for the colonic J-pouch using the descending colon, not the sigmoid colon, at two-years of follow-up. This suggests that in patients in whom a straight coloanal anastomosis could be performed without an ileostomy, this may be a reasonable alternative to constructing a J-pouch with a protecting loop ileostomy. On the other hand, it also may suggest that a colonic J-pouch without an ileostomy may be an alternative. The answer is yet unknown. For now, recommendations for loop ileostomy for diversion after either a low coloanal or colonic J-pouch anal anastomosis are very liberal.

J.W. Fleshman, Jr., M.D.

Omentoplasty in the Prevention of Anastomotic Leakage After Colonic or Rectal Resection: A Prospective Randomized Study in 712 Patients

Merad F, and the French Associations for Surgical Research (Hôpital Louis Mourier, Colombes, France; et al)

Ann Surg 227:179-186, 1998 5–117

Background.—Omentoplasty (OP) involves wrapping the omentum around the colonic or rectal anastomosis. Although some authorities have proposed that OP reinforces intestinal sutures and reduces the rate of anastomotic leakage, no prospective, randomized studies have proved it. The value of OP in preventing anastomotic leakage after colonic or rectal resection was investigated in a multicenter study.

Methods.—Between 1989 and 1994, 705 patients, aged 15 to 101 years, were randomly assigned to undergo OP to reinforce the colonic anastomosis after colectomy or not to undergo OP. Randomization was done after the resection and anastomosis had been performed, the anastomosis had been tested for airtightness, and the omental flap was judged feasible.

Findings.—Overall, 4.9% of the patients had anastomotic leakage after surgery, including 4.7% in the OP group and 5.2% in the control group. The mortality rates in the OP and control groups were 4.9% and 4.2%, respectively. Five patients (0.8%) with anastomotic leakage died, including 2 undergoing OP. Repeat surgery was needed in 30% of the patients. Twelve repeat operations (6 in each group) were for anastomotic leakage. Repeat surgery resulted in death in 14% of the patients. This rate, as well as the rate of other intra-abdominal and extra-abdominal complications, did not differ significantly between the 2 groups.

Conclusion.—Performing OP to reinforce colorectal anastomosis does not reduce the rate or severity of anastomotic failure. On the contrary, this procedure reportedly carries the potential risks of infection from necrosis of the pedicled graft and late intestinal obstruction.

▶ The use of the omentum to wrap a colorectal anastomosis or colocolonic anastomosis has been attractive to surgeons for many years. This is a randomized prospective trial using multicenters and a large group of patients. It suggests that OP does not prevent anastomotic leaks nor the complications of anastomotic leaks. However, other factors influencing the anastomotic leak rate were identified in this study. Distal colorectal anastomoses and those performed for diverticulitis were found to be at higher risk to leak. Proximal diversion actually increased the risk of a leak but prevented the complications of an anastomotic leak.

Final recommendations from the article can be that all patients should be tested for a leak at the time of operation, using insufflation of either air or Betadine. If there is a suggestion of a leak, proximal diversion should be used because even after suturing to reinforce the staple line, 20% of anastomoses will leak. Proximal diversion will reduce the complications associated with an anastomotic leak and allow the patient to eventually undergo colostomy or ileostomy closure. OP is not suggested, but not contraindicated, based on these findings. Again, surgeon preference and judgment remain important in the decision to use this technique.

J.W. Fleshman, Jr., M.D.

Colonoscopy

Is Colonoscopy Indicated for Small Adenomas Found by Screening Flexible Sigmoidoscopy?

Wallace MB, Kemp JA, Trnka YM, et al (Harvard Pilgrim Health Care, Boston; Brockton/West Roxbury Veterans Affairs Med Ctr, Mass)

Ann Intern Med 129:273-278, 1998 5–118

Background.—Authorities disagree about whether colonoscopic examination of the proximal colon should be done in patients with a small tubular adenoma on screening flexible sigmoidoscopy. The prevalence of advanced polyps in the proximal colon among such patients was reported.

Methods.—This prospective cohort study included 4,490 patients undergoing sigmoidoscopy. All were older than 50 years and asymptomatic; none had risk factors for colon cancer. Biopsies were performed on all polyps found at sigmoidoscopy, and all polyps were characterized. Patients with distal adenomas were offered colonoscopy.

Findings.—A neoplastic lesion was found in 401 patients (8.9%). Colonoscopy was performed in 301 (75%) of these patients. None of the 90 patients with a single tubular adenoma 1 to 5 mm in diameter in the distal colon had an advanced proximal polyp, vs. 5.4% of the patients with multiple distal polyps 1 to 5 mm or 6 to 10 mm in diameter and 7.9% of those with polyps larger than 10 mm (advanced). Patients at low risk, with a single tubular adenoma 1 to 5 mm in diameter, made up 44% of the group with distal adenomas or cancers detected at flexible sigmoidoscopy.

Conclusions.—Patients undergoing screening sigmoidoscopy with single tubular adenomas of 5 mm or less had a low prevalence of advanced proximal polyps. Colonoscopy may not be beneficial in such patients.

Colonic Chicken Skin Mucosa: An Endoscopic and Histological Abnormality Adjacent to Colonic Neoplasms

Shatz BA, Weinstock LB, Thyssen EP, et al (Washington Univ Med Ctr, St Louis; West Central Pathologists, St Louis)

Am J Gastroenterol 93:623-627, 1998 5–119

Background.—In a previous study, the authors described the endoscopic finding of pale yellow-speckled mucosa, resembling chicken skin, adjacent to colonic neoplasms. This "chicken skin mucosa" (CSM) differs from gastrointestinal xanthelasmas in that it is always associated with colonic neoplasms. The prevalence, endoscopic features, clinical significance, and possible causes of CSM were further studied.

Methods and Findings.—Eight hundred fifty-two consecutive colonoscopies were assessed prospectively for the presence of CSM associated with cancer or adenomas of 1 cm or larger. CSM was found adjacent to 8 of 10 distal colorectal cancers, 1 of 4 proximal colon cancers, 16 of 42 distal adenomas, and 3 of 44 proximal adenomas. Histologic evidence of CSM was observed in 4 of 7 resected distal cancers. Biopsy specimens of the CSM demonstrated that lipid-filled macrophages in the lamina propria caused this endoscopic finding. On electron microscopy, the surface epithelial cells had small intestine-like microvilli. CSM was not associated with other colonic conditions nor with the laxative preparation. In 4 patients, the CSM finding alerted the endoscopist to the presence of polyps in places that were diffiuclt to see (Fig 1).

Conclusion.—CSM is an endoscopic finding caused by fat accumulation in macrophages in the lamina propria of the mucosa adjacent to colonic neoplasms. The pathophysiologic implications of CSM have yet to be defined.

▶ The authors of this interesting report have identified a visual signal on colonoscopy to identify neoplastic lesions. The appearance of CSM around neoplasms has induced them to biopsy and remove numerous lesions that might have otherwise been missed. The presence of CSM on the left side of the colon, as opposed to the right, is something that needs to be evaluated. The observation of CSM may actually become a signal that an individual should be screened colonoscopically on a more frequent basis. The authors are to be congratulated on identifying something that is clinically helpful and may change clinical practice in the future. Readers should be aware of its presence if they do colonoscopy on a regular basis for patients with cancer.

J.W. Fleshman, Jr., M.D.

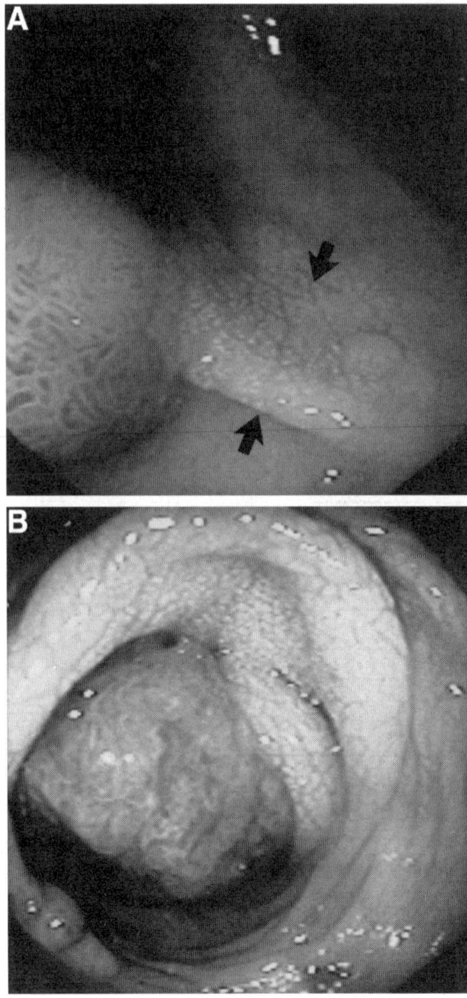

FIGURE 1.—A, sessile sigmoid adenoma with chicken skin mucosa adjacent to the polyp (*arrows*); B, rectal carcinoma with chicken skin mucosa. (Reprinted by permission of the publisher from Shatz BA, Weinstock LB, Thyssen EP, et al: Colonic chicken skin mucosa: An endoscopic and histological abnormality adjacent to colonic neoplasms. *Am J Gastroenterol* 93:623-627. Copyright 1998 by Elsevier Science Inc.)

Laparoscopy

Laparoscopic Management of Acute Small Bowel Obstruction

Bailey IS, Rhodes M, O'Rourke N, et al (Royal Brisbane Hosp, Australia)
Br J Surg 85:84-87, 1998 5–120

Background.—Although laparoscopic management of acute bowel obstruction is an attractive option, its clinical potential has not been well defined. The outcomes of laparoscopic treatment of acute small-bowel obstruction at 1 center were analyzed.

Methods and Findings.—Sixty-nine patients with acute small-bowel obstruction managed in a laparoscopic unit and 70 managed in a general unit were compared retrospectively. Eighty percent of the patients in the laparoscopic unit underwent laparoscopy, compared with 14% in the general unit. Laparoscopy completed treatment in 45% of the laparoscopic unit patients and assisted in an additional 22%. Patients undergoing laparoscopy were discharged sooner than those undergoing laparotomy, with median hospital stays of 3 and 8 days, respectively. However, patients undergoing laparoscopy had a greater chance of early, unplanned reoperation.

Conclusion.—Performing laparoscopy is feasible in a high percentage of patients needing surgery for acute small-bowel obstruction. Although the length of stay was decreased for such patients, their risk of early, unplanned reoperation was increased.

► The management of small-bowel obstruction is a difficult problem in an open operation in the majority of cases. Use of laparoscopic techniques in this disease should be undertaken only by the most experienced surgeons. This article illustrates the potential usefulness of laparoscopic techniques in approximately 50% of patients presenting with small-bowel obstruction caused by adhesions. The authors rightly emphasize the care that must be taken to avoid injury to the bowel. The reoperation rate in patients treated with laparoscopic techniques is higher, but the mortality and complication rates are essentially the same as for an open technique.

One must remember that a large number of patients who undergo exploration for small-bowel obstruction do so in the emergency, after-hour, time period. This often means that the standard operating team is not together, and this may make the procedure more difficult. Certainly, laparoscopic technique should be able to manage those patients with a single band-like adhesion causing obstruction and result in improved recovery. Patients should be followed closely because there is a 10% reoperation rate for those individuals.

J.W. Fleshman, Jr., M.D.

Laparoscopic Colectomy

Laparoscopic Management of Acute Peritonitis

Navez B, Tassetti V, Scohy JJ, et al (Hôpital Saint-Joseph, Gilly (Charleroi), Belgium; Hôpital Civil, Strasbourg, France)
Br J Surg 85:32-36, 1998 5–121

Purpose.—Peritonitis was previously regarded as a contraindication to laparoscopy. The reason for this contraindication was a theoretical risk of malignant hypercapnia or toxic shock syndrome. The feasibility, safety, and efficiency of laparoscopy for the management of peritonitis were determined.

Patients.—Two hundred thirty-one patients (mean age, 49 years) who underwent laparoscopy during episodes of acute peritonitis were included in the retrospective study. The patients (121 females and 110 males; mean age, 54 years) were treated at 2 centers over a 5-year period. Diagnoses included appendicular peritonitis (91 patients), perforated gastroduodenal ulcers (69), colonic perforations (35), and miscellaneous diagnoses (36). Peritonitis was generalized in 54% of the patients.

Outcomes.—The postoperative mortality rate was 4%. In 85% of the patients, laparoscopy enabled the identification of the exact cause of peritonitis; in 25%, laparoscopy led to a change in the preoperative diagnosis. Because of laparoscopy, unnecessary laparotomy was avoided in 7% of the patients, and the incision site was modified in 9%. Conversion to laparotomy was necessary in 15% of the patients overall: 25% of those with appendicular peritonitis, 16% of those with gastroduodenal perforation, and 83% of those with colonic perforation. There were no cases of malignant hyperthermia but 2 of postoperative septic shock; both patients survived.

Conclusions.—Laparoscopy can be safely carried out in patients with peritonitis. Laparoscopy can confirm the preoperative diagnosis and clarify treatment planning, sometimes avoiding the need for laparotomy. It is particularly useful for patients with appendicular or gastroduodenal perforation. Patients with colonic perforation are more likely to require laparotomy, but even colonic perforation may be managed laparoscopically with increasing surgical experience.

▶ This article is interesting, in that it presents a large group of patients with acute peritonitis from multiple causes and their outcome after laparoscopic management. The patients with colonic sources of peritonitis were the least likely to have laparoscopic management, and a conversion to open laparotomy was required in 83% of instances. This was thought to be due to the inexperience and learning curve on the part of the laparoscopic surgeon. However, I would suggest that it is more likely good judgment and the nature of the problem in the colon that required conversion. The repair of a perforation after colonoscopy is certainly a reasonable procedure to be performed laparoscopically. However, gross fecal peritonitis from diverticulitis or ischemic bowel certainly would tax even the most experienced and aggressive laparoscopic colorectal surgeon. Again, we find that laparoscopy may be useful in selected cases but should not be applied generally to perforations and free peritonitis from the colon.

J.W. Fleshman, Jr., M.D.

Outcome Following Laparoscopic Resection for Colorectal Cancer

Psaila J, Bulley SH, Ewings P, et al (Yeovil District Hosp, England)

Br J Surg 85:662-664, 1998 5–122

Background.—For several reasons, the use of laparoscopic techniques for resecting colorectal cancer has not been widely accepted. However, provided that minimal access techniques do not compromise cancer cure, laparoscopic colorectal resection may be of value in improving recovery compared with conventional surgery.

Methods and Findings.—In this prospective study, 25 patients with colorectal cancer undergoing elective laparoscopic resection and 29 undergoing open resection were compared. The mean lengths of stay in the 2 groups were 10.7 and 17.8 days, respectively, a significant difference. Mean morphine requirements were also reduced in patients undergoing laparoscopic resection. Recovery, determined by dynamometer hand grip and the SF-36 symptom score, was more rapid in the laparoscopic group. Tumor clearance was adequate in patients undergoing laparoscopic resection. The number of lymph nodes harvested was comparable in the 2 groups. No port site or wound recurrence was observed at a median 28 months' follow-up.

Conclusion.—When laparoscopic colorectal resection is feasible, it can provide early benefits compared with conventional surgery. In this series, these benefits were noted for 4 months after surgery, which is longer than has been described previously.

▶ Larparoscopic colectomy continues to be used by a number of groups around the world with varying results. This study represents a prospective, consecutive series, and not a randomized trial, looking at the use of laparoscopic colectomy for cancer. The authors have shown no adverse effect from the laparoscopic approach after a short follow-up in this group of patients. They have shown some early benefits from shortened length of stay and decreased pain after the laparoscopic procedure. However, they do not tell us how the patients were treated in the postoperative period and, therefore, cannot conclude that the laparoscopic approach alone affected the length of stay.

The total cost of treatment was somewhat lower for the laparoscopic group, and this bears some attention as it may be a future reason for using a laparoscopic approach for patients with colorectal disease. Until a randomized, prospective trial is completed on the use of laparoscopic technique for colon and rectal cancer, it is still advisable for individuals to participate in either a local prospective trial or a national, multicenter, randomized trial looking at this technique.

J.W. Fleshman, Jr., M.D.

A Prospective, Randomized Trial Comparing Laparoscopic Versus Conventional Techniques in Colorectal Cancer Surgery: A Preliminary Report

Milsom JW, Böhm B, Hammerhofer KA, et al (Cleveland Clinic Found, Ohio; Humboldt Univ, Berlin)

J Am Coll Surg 187:46-57, 1998 5–123

Background.—Previous uncontrolled studies of laparoscopic techniques in colorectal surgery have not shown clear advantages compared with conventional approaches. In addition, concerns have been raised about an unusual rate of early recurrences after laparoscopic procedures for colorectal cancer. Laparoscopic and conventional techniques were compared in a prospective, randomized study of patients undergoing bowel resection for colorectal cancers or polyps.

Methods and Findings.—Fifty-five patients were assigned to laparoscopy and 54 to conventional surgery. Forty-two and 38, respectively, had cancer, and the rest had large adenomas. Overall recovery of 80% of forced expiratory volume in 1 second and forced vital capacity occurred at a median of 3 days in the laparoscopy group and 6 days in the conventional group. Patients undergoing laparoscopy required significantly less morphine than those undergoing conventional surgery for up to 2 days after surgery. Flatus returned at a median 3 and 4 days in the laparoscopic and conventional procedure groups, respectively. All patients had clear tumor margins. No port site recurrences were noted in the laparoscopic group at a median follow-up of 1.5 years. Seven patients have died from cancer, 3 in the laparoscopy group and 4 in the conventional surgery group.

Conclusion.—Laparoscopic techniques appear to be as safe as conventional surgery in selected patients undergoing large bowel resection for cancer or polyps. Laparoscopy was associated with a faster recovery of pulmonary and gastrointestinal function, apparently without compromising cancer outcomes in the short term. Longer follow-up is needed to more fully determine outcomes.

▶ An interim analysis in a randomized prospective trial is difficult to interpret. The group of patients presented in this article is a very small group of patients and essentially shows an early advantage for the laparoscopic group in terms of pulmonary and gastrointestinal function. Interestingly, there was no significant difference in length of hospital stay between the laparoscopic and the open group. This most likely reflects the inclusion of patients who had complications in both groups.

A small trial such as this is unable to document oncologic advantages or disadvantages. Short-term follow-up certainly limits the ability of the trial to make a conclusion on these issues. Indeed, Dr. Milsom himself has recommended that support be given to the current multicenter, randomized, prospective trial being performed by the Clinical Outcomes of Surgical Therapy Group. This small randomized trial showed no increase in wound complications or implantation at trochar sites of the tumor. As noted in the commentary for Abstract 5–122, the need for randomized, prospective trial results is still paramount.

J.W. Fleshman, Jr., M.D.

Laparoscopically Assisted Anterior Resection for Diverticular Disease: Follow-up of 100 Consecutive Patients

Stevenson ARL, Stitz RW, Lumley JW, et al (Royal Brisbane Hosp, Australia)

Ann Surg 227:335-342, 1998 5–124

Background.—The increased complexity of laparoscopic techniques applied to dissection or resection of the colon and rectum may be one reason for their lack of acceptance. The outcomes of modified laparoscopically assisted anterior resection for diverticular disease were analyzed.

Methods and Findings.—One hundred twenty consecutive patients were treated for symptomatic diverticular disease. The median duration of surgery was 180 minutes. The median length of stay was 4 days, and median time to passage of flatus was 2 days. Overall morbidity was 21%, with a 5% rate of wound infection. None of the patients died. The complication rate was significantly greater in 8 patients undergoing open laparotomy than in those undergoing laparoscopy, at 75% and 16%, respectively. Over time, length of surgery and length of hospital stay declined significantly. Ninety patients were followed for 37 months. Ninety-three percent reported symptomatic improvement. None of these patients was hospitalized again, and no one needed antibiotic therapy for recurrent symptoms.

Conclusion.—The morbidity and mortality associated with laparoscopically assisted anterior resection for diverticular disease are acceptable. The median postoperative hospital stay was only 4 days. The patients were free of diverticulitis recurrence during follow-up and were satisfied with their cosmetic and functional results.

► Laparoscopic management of diverticulitis has been the training ground for most laparoscopic surgeons as malignant disease is still relegated to randomized trials. This article from Brisbane, Australia reveals the excellent results obtainable with laparoscopic approaches for diverticulitis. This disease is uniquely suited for this technique as it results in shortened length of stay, smaller incisions, less pain, and all the benefits that one would expect from laparoscopic treatment. The complication rate and recurrence rate are unchanged from those of open operations. There is apparently a learning curve but once obtained, the performance of an anterior resection through the laparoscopic approach should be possible in most circumstances.

J.W. Fleshman, Jr., M.D.

Minilaparotomy Approach to Tumors of the Right Colon

Fürstenberg S, Goldman S, Machado M, et al (Ersta Hosp, Stockholm)
Dis Colon Rectum 41:997-999, 1998 5–125

Background.—A previous comparison of minilaparotomy with laras-copic-assisted surgery for colorectal diseases found no significant differences in time to return of bowel function, transfusion requirements, or postoperative complications. The authors concluded that early return of function and discharge depends on the use of small incisions, by minilaparotomy or laparoscopy. In this study, the minilaparotomy approach to right colonic tumors was reported.

Methods and Findings.—Forty-seven patients, aged 52 to 88 years, with tumors in the right colon underwent resection of the right colon by minilaparotomty between 1994 and 1997. Bowel function returned after a mean of 2 days. Passage of stools resumed after 4 days. Pain medication was required only in the first 3 days after surgery. There were no postoperative deaths and few major complications. No tumors recurred locally in the early postoperative period.

Conclusion.—The minilaparotomy technique appears to be an attractive alternative to conventional colon surgery in the treatment of right colon tumors. Tumors of 10 cm or smaller could be resected by minilaparotomy. A significant number of lymph nodes could also be removed during the procedure.

▶ The laparoscopic-assisted approach to colorectal disease requires a small incision for specimen extraction and construction of an anastomosis. The incision is usually 6 cm to 10 cm in length and is variably placed throughout the abdomen, depending on the surgeon's preference. A minilaparotomy approach provides the same reduction in incision length and improvement in pain and bowel function. The use of the minilaparotomy approach, however, is the main reason that laparoscopy was developed to provide broader view. "Keyhole" surgery can be done, but this limits abdominal exploration and the overall view of the abdominal cavity during the procedure.

If the patient is ideally suited for a minilaparotomy approach, there is very little contraindication to this method. However, if the abdominal wall is very thick, or the tumor or disease results in a large area of tissue, the minilaparotomy approach may not be possible. Certainly, a combination of a minilaparotomy and laparoscopy are essential in some cases, and the surgeon should be able to perform both. In choosing the approach, however, one must remember not to compromise the patient's care. If the surgeon is more comfortable with a standard laparotomy technique and can perform the minilaparotomy approach, this may be an excellent alternative to the open standard wide excision.

J.W. Fleshman, Jr., M.D.

Prospective Multicenter Study of the Quality of Oncologic Resections in Patients Undergoing Laparoscopic Colorectal Surgery for Cancer

Köckerling F, and the Laparoscopic Colorectal Surgery Study Group (Univ of Erlangen, Germany)

Dis Colon Rectum 41:963-970, 1998 5–126

Background.—The role of laparoscopic colorectal surgery for cancer has not been established, and the results of large, randomized studies will not be available for several years. This study analyzed the results of such resections in consecutive patients treated by unselected surgeons.

Methods.—Data on 231 operations for cancer, 167 with a curative intent, performed in the German-speaking countries of Europe since 1995 were analyzed. The curative resections included 63 sphincter-sparing proctectomies, 51 sigmoid resections, and 27 abdominoperineal resections. Twenty patients underwent segmental resections.

Findings.—Intraoperative tumor spillage was reported in 2% of the procedures. The mean number of lymph nodes harvested was 13, and the mean number of positive lymph nodes harvested was 2.2. The number of resected lymph nodes differed significantly among participating centers. In every patient, distal and proximal resection margins were free of tumors. Lateral margins examined were also tumor free. Among the 63 curative low anterior resections, the mean distal resection margin was 39 mm. In 8 of these resections, it was less than 20 mm. The mean blood loss was 344 mL. Twenty-one percent of the patients needed blood transfusions.

Conclusion.—The quality of laparoscopic colorectal procedures for cancer is, on average, satisfactory. However, it differs among surgeons. This study does not address the issues of local recurrence, long-term survival rates, or the incidence of port site metastases.

► In lieu of a randomized, prospective trial, the German surgeons have established a registry of laparoscopic colorectal surgery. In some ways, this is an excellent method of evaluating the technique because the study group is made up of multiple centers and multiple surgeons performing procedures of their preference. Through the database, a clear picture of the pathologic and technical outcome can be obtained. Unfortunately, a true evaluation of the technique as an oncologic method is not really possible as comparing 2 techniques does not produce a randomized, prospective study.

This article demonstrates the variability in evaluating lymph node harvest as a possible means of determining adequate oncologic response. Different centers showed different detection rates of lymph nodes. The article also shows that clear margins can be obtained by nearly every laparoscopic surgeon. It is possible to perform an oncologic procedure in the majority of cases. Although the surgeon's evaluation of the procedure is very subjective, the pathologist can identify areas of break in technique. Positive lateral margins or perforation of the tumor are used to objectively determine the adequacy of the resection. Clearly, the final judgment regarding oncologic resection will have to reside in a randomized, prospective trial comparing laparoscopic colectomy with open colectomy for curable cancer.

J.W. Fleshman, Jr., M.D.

Trauma

Rectal Trauma: Management Based on Anatomic Distinctions

McGrath V, Fabian TC, Croce MA, et al (Univ of Tennessee, Memphis)
Am Surg 64:1136-1141, 1998 5–127

Background.—Although the incidence of rectal injuries has increased over the last 2 decades, treatment remains controversial and morbidity high. There are 4 main management procedures for rectal injuries: fecal diversion, presacral drainage, injury repair, and distal rectal washout. The 5-year experience at 1 institution was analyzed to determine which treatment options contributed to reducing morbidity and whether treatment should vary by injury location.

Study Design.—All 58 consecutive, penetrating, full-thickness rectal injuries treated at the Regional Medical Center in Memphis from October 1991 to July 1996 were included in this study. Of the 58 patients, 57 were male, with an average age of 29 years. The injury mechanism was gunshot in 92% of patients. Age, race, sex, injury mechanism, vital signs, method of diagnosis, and digital rectal and sigmoidoscopy examination results were recorded for each patient. Complications were assessed. Injuries to the anterior and lateral surfaces of the upper two thirds of the rectum were classified as intraperitoneal (IP), injuries to the lower one third were classified as extraperitoneal (EP), and injuries to the posterior surface were also classified as EP.

Findings.—Of the 58 rectal wounds managed in this series, 16 were classified as IP and 42 as EP. Of these 58 wounds, 6 IP and 4 EP wounds underwent repair without diversion. There were no leaks. In the remaining 48 wounds there were 10 septic complications. There were 38 patients with diverted EP wounds. There was no statistically significant association between repair and infection. There was also no significant association between washout and infection.

Conclusion.—This small study suggests that most IP rectal injuries can be managed with primary repair. EP injuries should be explored and then repaired. EP wounds to the lower third of the rectum that are explored and repaired do not require presacral drainage. Unexplored EP injuries should be managed with presacral drainage to minimize abscess formation. Distal rectal washout had no effect on outcome. Larger studies are necessary to definitively determine the optimal management of rectal wounds.

▶ Rectal trauma has classically been treated with diversion, rectal washout, and primary repair or presacral drainage. This relatively large series of patients with rectal trauma has been treated with selective methods with respect to the anatomical position of the trauma. Upper rectal lesions or IP lesions have been repaired primarily with low morbidity and mortality. EP lesions have been repaired or drained, and colostomy was not always closed. Apparently, distal rectal washout does not influence outcome. Fortunately, rectal trauma is rare; but in civilian emergency rooms the occasional lesion will be seen and a selective management is indicated, as this article has shown.

J.W. Fleshman, Jr., M.D.

Miscellaneous

Why Do Children Have Chronic Abdominal Pain, and What Happens to Them When They Grow Up? Population Based Cohort Study

Hotopf M, Carr S, Mayou R, et al (King's College School of Medicine and Dentistry and Inst of Psychiatry, London; Royal Free Hosp, London)
BMJ 316:1196-1200, 1998 5–128

Background.—In most cases of recurrent abdominal pain in children, no defined organic disease is found, and this has led clinicians and researchers to look for psychosocial reasons for the pain. There is little information on the long-term outcome of children with persistent abdominal pain. A study was devised to test the hypothesis that children with recurrent abdominal pain tend to have anxious parents, come from families with high rates of physical illness, and have high rates of medically unexplained symptoms and psychiatric disorders as adults.

Methods.—Data were collected from participants in the Medical Research Council national survey of health and development, a national birth cohort study established in 1946. Abdominal pain throughout childhood with no defined organic disease, and measures of physical symptoms and psychiatric disorders at age 36 years were examined.

Results.—The parents of children with recurrent abdominal pain had high rates of complaints about physical health. The mothers of these children had higher neuroticism scores. The association of childhood personality with persistent abdominal pain is shown in Table 2. Children with persistent abdominal pain were more likely to have psychiatric disorders as adults, but, after psychiatric disorders were controlled, these subjects did not have much increased risk of physical symptoms as adults (Table 3).

Discussion.—These findings indicate that chronic abdominal pain in children is associated with poor health and emotional disorder in the parents. Children with chronic abdominal pain do not necessarily continue to have physical symptoms as adults, but they do have a higher risk of psychiatric disorders in adulthood.

► This important population-based cohort study evaluates the outcomes in adulthood of abdominal pain throughout childhood in children without defined organic disease. With an increasingly health-conscious population, parents of children with abdominal pain may be less readily reassured than they would have been in the past. This leads to more extensive investigation today than in the past. Modern medical advances might avoid unnecessary

TABLE 2.—Relation Between Abdominal Pain and Childhood Personality and Behavior and School Absences

Risk Factor (Assessor)	No Exposed	No (%) Affected	Odds Ratio (95% CI)*	LR χ^2 for Trend; *P* Value
Neuroticism on Pintner personality inventory				
Non-neurotic	1183	21 (1.8)	1.00	0.99; 0.32
Mid-neurotic	1042	19 (1.8)	1.07 (0.50 to 2.25)	
Neurotic	1026	23 (2.2)	1.34 (0.67 to 2.68)	
Introversion on Pintner personality inventory				
Introvert	975	24 (2.5)	1.00	0.57; 0.45
Ambivert	1104	17 (1.5)	0.83 (0.40 to 1.68)	
Extravert	1172	22 (1.9)	0.79 (0.39 to 1.60)	
Energy level at age 13 (teacher)				
Never tired	233	1 (0.4)	1.00	1.82; 0.18
Normally energetic	3026	62 (2.1)	2.48 (0.34 to 18.12)	
Always tired	187	5 (2.7)	3.33 (0.37 to 30.08)	
Day dreaming in class at age 13 (teacher)				
Seldom or never	1664	25 (1.5)	1.00	4.77; 0.03
Sometimes	1602	36 (2.3)	1.55 (0.84 to 2.87)	
Frequently	212	8 (3.8)	2.37 (0.88 to 6.33)	
Disobedience in class at age 13 (teacher)				
Seldom or never	3145	64 (2.0)	1.00	0.74; 0.4
Sometimes	321	321 (0.9)	0.45 (0.19 to 1.02)	
Frequently	26	2 (7.7)	2.90 (0.77 to 10.93)	
Lying in class at age 13 (teacher)				
Seldom or never	2926	55 (1.9)	1.00	0.04; 0.83
Sometimes	483	13 (2.7)	1.36 (0.61 to 2.60)	
Frequently	49	1 (2.0)	0.36 (0.05 to 2.71)	
Periods of absence (weeks) at ages 6-10 (school doctor)				
0-2	855	14 (1.6)	1.00	5.3; 0.02
3-4	717	9 (1.3)	0.61 (0.22 to 1.69)	
5-8	851	22 (2.6)	1.66 (0.76 to 3.66)	
≥9	622	19 (3.1)	1.75 (0.77 to 4.01)	
School absence at age 13 (teacher)				
Seldom or never	824	12 (1.5)	1.00	2.24; 0.13
Sometimes	888	13 (1.5)	1.07 (0.41 to 2.79)	
Frequently	851	24 (2.8)	1.71 (0.70 to 4.14)	

Abbreviation: LR, likelihood ratio test.
*Odds ratios corrected for sex and father's social class, weighted for sampling.
(This table was first published in the *BMJ* from Hotopf M, Carr S, Mayou R, et al: Why do children have chronic abdominal pain, and what happens to them when they grow up? Population based cohort study. *BMJ* 316:1196-1200, 1998. Reproduced by permission of the *BMJ*.)

operations today more than in the past, but they might also enforce illness beliefs in the patient. The authors conclude that the outcome in terms of symptoms of persistent pain is good. Their data suggest that medically unexplained persistent abdominal pain in childhood might be a predictor of adult psychiatric disorders more than of abdominal symptoms in adulthood.

G. Aliperti, M.D.

TABLE 3.—Relation Between Childhood Abdominal Pain and Adult Psychiatric Disorder and Physical Symptoms at Age 36 Years

Outcome	No of Children	No (%) With Abdominal Pain	Odds Ratio* (95% CI)
Persistent abdominal pain			
No	2383	45 (1.9)	1.30 (0.50 to 3.38)
Yes	226	7 (3.1)	1.03 (0.39 to 2.73)†
Persistent headache			
No	2045	38 (1.9)	1.51 (0.73 to 3.13)
Yes	563	14 (2.5)	1.20 (0.57 to 2.56)|
Index of definition on present state examination			
1	1239	13 (1.1)	2.72 (1.65 to 4.49)‡
2	811	19 (2.3)	
3	225	9 (4.0)	
4	158	5 (3.2)	
5	129	1 (0.8)	
6	24	4 (16.7)	
7	6	1 (16.7)	
No of common somatic symptoms			
0	1312	20 (1.5)	1.74 (1.04 to 2.92)‡
1	786	16 (2.0)	1.39 (0.83 to 2.36)†‡
2	345	9 (2.6)	
3	130	5 (3.9)	
4	30	1 (3.3)	
5	7	1 (14.3)	

*Derived by logistic regression unless marked otherwise.

†Corrected for psychiatric disorder at age 36 (see text).

‡Ordinal regression, corrected for sex, father's social class, marital status at age 36, and educational status. Note that ordinal regression derives single odds ratio describing increased risk of having outcome in abdominal pain group compared with "no pain" group, independent of level of severity of outcome.

(This table was first published in the *BMJ* from Hotopf M, Carr S, Mayou R, et al: Why do children have chronic abdominal pain, and what happens to them when they grow up? Population based cohort study. *BMJ* 316:1196-1200, 1998. Reproduced by permission of the *BMJ*.)

Cyclooxygenase 2 Is Induced in Colonic Epithelial Cells in Inflammatory Bowel Disease

Singer II, Kawka DW, Schloemann S, et al (Merck Research Labs, Rahway, NJ; Washington Univ, St Louis)

Gastroenterology 115:297-306, 1998 5–129

Objective.—Cyclooxygenase (COX)-1 and COX-2 are the key enzymes in prostaglandin (PG) synthesis. PG levels are highly elevated in mucosa from patients with inflammatory bowel disease (IBD), but the origins of these PGs and the relative roles of COX-1 and COX-2 remain unclear. This immunohistochemical study examined the expression and distribution of COX-1 and COX-2 in normal colon and colon from patients with IBD.

Methods and Findings.—On Western blotting and immunohistochemistry, comparable levels of COX-1 protein were found in epithelial cells from normal colon, Crohn's disease colon, and ulcerative colitis colon. Normal epithelial cells showed no COX-2 protein, but epithelial cells from Crohn's disease and ulcerative colitis colon did. The 3 tissue types showed similar COX-1 expression in epithelial cells in the lower half of the colonic crypts. Normal colon expressed no COX-2, but this protein was found in apical epithelial cells and lamina propria mononuclear cells from Crohn's colitis and ulcerative colitis tissue. Villus epithelial cells of Crohn's ileitis tissue demonstrated COX-2. COX-2–expressing colonic epithelial cells in ulcerative colitis tissue also expressed inducible nitric oxide synthase.

Conclusions.—This study demonstrates the expression of COX-2 in surface epithelial cells in Crohn's colitis and ulcerative colitis, as well as in villus epithelial cells in Crohn's ileitis. In IBD, as in normal colon and ileum tissue, COX-1 is localized to the crypt epithelium. Several lines of evidence suggest that epithelial expression of COX-2 in IBD may represent a protective response of the wound healing process.

▶ The identification of 2 distinct isoforms (COX-1 and COX-2) has been an important development, which has led to an understanding of mucosal injury and repair. The inhibition of COX-1 is central to nonsteroidal anti-inflammatory drug (NSAID)-related mucosal injury. The role of cyclooxygenase in the development of IBD has not been well studied. In addition, the clinical relevance is important both in the design of new therapeutic approaches as well as in understanding the recognized risk of exacerbations of UC and Crohn's disease by NSAIDs. This study identifies COX-2 expression predominantly in epithelial cells in association with active Crohn's and ulcerative colitis. COX-2 expression was weakest in normal mucosa. The role of COX-2 in the pathogenesis IBD is likely through PGs (PGE2 in particular), which may increase the diarrhea by inducing chloride secretion, but it also serves to regulate other cytokine and, perhaps, mucosal protection. As COX-2 induction may be important in mucosal repair as a response to injury, the newly available selective COX-2 inhibitors, although perhaps having a lower risk of gastrointestinal injury in healthy patients, may still cause IBD to worsen and currently cannot be recommended as a safe alternative in patients with IBD.

G. Aliperti, M.D.

Use of Mesalazine Slow Release Suppositories 1 g Three Times per Week to Maintain Remission of Ulcerative Proctitis: A Randomised Double Blind Placebo Controlled Multicentre Study

Marteau P, Crand J, Foucault M, et al (Saint-Lazare Hosp, Paris)

Gut 42:195-199, 1998 5–130

Background.—Previous studies have shown that the daily use of suppositories containing 500 mg of mesalazine (5-aminosalicylic acid, or 5-ASA) is effective in maintaining remission in patients with ulcerative proctitis. Slow-release mesalazine suppositories contain 1 g of mesalazine and have the advantage that they need not be used every day. This study compared the effectiveness of slow-release mesalazine suppositories in preventing relapses in patients with ulcerative proctitis.

Methods.—The subjects were 95 adults (mean age, 41 years) with cryptogenetic proctitis. All patients had experienced 2 or more recurrences in the preceding 12 months, but were in remission (for less than 14 days) at the time of enrollment. Patients were randomized to receive suppositories consisting of either placebo (n = 47; 19 men and 28 women) or slow-release mesalazine (n = 48; 25 men and 23 women). Suppositories were used 3 days per week for 12 months or until relapse occurred, at which point they were used daily until remission was achieved or (after 30 days of daily suppositories) treatment was deemed a failure. Relapse was defined as an increase in the endoscopy score of 1 or more compared with baseline or the occurrence of rectal bleeding 2 or more times in 1 day. Clinical and rectoscopic examinations were performed at regular intervals.

Findings.—The thrice-weekly suppository regimen successfully prevented recurrences in 25 patients (52%) who were taking slow-release mesalazine and in 18 patients (38%) who were taking placebo. Up to 270 days, the relapse rate was significantly lower in the mesalazine group than in the placebo group (38% vs. 60%). At some point during the 12-month study, 18 patients taking mesalazine and 26 taking placebo switched to a once-daily regimen because of recurrence. Significantly more patients with recurrence who took mesalazine (11, or 61%) were able to achieve remission with this protocol and stayed in the study than those who took placebo (22, or 8%). Thus, overall, withdrawals due to failure, pregnancy, or other factors (55 patients total) were significantly more common in the placebo group (36 patients, or 77%) than in the mesalazine group (19 patients, or 40%). Adverse events were experienced by 6 patients in the mesalazine group (13%) and by 5 patients in the placebo group (11%). Most of these were mild (including anal or rectal pain or difficulty with insertion of the suppository, asthenia, hypotension, moderate leukopenia, mild hair loss), and only 3 patients (1 receiving mesalazine, 2 receiving placebo) dropped out because of intolerance (anal or rectal burning).

Conclusions.—Slow-release mesalazine suppositories administered 3 times a week were effective in maintaining remission in about half of these patients with cryptogenetic proctitis. After about 9 months, however, this regimen was no longer significantly more effective than placebo, which suggests that perhaps maintenance treatment could be stopped after a few months. For subjects who experienced relapse, almost two thirds were able to achieve remission by switching to once-daily insertion of slow-release mesalazine suppositories.

Maintenance Treatment of Ulcerative Proctitis With Mesalazine Suppositories: A Double-blind Placebo-controlled Trial

d'Albasio G, and the Italian IBD Study Group (Ospedale Careggi, Firenze, Italy; et al)

Am J Gastroenterol 93:799-803, 1998 5–131

Background.—Although studies have shown that mesalazine (5-aminosalicylic acid, or 5-ASA) suppositories can help maintain remission in patients with ulcerative proctitis, the optimum dose and dosing schedule have yet to be defined. These authors compared 2 different dosages of mesalazine suppositories in patients with ulcerative proctitis.

Methods.—The subjects were 111 adults (mean age 41) with ulcerative proctitis whose disease was in remission but who had experienced a relapse within the past 6 months. Patients were randomized into 3 groups to receive suppositories consisting of placebo (n = 35, 25 men and 10 women) or mesalazine, 500 mg, at daily dosages of 500 mg (n = 40, 23 men and 17 women) or 1 g (i.e., 2 suppositories; n = 36, 21 men and 15 women). Treatment continued for 12 months, and clinical, physical, and endoscopic examinations were performed at regular intervals. Relapse was defined as a Baron's score of more than 1 (i.e., at least hyperemic mucosa with indistinct vascular pattern).

Findings.—By the end of treatment, relapse had occurred in 10% of the patients taking 1 g of mesalazine per day, 32% of those taking 500 mg/day, and 47% of those taking placebo (mesalazine 1 gm/day vs. placebo, P = 0.007) (Fig 2). Adverse events prompting withdrawal were experienced by 2 patients in the 1 g/day group (anal canal irritation and abdominal pain

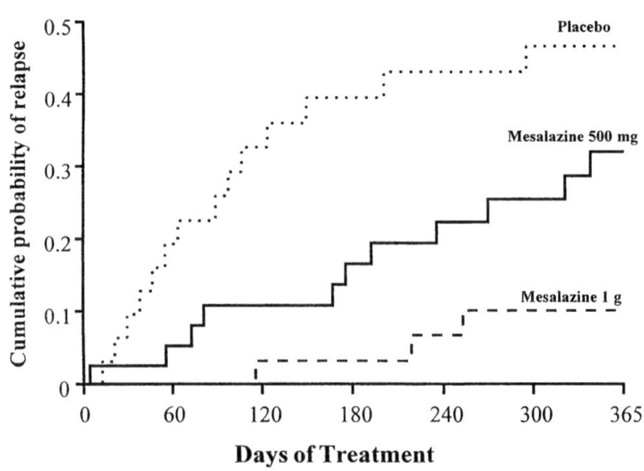

FIGURE 2.—Cumulative relapse rate: 5-ASA 1 g vs. placebo (log rank test): (1df) = 11.6225 (P = 0.007); 5-ASA 1 g vs. 5-ASA 500 mg (log rank test): (1df) = 4.5275 (P = 0.0334); 5-ASA 500 mg vs. placebo (log rank test): (1df) = 2.4497 (P = 0.1175). (Reprinted by permission of the publisher from d'Albasio G, and the Italian IBD Study Group: Maintenance treatment of ulcerative proctitis with mesalazine suppositories: A double-blind placebo-controlled trial. *Am J Gastroenterol* 93: 799-803. Copyright 1998 by Elsevier Science Inc.)

with constipation), by 2 patients in the 500 mg/day group (abdominal pain and constipation with swelling), and by 1 patient in the placebo group (tenesmus and swelling). In addition, 4, 3, and 4 patients in the 3 groups, respectively, withdrew because of poor compliance.

Conclusions.—Mesalazine suppositories were effective in maintaining remission in these patients with ulcerative colitis. This approach was safe and was generally accepted by the patients. The more effective dosage was 500 mg twice a day.

► Mesalazine is well established for treatment of active disease as well as for maintenance of remission. However, numerous refinements in their use continue to improve their clinical use. These two studies (Abstracts 5–130 and 5–131) on the use of topical therapy to maintain remission in ulcerative proctitis represent attempts to determine optimal dosing and whether lower dosing of suppositories may allow for better compliance without diminished efficacy. As is known for oral mesalazine preparations, more is better. The higher dosing (500 mg bid) used in the trial by d'Albasio et al. was highly effective and better than the lower dose (500 mg qd). Although the patient populations may differ, the low-dose regimen studied by Marteu et al (1 g 3 times a week) was even less effective, with efficacy not statistically significant beyond 9 months, although still with a trend toward maintenance of remission. However, one should not conclude that all patients need the highest dose. Although neither study identified a subgroup that did better at a higher dose on the basis of clinical or histologic characteristics, therapy can be individualized, according to clinical history and the dose the patients were receiving when their conditions flared, to determine the optimal dosing for a particular patient.

G. Aliperti, M.D.

Risk Factors for Self-Reported Colon Polyps

Kahn HS, Tatham LM, Thun MJ, et al (American Cancer Society, Atlanta, Ga; Emory Univ, Atlanta, Ga)

J Gen Intern Med 13:303-310, 1998 5–132

Background.—Given its cost and potential adverse effects, screening for colon polyps is generally not performed in individuals who are not considered at increased risk. But are there risk factors for colon polyps other than diet and a personal or family history of colorectal neoplasia or inflammatory bowel disease? These authors studied a large population to determine whether other factors increase one's risk of colon polyps.

Methods.—The subjects were 72,868 men and 81,356 women who completed the American Cancer Society's Cancer Prevention Study II survey in 1982 (baseline) and a follow-up survey in 1992. None of the subjects had colon polyps at baseline, but colon polyps had developed in 7,504 men (10.3%) and 5,111 women (6.3%) by 1992. Personal and clinical data were reviewed to determine any significant associations with the development of colon polyps; data were adjusted for age, family history of colorectal cancer, and diet.

Findings.—The development of colon polyps was significantly more likely in subjects with baseline reports of smoking (odds ratio [OR] depending on level of smoking, 1.20 to 1.34 for men and 1.21 to 1.50 for women), high alcohol intake (2 or more drinks per day; OR, 1.24 for men and 1.13 for women), and a body mass index more than 26 (OR, 1.06 for men and 1.07 for women). In addition, compared with subjects with no gallbladder disease, risks were significantly increased in subjects who had undergone gallbladder surgery up to 1982 (OR, 1.27 for men and 1.57 for women) and in subjects with gallbladder disease or gallstones (OR, 2.74 for men and 2.72 for women). The development of colon polyps was significantly less likely in subjects with baseline reports of a high exercise level (OR, 0.83 for men and 0.90 for women), frequent aspirin use (10 or more times a month; OR, 0.85 for women), and high parity (4 or more births; OR, 0.84 for women). Interestingly, in subjects with diseased gallbladders or whose gallbladders had been removed, there was a significantly weaker association between the development of colon polyps and both baseline smoking status and high body mass index.

Conclusions.—Patients who smoke or who drink 2 or more drinks per day, those with a high body mass index, and those with gallbladder disease, gallstones, or gallbladder surgery are at a modestly increased risk of colon polyps. Thus, screening for polyps in these individuals could prove beneficial. Why a diseased or missing gallbladder has a protective effect on the development of colon polyps is unknown and deserves further study.

6 The Liver

Hepatitis A

Serious Hepatitis A: An Analysis of Patients Hospitalized During an Urban Epidemic in the United States

Willner IR, Uhl MD, Howard SC, et al (Univ of Tennessee, Memphis)

Ann Intern Med 128:111-114, 1998 6–1

Background.—In 1994 and 1995, Tennessee's Shelby County (which contains Memphis) experienced an epidemic of hepatitis A, with more than 1,700 reported cases. The clinical features of 256 patients who were hospitalized with acute hepatitis A are described.

Methods.—In 1994 and 1995, medical records identified 256 patients (136 men and 120 women; mean age, 26 years; 82% black) who were hospitalized for acute hepatitis A. Data were gathered on demographics, risk factors, laboratory findings, underlying medical conditions, severe complications, and outcomes.

Findings.—The most common symptom at admission was prolonged nausea or vomiting (89%); coagulopathy (26%), jaundice (21%), and abdominal pain (18%) were also common. Thirty-nine serious complications occurred in 35 patients (14%); 19 were hepatobiliary and 20 were extrahepatic. According to current guidelines, only 2 of these 35 patients would have been advised to receive hepatitis A virus (HAV) vaccination. Of the 20 patients with extrahepatic complications, 5 died (2 because of fulminant hepatic failure, 2 because of autoimmune hepatitis, and 1 because of progressive liver failure). Age 40 years or older was significantly associated with a greater risk of severe complications, including death: 25% of patients 40 years or older had 1 or more serious complications compared with 11% of patients younger than 40 years. Additionally, 3 of 53 patients (5.7%) who were 40 years or older died, whereas only 2 of 203 patients (1%) who were younger than 40 years died. Forty-four patients (17%) had pre-existing disease, but there was no association between underlying disease and serious complications.

Conclusions.—In these patients with hepatitis A, age was associated with the occurrence of severe complications and death. The 5 patients who died had a median age of 40 years, and only 1 had chronic liver disease. Nonetheless, 2 patients (23 and 28 years old, respectively) also died because of hepatitis A, so younger patients are also at risk. The current guidelines for HAV vaccination would not have applied to most of the patients in whom severe complications developed. Thus, measures should be taken to increase Americans' immunity to hepatitis A.

Fulminant Hepatitis Associated With Hepatitis A Virus Superinfection in Patients With Chronic Hepatitis C

Vento S, Garofano T, Renzini C, et al (Univ of Verona, Italy; A. Pugliese Hosp, Catanzaro, Italy; San Marino State Hosp)

N Engl J Med 338:286-290, 1998 6–2

Background.—Fulminant hepatic failure is not usually associated with hepatitis A virus (HAV) infection—unless the patient has chronic liver disease, in which case mortality rates are significantly higher. The effects of superinfection with HAV were evaluated in patients with chronic hepatitis B or C virus infections (HBV, HCV).

Methods.—Over 7 years, 595 patients (405 men and 190 women; mean age, 29.1 years) with HBV (n = 163) or HCV (n = 432) who were seronegative for anti-HAV at enrollment were evaluated. Every 4 months, all patients underwent tests to detect serum IgM and IgG antibodies to HAV. Within 1 year of enrollment, each patient underwent a liver biopsy to determine the extent of the cirrhosis.

Findings.—In all, 27 patients (10 patients with HBV and 17 with HCV) acquired HAV superinfection. Nine of the 10 patients with HBV and HAV superinfection had an unaffected course; 1 patient with cirrhosis had marked cholestasis. In these patients, before HAV superinfection HBV DNA had been present, but it disappeared during the infectious HAV period and reappeared after recovery. Ten of the 17 patients with HCV and HAV superinfection had an uncomplicated course. Similarly, HCV DNA was present before the superinfection, disappeared or decreased during the infectious HAV period, and reappeared after recovery. However, in 7 of the 17 patients with HCV and HAV superinfection fulminant liver failure developed. All but 1 of the patients died within 12 days of admission, and autopsies revealed massive necrosis of liver cells. The patient who survived was treated with methylprednisolone for 3 weeks, and 9 months later she was negative for serum IgM anti-HAV and fecal HAV RNA. During the early HAV infection stage in all 7 of these patients, HCV RNA was not detectable in serum.

Conclusions.—All but 1 patient with HBV and HAV superinfection had an uncomplicated course. However, in 47% of the patients with HCV in whom HAV superinfection developed, fulminant hepatitis also developed, and 6 of these 7 died. Thus, to avoid life-threatening severe liver damage, HAV vaccination is recommended for patients with HCV who are at risk of acquiring HAV superinfection.

Safety and Immunogenicity of Hepatitis A Vaccine in Patients With Chronic Liver Disease

Keeffe EB, Iwarson S, McMahon BJ, et al (Stanford Univ Med Ctr., Calif; Göteborg Univ, Sweden; Centers for Disease Control, Anchorage, Alaska; et al)

Hepatology 27:881-886, 1998 6–3

Background.—Patients with chronic liver disease who become infected with hepatitis A are at increased risk of death. Whether an inactivated hepatitis A vaccine could be safely used in patients with chronic hepatitis was studied.

Methods.—The study involved 188 healthy research subjects (47.8% men; mean age, 39.8 years) and 287 patients with chronic liver disease. The hepatitis A vaccine was administered to the 46 patients with chronic hepatitis B (71.7% men; mean age, 38.3 years) and the 70 patients with chronic liver disease not caused by viral hepatitis (53.6% men; mean age, 43.1 years). Of the patients with chronic hepatitis C, 104 (63.8% men; mean age, 40.9 years) were treated with the hepatitis A vaccine and 67 (68.7% men; mean age, 45 years) were treated with the hepatitis B vaccine (which has low reactogenicity) so that the safety of the 2 vaccines could be compared. The 2 doses of hepatitis A vaccine were injected 6 months apart, and the 3 doses of hepatitis B vaccine were injected at study enrollment and at 1 and 6 months later.

Findings.—After vaccination, local symptoms occurred in about one third (35.5%) of all doses administered to all participants. Symptoms at the injection site were significantly less with the hepatitis B vaccine than with the hepatitis A vaccine (19.8% vs. 37.5%), although the frequency of systemic symptoms did not differ according to vaccine. General symptoms were significantly more likely with either of the vaccines in the patients than in the controls (16.5% to 27.9% vs. 11.1%). All symptoms were typically mild to moderate, and all resolved without treatment. Serum levels of total bilirubin, albumin, alkaline phosphatase, and liver enzymes did not change nor did prothrombin times. Seroconversion after the first hepatitis A vaccination occurred to a greater extent in the controls (93% of controls seroconverted) than in the patients with chronic hepatitis B (83.7%), the patients with chronic nonviral liver disease (83.1%), and the patients with chronic hepatitis C (73.7%). After the second hepatitis A vaccination, however, 94% of all recipients were seropositive for antibodies to hepatitis A. In comparison, after the last dose of hepatitis B vaccine, 100% of patients had seroconverted.

Conclusions.—The administration of hepatitis A vaccine to patients with chronic hepatitis B or C or chronic nonviral liver disease produced a satisfactory antibody response. The side effects were generally mild or moderate and self-limited, and there was no notable effect on hepatic functioning. Thus, hepatitis A vaccination can be safely recommended for this patient population.

► A large segment of the U.S. adult population is susceptible to hepatitis A. It is becoming rare in children as a result of improved hygiene and now affects mainly adults. While it is usually self-limited (approximately 85%), there is an increased risk for older individuals and patients with chronic liver disease.

Willner et al. (Abstract 6–1) reported an outbreak of hepatitis A and found that the median age of the patients who died was 40 years and that complications and mortality were more common in patients 40 years or older.

Vento et al. (Abstract 6–2) compared the course and the outcome of acute hepatitis A between patients with chronic hepatitis C and those with chronic hepatitis B. They found a high fatality rate among patients with chronic hepatitis C; also, HAV infection does not cause severe liver injury in patients with chronic HBV infection.

The safety of inactivated hepatitis A vaccine was evaluated by Keeffe et al. (Abstract 6–3). They found that it was safe when administered to patients with chronic liver disease originating from hepatitis B or C and other chronic liver disease not caused by viral hepatitis.

Thus, we need to reinforce to our patients who are older than age 40 years and who are at an increased risk for acquiring hepatitis A (travelers to areas in which hepatitis A is endemic, those with occupational exposure, IV drug users, gay men, and persons in communities with cyclic epidemics)[1] the importance of receiving the inactivated hepatitis vaccine. In addition, it should be administered to patients with chronic hepatitis C who are at risk for HAV infection as recommended by the World Health Organization.

J.S. Barkin, M.D.

Reference

1. Centers for Disease Control and Prevention: Prevention of hepatitis A through active or passive immunization: Recommendations of the Advisory Committee on Immunization Practices (ACIP). *MMWR Morb Mortal Wkly Rep* 45S(RR-15):1-30, 1996.

Hepatitis B

Long-term Follow-up of Patients With Chronic Hepatitis B Treated With Interferon Alfa

Lau DT-Y, Everhart J, Kleiner DE, et al (Natl Inst of Diabetes and Digestive and Kidney Diseases, Bethesda, Md; Natl Cancer Inst, Bethesda, Md; Natl Institutes of Health, Bethesda, Md; et al)
Gastroenterology 113:1660-1667, 1997 6–4

Background.—Although no therapy for hepatitis B virus (HBV) infection is completely satisfactory, interferon alfa (IFN-α) does cause disease remission in 25% to 40% of patients. However, is the long-term prognosis any better for patients with HBV who receive IFN-α? This question was addressed in patients with HBV who had received IFN-α up to 11 years earlier.

Methods.—Overall, 103 patients with chronic HBV who were treated with IFN-α were enrolled in 3 clinical trials between 1984 and 1991. Patients were followed up at least yearly through 1994, and follow-up evaluations included serologic testing, biochemical tests to identify liver disease, and biopsy specimens. The mean follow-up was 6.2 years (range, 0.9 to 11.1 years). A response to IFN-α was defined as the loss of HBV DNA during therapy and the clearance of hepatitis B early antigen (HBeAg) less than 1 year after IFN-α therapy began.

Findings.—Most of the patients with HBV who were treated with IFN-α did not respond (70%), but 31 patients did respond (30%). Women and blacks were significantly more likely to respond to IFN-α therapy, as were patients with more severe liver disease (including cirrhosis). During follow-up, most patients who responded to therapy were still negative for HBeAg (94%) and hepatitis B surface antigen (HBsAg; 71%). However, significantly fewer of those who did not show a response were negative for HBeAg (40%) or HBsAg (8.3%). Patients who did and did not show a response to therapy did not differ significantly in the rate of complications related to liver disease (13% vs. 27%) or in mortality rates (at 9 years, 29% vs. 33%). However, because patients who had cirrhosis were more likely to be treated with IFN-α, the data were corrected on the basis of cirrhosis in the pretreatment liver biopsy sample. Seventeen patients had pre-existing cirrhosis; 10 did not show a response to therapy, and all 10 experienced liver-related complications or death. In contrast, 10 patients with pre-existing cirrhosis responded to IFN-α, and only 4 of them experienced liver-related complications or death. Multivariate analysis indicated that cirrhosis and nonresponse status were associated with hazard ratios for liver complications or death of 30.0 and 13.7, respectively.

Conclusions.—Patients with chronic hepatitis B who respond initially to IFN-α typically retain their improvements in immunologic status over time. Patients with pretreatment cirrhosis were particularly likely to respond to IFN-α. Also, patients with pretreatment cirrhosis who responded to IFN-α had significantly fewer liver-related complications and significantly lower mortality rates compared with those with cirrhosis who did not respond to therapy. Black patients were more likely to respond to therapy (5 of 6, or 87%) than white patients (26 of 97, or 27%); further studies are needed to examine these race differences in IFN-α response rates.

► Chronic infection with HBV affects an estimated 1 million Americans[1] and is a major cause of cirrhosis and hepatocellular carcinoma. IFN-α induces remission in 25% to 40% of patients with a follow-up duration of up to 2 years.

Lau et al. evaluated the long-term survival and clinical outcome of patients treated with INF-α. Overall, they had a 30% response rate. Long-term follow-up to 11 years showed that liver-related complication-free survival was better among patients who responded to IFN-α therapy than among nonresponders. Thus, we need to treat patients with HBV infection, for if they respond, their long-term survival will be altered.

J.S. Barkin, M.D.

Reference

1. Alter MJ, Mast EE: The epidemiology of viral hepatitis in the United States. *Gastroenterol Clin North Am* 23:437-455, 1994.

Hepatitis C

Early HCV RNA Values After Interferon Predict Response

Wiley TE, Briedi L, Lam N, et al (Univ of Illinois, Chicago)

Dig Dis Sci 43:2169-2172, 1998 6–5

Background.—In patients with chronic hepatitis C virus (HCV) infection who are treated with interferon-α (INF-α), numerous studies have suggested that the extent of HCV RNA clearance at 1 or 3 months can predict the patient's response at the end of therapy. These authors examined whether the extent of HCV RNA clearance at 48 hours can predict the response to 6 months of INF-α therapy.

Methods.—The subjects were 23 patients with HCV (16 men and 7 women, mean age 46) who had never received INF-α before. One patient had HCV genotype 2b, 2 patients had genotype 3a, and the remaining 20 patients had genotype 1a or 1b. Patients were treated with a standard intravenous dose of INF-α (3×10^6 IU) 3 times a week for 6 months. At baseline, 24 and 48 hours, and 1, 3, and 6 months after the first injection, blood samples were drawn for measuring serum HCV RNA levels by branched-chain DNA analysis and polymer chain reaction.

Findings.—Compared with baseline (6.0 ± 1.6 mEq/mL), HCV RNA levels were significantly lower at 24 hours (2.4 ± 0.7 mEq/mL) and 48 hours (4.3 ± 1.1 mEq/mL); although levels rose by 48 hours, this increase was not statistically significant compared with the 24-hour level. Compared with 48-hour levels, HCV RNA levels at 1 and 6 months did not decrease significantly. At 48 hours, 17 patients were positive for HCV RNA; all 17 were still positive for HCV RNA at 1 and 3 months. All of these patients had HCV genotype 1a or 1b. Eight of these patients discontinued therapy after 3 months because of lack of HCV RNA clearance. In the remaining 9 patients who completed 6 months of INF-α therapy, no further clearance of HCV RNA occurred. At 48 hours, 6 patients were negative for HCV RNA; 3 were still negative at 6 months. All 3 of these patients had genotypes other than 1a or 1b, and all had baseline HCV RNA levels of 1.0 mEq/mL or less.

Conclusions.—HCV RNA levels measured 48 hours after the first dose of INF-α can predict levels after 1, 3, and 6 months of therapy. None of the patients in whom branched-chain DNA analysis detected HCV RNA at 48 hours had a further lowering of HCV RNA levels after up to 6 months of therapy. Furthermore, none of the patients with HCV genotype 1a or 1b responded to standard INF-α therapy.

► The authors of this study use a small patient population to suggest that "if HCV (hepatitis C virus) RNA levels are not rapidly reduced to levels that are undetectable by bDNA by 48 hours, the levels will not be further lowered during 6 months of standard IFN-α (interferon-α)." This seems to represent, in part, an especially poor response to IFN treatment for patients infected with genotypes 1a and 1b. A review of their data shows that none of twenty patients with genotype 1 HCV cleared the virus during 6 months of standard IFN dosing. This might suggest that treatment of patients with genotype 1 HCV is futile; however, even though genotype 1 is the most recalcitrant to IFN, common experience suggests a response rate of 10% to 15%. Although this paper is intriguing, the small study size and the results that superficially conflict with previously published data minimize its applicability to clinical practice.

M.J. Bernstein, M.D.

Interferon Alfa-2b Alone or in Combination With Ribavirin as Initial Treatment for Chronic Hepatitis C

McHutchison JG, for the Hepatitis Interventional Therapy Group (Scripps Clinic and Research Found, La Jolla, Calif; et al)

N Engl J Med 339:1485-1492, 1998 6–6

Background.—Interferon therapy is often used to treat patients with chronic hepatitis C virus (HCV) infection, but in at least 15% of these patients cirrhosis will develop. Thus, methods to improve the effectiveness of interferon therapy are needed, and some studies suggest that the combination of interferon and ribavirin is more effective than interferon therapy alone. This study compared interferon alone and in combination with ribavarin to determine safety, efficacy, and optimal dosing scheme.

Methods.—The participants were 912 patients with chronic HCV infection who were randomized into 4 groups. In the interferon alone groups (n = 456), patients received recombinant interferon alfa-2b (3×10^6 U 3 times a week) plus placebo for either 24 weeks (n = 231) or 48 weeks (n = 225). In the combination groups (n = 456), patients received recombinant interferon alfa-2b (same dosage) plus ribavarin (1,000 or 1,200 mg/day, depending on the patient's weight) for either 24 weeks (n = 228) or 48 weeks (n = 228). All 4 groups were similar in age, gender, weight, pretreatment serum HCV RNA levels, HCV genotype, and incidence of cirrhosis. Patients were evaluated regularly to measure serum levels of HCV RNA and aminotransferases, and 24 weeks after the end of treatment a liver biopsy was performed.

Findings.—Based on serum HCV RNA levels, patients receiving combination therapy for 48 weeks had a significantly better response than those receiving combination therapy for 24 weeks (38% vs. 31%, respectively) (Table 3). Both of these groups had a significantly better response than patients receiving interferon alone for 48 weeks (13%), and all 3 groups had a significantly better response than patients receiving interferon alone for 24 weeks (6%). The same pattern was seen in biochemical responses, with significant differences among combination therapy for 48 weeks (34%), combination therapy for 24 weeks (26%), interferon alone for 48 weeks (12%), and interferon alone for 24 weeks (5%). Based on liver biopsy findings, patients taking combination therapy for 24 or 48 weeks had a significantly better response than those receiving interferon alone for 24 or 48 weeks (57% and 61% vs. 44% and 41%). In the 72% of patients with HCV genotype 1 infection, combination treatment for 48 weeks was 4 times as effective as interferon alone for 48 weeks (28% vs. 7%). Adverse events, however, were more common with combination therapy, and in 8% of patients the dose of ribavarin was reduced because of the development of anemia. With either combination therapy or inter-

TABLE 3.—Rates of Histologic Response

Variable	Interferon		Interferon and Ribavirin	
	24 Wk (N=176)	48 Wk (N=158)	24 Wk (N=179)	48 Wk (N=157)
Change in inflammation score†				
All patients				
Percent with improvement	44	41	57	61
Mean change	−0.6	−1.0	−1.8‡	−2.4§
Patients with a response				
Percent with improvement	89	78	88	86
Mean change	−3.8	−5.2	−4.4	−4.5
Patients with a relapse or no response				
Percent with improvement	41	35	41	39
Mean change	−0.4	−0.3	−0.6	−0.5
Change in fibrosis score¶				
All patients				
Percent with improvement	11	17	16	14
Mean change	0.1	−0.1	0.0	0.0
Patients with a response				
Percent with improvement	11	26	24	16
Mean change	−0.2	−0.2	−0.2	−0.1
Patients with a relapse or no response				
Percent with improvement	11	16	12	12
Mean change	0.1	0.0	0.2	0.2

*The numbers of patients are the numbers with pretreatment and posttreatment biopsy specimens.

†Scores could range from 0 to 18, with higher scores indicating more severe abnormalities. Improvement was defined as a decrease in the inflammation score of at least 2 points, no change as an increase or decrease of 1 point, and worsening as an increase of at least 2 points.

‡P = 0.0005 for the comparison with 48 weeks of treatment with interferon alone.

§P less than 0.001 for the comparison with 48 weeks of treatment with interferon alone.

¶Scores could range from 0 (no fibrosis) to 4 (cirrhosis). Improvement was defined as a decrease of at least 1 point in the score.

(Reprinted by permission of The New England Journal of Medicine from McHutchison JG, for the Hepatitis Interventional Therapy Group: Interferon Alfa-2b alone or in combination with ribavirin as initial treatment for chronic hepatitis C. *N Engl J Med* 339:1485-1492.)

feron alone, adverse events were higher after 48 weeks of treatment than after 24 weeks.

Conclusions.—Based on virologic, biochemical, and histologic end points, combination therapy with interferon alfa-2b and ribavirin is more effective in treating chronic HCV infection than is interferon alone. Treatment for 48 weeks was more effective than treatment for 24 weeks, but the incidence of adverse events was higher with longer dosing.

Treating Histologically Mild Chronic Hepatitis C: Monotherapy, Combination Therapy, or Tincture of Time?

Levine RA (State Univ of New York)

Ann Intern Med 129:323-326, 1998 6–7

Background.—Of the approximately 4 million cases of hepatitis C virus (HCV) infection, only about 25% will progress to cirrhosis, and the risk of progression is even less in those individuals with histologically mild disease. In this editorial, the author argues for deferring interferon monotherapy in appropriate patients until combination treatments become available.

Selecting Which Patients to Treat.—Interferon-α monotherapy is expensive, causes significant adverse effects, and frequently is ineffective. Recent trials comparing interferon monotherapy with interferon plus ribavirin show that the combination is more effective and more likely to cause clearance of HCV RNA. Therefore, unless the patient is at risk of progression to cirrhosis, why subject him or her to interferon monotherapy when combination therapies are more effective? The greatest risk of progression to cirrhosis occurs in patients who have portal or bridging fibrosis or moderate inflammation and necrosis on biopsy. Patients with histologically mild HCV (stage 1 fibrosis, grade 1 necroinflammatory activity) are not likely to progress to cirrhosis, and thus they may not need immediate treatment. These patients are much more likely to receive more benefit from the increased effectiveness of newer therapies under evaluation. Patients with mild HCV and persistently normal alanine aminotransferase (ALT) levels offer a particular treatment challenge. These patients often respond to interferon monotherapy with a persistent elevation in ALT levels and no improvement in HCV RNA clearance. However, they rarely progress to cirrhosis; therefore, delaying interferon monotherapy until more effective treatments become available seems prudent. But it must be mentioned that some patients (i.e., pregnant women, surgeons) may want to undergo interferon monotherapy in the hope of clearing active HCV infection, and in these circumstances treatment seems warranted.

Advances in Treatment.—On the basis of current experience, patients with mild HCV who respond to a 6- or 12-month course of interferon-α with clearance of HCV RNA can generally be expected to maintain this response. More recently it has been discovered that the sustained virologic response rate can be improved with the addition of ribavirin to interferon-α therapy. In addition, consensus interferon, a new synthetic type 1 interferon, is useful in treating relapses after interferon monotherapy. Thus, newer drugs and regimens are more appropriate than interferon monotherapy for treating patients with mild HCV. The near future promises to refine treatment strategies for optimal effectiveness, such as higher or daily doses of interferon and gradual drug withdrawal or maintenance therapies. Other strategies under investigation include conjugating interferon to polyethylene glycol to improve its efficacy, immunotherapies such as adding interleukin-10 to boost the host immune response, interfering with serine protease or RNA polymerase activity with protease inhibitors, and blocking viral gene expression with antisense nucleic acids.

▶ In anticipation of FDA approval of ribavirin/interferon combination therapy for hepatitis C virus (HCV), many hepatologists advocated deferring interferon monotherapy. These doctors justified this along 3 major points. Most important, combination therapy would maximize the number of patients who would achieve a sustained response. Second, the use of combination therapy as initial therapy would limit the number of patients forced to endure an incompletely successful course of monotherapy followed by a second interferon-containing regimen. Finally, because liver failure or hepatocellular carcinoma develops in only 20% to 25% of patients with chronic HCV and the progression of these complications occurs over decades, waiting for improved therapy might have a small price with respect to overall clinical outcome. Although not specifically addressing the issues surrounding monotherapy and combination therapy, the ideas behind the foregoing arguments are well communicated in a perspective editorial written by Dr. Robert Levine from Syracuse.

For those who chose to delay interferon monotherapy until combination therapy became widely available, a paper produced by the Hepatitis Interventional Therapy Group (Abstract 6–6) seems to have justified their decision. The article convincingly demonstrates that treatment with ribavirin/interferon, when compared with interferon monotherapy, produced a higher percentage of patients who responded to treatment and maintained a sustained response. Furthermore, combination therapy was complicated by only a modest increase in adverse effects. For patients with genotype 1, 48 weeks of therapy has a significant advantage over 24 weeks of treatment. For patients with genotype 2 or 3, 24 weeks of therapy was as effective as more prolonged treatment. Furthermore, as might be expected, the response in patients with HCV genotype 2 or 3 was much more consistent than in those with genotype 1. Whether patients with genotype 2 or 3 should receive only 6 months of treatment is debatable, because up to one out of three patients will experience relapse and individual physicians and their patients might reasonably desire subsequent re-treatment with a full year of therapy.

Let us now return our attention to Dr. Levine's position statement (Abstract 6–7). Dr. Levine by no means rejects current interferon-based therapies, but he does suggest the validity of deferring therapy in a subset of patients who have histologically mild hepatitis C. Even with the recent FDA approval of combination therapy for the treatment of interferon-naïve HCV patients, Dr. Levine's arguments remain sound. According to genotypes, most patients treated with combination therapy for HCV will not have a sustained response. These patients will nonetheless be exposed to the adverse effects and the expense of interferon-based regimens. Selecting those patients who would be best served by deferring therapy and waiting for the inevitable availability of new treatments against HCV should be a cogent field for discussion.

M.J. Bernstein, M.D.

Re-treatment of Chronic Hepatitis C With Consensus Interferon

Heathcote EJL, and the Consensus Interferon Study Group (Univ of Toronto; et al)

Hepatology 27:1136-1143, 1998 6–8

Background.—With interferon-alfa (IFN-α) treatment for hepatitis C virus (HCV) infection, the overall sustained response rate is only 15% to 20%. This may be improved through the use of consensus interferon (CIFN), a genetically engineered novel type 1 interferon developed by use of the most frequent amino acid of several natural IFN-α subtypes. This study examined the use of CIFN for retreatment of patients with nonresponse or relapse after previous treatment with CIFN or IFN-α.

Methods.—The multicenter, open-label, phase 3 trial including 337 patients requiring retreatment for chronic HCV infection. Initial treatment consisted of 3 or 9 μg of CIFN or 3 million U of IFN-α-2b in a previous trial. The patients were randomly assigned to receive 24 or 48 weeks of CIFN, 15 μg subcutaneously. Both groups were then followed up for an additional 24 weeks. Response was assessed by measurement of alanine aminotransferase (ALT) and of HCV RNA.

Results.—The sustained response rate to retreatment was higher for patients who had relapses after initial therapy than for those who had no initial response. Among relapsers, the rate of sustained HCV RNA response was 58% in the 48-week treatment group vs. 28% in the 24-week

TABLE 6.—Predictive Factors of Retreatment Response

	Sustained Virologic Responders to Retreatment (n = 12)	Relapsers to Retreatment (n = 28)	Nonresponders to Retreatment (n = 62)
Median baseline viral value (PCR)*	0.5×10^6	5.0×10^6	4.8×10^6
% genotype 1	50%	67%	85%
Median baseline HAI score	5.0	5.5	6.5

NOTE: Predictive factors of response were calculated for patients retreated for 48 weeks with 15 μg of CIFN and excludes patients previously treated with 3 μg of CIFN.

(Courtesy of Heathcote EJL, and the Consensus Interferon Study Group: Re-treatment of chronic hepatitis C with consensus interferon. *Hepatology* 27:1136-1143, 1998.)

treatment group. The rate of sustained ALT response was 52% vs. 39%. Among patients with no initial response, the rate of sustained HCV RNA response was 13% in the 48-week group vs. 5% in the 24-week group; the rate of sustained ALT response was 17% vs. 12%, respectively. Retreatment with the higher dose of CIFN was well tolerated, with no increased rate of adverse effects. Baseline viral load and HCV genotype were significant predictors of virologic response to retreatment (Table 6).

Conclusions.—Patients with chronic HCV infection with relapse or nonresponse to initial interferon therapy may be safely and effectively retreated with a higher dose of CIFN. The chances of sustained response, as assessed by HCV RNA or ALT, are better for patients who responded than those who had relapses, compared with those who did not respond to initial treatment. The response rate is better with 48 weeks than with 24 weeks of CIFN retreatment.

Interferon-α-2B and Ribavirin in Combination for Chronic Hepatitis C Patients Not Responding to Interferon-α Alone: An Italian Multicenter, Randomized, Controlled, Clinical Study

Barbaro G, Di Lorenzo G, Soldini M, et al (Univ "La Sapienza," Rome; Univ of Torino, Italy; Univ of Pavia, Italy; et al)

Am J Gastroenterol 93:2445-2451, 1998 6–9

Introduction.—A long-term response to interferon alfa (IFN-α) is achieved in 10% to 20% of patients with chronic hepatitis C virus (HCV) infection. The nucleoside analog ribavirin may help to achieve a response in patients who do not respond to IFN-α alone. The combination of ribavirin and IFN-α2b was studied for use in patients with chronic hepatitis C who did not respond to treatment with IFN-α2b alone.

Methods.—The multicenter, randomized trial included 303 patients with chronic hepatitis C who had no serologic and histologic response to previous IFN-α2b therapy at the standard dosage of 3 MU 3 times weekly. One group received recombinant IFN-α2b at the standard dosage plus oral ribavirin, 1,000 to 1,200 mg/d; the other group received recombinant IFN-α-2b at a dosage of 6 MU 3 times weekly. Both treatments continued for 24 weeks, with an additional 24 weeks of follow-up after treatment. Response was assessed in terms of alanine aminotransferase (ALT) level and HCV RNA titer.

Results.—At the end of the treatment period, the ALT concentration was normal in 65% of patients receiving IFN-α plus ribavirin vs. 23% of those receiving IFN-α only. The rate of sustained biochemical response at 48 weeks was 39% vs. 10%. For patients receiving the combination therapy, HCV RNA became undetectable in 41% of patients with a biochemical response at 24 weeks, and remained undetectable in 23 patients with sustained biochemical responses at 48 weeks. For patients receiving IFN-α only, HCV RNA became undetectable in 24% of patients with a biochemical response at 24 weeks and remained undetectable in 2 patients with a sustained biochemical response at 48 weeks. Compliance was high in both groups.

Conclusions.—For patients with chronic hepatitis C with no response to standard IFN-α therapy, a combination of IFN-α and ribavirin provides a chance of a sustained biochemical and virologic response. The results of retreatment with a higher dose of IFN-α are not satisfactory. Further study is needed to determine the ability of long-term combination therapy to induce prolonged remission.

▶ Previously established interferon dosing schedules for the treatment of chronic hepatitis C have a poor therapeutic index. More than half of patients either do not have a biochemical or virologic response. Of the patients with initial response, many experience relapse after interferon therapy is discontinued. Treatment options for these patients are being developed. These articles (Abstracts 6–8 and 6–9) describe 2 studies among many others that describe alternative interferon regimens and combination regimens as management options for patients who have not experienced sustained response after initial interferon treatment.

Abstract 6–8 represents the work of the Consensus Interferon Study Group. The article validates the use of high-dose consensus interferon (15 μg) 3 times a week in the treatment of patients with hepatitis C with either no response to, or relapse after 24 weeks of prior lower-dose interferon therapy. This multicenter North American study randomly assigned patients to receive either 24 weeks or 48 weeks of CIFN and demonstrated especially favorable responses among patients who had relapses after therapy. Still, a significant response rate was seen among patients who were nonresponders to initial treatment regimens. From the data presented here, it seems that the improved response resulted from the dosage increment, but contributions from unique characteristics of CIFN cannot be excluded.

Abstract 6–9 was based on data obtained in Italy. The population differs from that used in the previously described article in 2 important ways. First, Barbaro and colleagues examined only patients who had not responded to initial interferon therapy; patients who had relapses were excluded from this analysis. Second, there was a notably lower percentage of patients with genotype 1, which is the subtype most refractory to interferon therapy. Patients were randomly assigned to receive either combination interferon-ribavirin therapy, or high-dose IFN-α2b. The importance of the study is its development of a significant role for combined interferon-ribavirin therapy in the management of patients with no response to monotherapy.

These are 2 of many investigations of a type that will be featured at meetings of hepatology specialists and discussion groups over the next few years. Although new drugs will always be developed, so far interferon alone or in combination has been at the foundation of hepatitis C therapy. New dosing regimens, different interferon types, and combination protocols will continue to evolve and will be tested for efficacy, safety, and tolerability. It seems likely, however, that for now both high-dose CIFN and combined interferon-ribavirin remain valid therapeutic options for patients in whom established front-line interferon therapy has previously failed.

M.J. Bernstein, M.D.

Retinal Complications and Plasma C5a Levels During Interferon Alpha Therapy for Chronic Hepatitis C

Sugano S, Suzuki T, Watanabe M, et al (Saiseikai Wakakusa Hosp, Yokohama, Japan)

Am J Gastroenterol 93:2441-2444, 1998 6–10

Background.—Patients receiving interferon alfa (IFN-α) therapy for chronic viral hepatitis may experience retinal complications, including retinal hemorrhage or cotton-wool spots. These complications are usually reversible, but their pathogenesis is uncertain. A previous study reported that patients treated with IFN-α with retinal hemorrhage have high levels of plasma-activated complement 5 (C5a), which induces intravascular granulocyte clumping. This study assessed the link between retinal complications and C5a levels in patients receiving IFN-α therapy for chronic hepatitis C.

Methods.—The study included 45 new patients with chronic hepatitis C (23 men and 22 women; age range, 32 to 65 years). Patients with diabetes mellitus or hypertension were excluded. Twenty-five patients were being treated with IFN-α2b, 10 MU/d for 2 weeks then 3 times weekly for 22 weeks. This group underwent optic fundus examination before the start of treatment and every 4 weeks thereafter, as well as whenever they developed visual symptoms. C5a levels were measured at frequent intervals from before to 24 weeks of treatment, or whenever a retinal complication was discovered. Regular optic fundus examinations were also performed in 20 control subjects who did not receive IFN, some of whom also underwent serial C5a measurements.

Results.—None of the patients had retinal hemorrhage or cotton-wool spots before the start of treatment. Twenty-four percent of patients receiving IFN-α therapy developed retinal hemorrhage, with 5 of the 6 episodes occurring within the first 8 weeks of treatment. Three of the 6 affected patients had visual symptoms, and 4 developed cotton-wool spots. Both retinal complications resolved over time, even though IFN-α therapy continued.

Before the start of IFN-α, and throughout the study in IFN-untreated controls, C5a levels were less than 7 ng/mL. The development of retinal hemorrhage was associated with increased C5a concentrations (mean, 27 ng/mL). This compared with mean C5a values of 5 to 6 ng/mL in the same patients before and after retinal hemorrhage, in IFN-treated patients without retinal hemorrhage, and in IFN-untreated controls.

Conclusions.—About one fourth of patients receiving IFN-α for chronic hepatitis C develop retinal hemorrhage or cotton-wool spots. These complications are associated with increased levels of C5a, which may play a pathogenetic role in retinal capillary infarction, hemorrhage, and cotton-wool spot formation. The retinal complications are symptomatic in half of affected patients and generally resolve over time.

▶ This study demonstrates retinal complications that seem associated with interferon treatment for chronic hepatitis C. The complications were usually minor and did not necessitate the discontinuation of therapy. The dose of interferon used in this study was higher than doses conventionally prescribed for hepatitis C in North American centers. Still, as higher doses and induction dosing are explored, we may need to be increasingly cautious to monitor patients for ophthalmologic complications.

M.J. Bernstein, M.D.

Hepatitis C Infection Risk Analysis: Who Should Be Screened? Comparison of Multiple Screening Strategies Based on the National Hepatitis Surveillance Program

Lapane KL, Jakiche AF, Sugano D, et al (Mem Hosp of Rhode Island, Pawtucket; Brown Univ, Providence, RI; Cleveland Clinic Found, Ohio; et al)
Am J Gastroenterol 93:591-596, 1998 6–11

Background.—Hepatitis C virus (HCV) is a public health problem. Most of those individuals infected with HCV are viremic and constitute a disease reservoir, even when they are asymptomatic. Identification of infected individuals could lead to the reduction of transmission of the virus, both through education and the elimination of viremia. Although universal blood testing is currently too expensive, a selective screening strategy would reduce both costs and viremia. Several selective screening strategies

TABLE 1.—Risk Factors for Hepatitis C Identified by Logistical Regression Model*

Risk Factors	Odds Ratio	95% Confidence Interval
Socially intrusive risk factors		
History of IV drug use	12.9	9.7-17.1
History of sex with IV drug user	4.4	3.2-6
Socially Nonintrusive risk factors		
History of transfusion	2.9	2.3-3.6
Age 30-49 yr	2.4	1.6-3.5
Male gender	2.2	1.8-2.7

*Other variables in the model and corresponding odds ratio (95% confidence intervals): Age > 50, 1.0 (0.7-1.6); gender missing, 3.1 (1.9-5.1); health professional, 0.56 (0.4-0.8); hemodialysis, 5.5 (2.3-13.0); history of transfusion missing, 0.5 (0.2-0.9); hemodialysis missing, 0.8 (0.4-1.3); history IV drug user missing 4.0 (2.6-6.2); hepatitis B vaccination, 0.6 (0.4-0.9); hepatitis B vaccination missing, 0.6 (0.4-0.8).

TABLE 2.—Performance Characteristics of Screening Strategies for Hepatitis C

Screening Strategy	Prevalence	Positive Predictive Value	Sensitivity	Negative Predictive Value	Specificity
Model 1*	20%	22%	65%	97%	84%
Model 2†	29%	16%	69%	97%	74%
Model 3‡	25%	14%	53%	96%	77%
Model 4§	12%	34%	63%	97%	92%

*Model 1, screening individuals with probability ≥7% using the mathematical predictive equation.

†Model 2, screening individuals with any socially intrusive risk factors (history of IV drug use, history of sex with IV drug user) or socially nonintrusive risk factors (history of blood transfusion, male gender, age 30-49 years).

‡Model 3, screening individuals with 2 or more socially nonintrusive risk factors.

§Model 4, performing ALT on all, followed by enzyme-linked immunosorbant assay on those with elevated ALT.

(Reprinted by permission of the publisher from Lapane KL, Jakiche AF, Sugano D, et al: Hepatitis C infection risk analysis: Who should be screened? Comparison of multiple screening strategies based on the National Hepatitis Surveillance Program. *Am J Gastroenterol* 93:591-596. Copyright 1998 from Elsevier Science Inc.)

were assessed with the use of the National Hepatitis Surveillance Program database to determine which one was the most cost-effective.

Study Design.—The National Hepatitis Surveillance Program database is composed of 13,997 individuals who self-referred themselves for viral hepatitis screening at 40 urban hospitals in the United States. Participants completed a risk profile questionnaire that included demographic, symptomatic, behavioral, and medical information. This study is based on the 9,269 of these questionnaires that contained sufficient information. Four strategies were considered: Model 1 employed a predictive equation with a cutoff; Model 2 employed a questionnaire that asked all questions; Model 3 omitted socially intrusive questions; and Model 4 was based on serum alanine aminotransferase (ALT) testing. Socially intrusive questions included those about the patient's history of drug use and history of sex with IV drug user. Socially nonintrusive questions were those that addressed age, gender and blood transfusion history. Cost per case was calculated for each of the 4 models.

Results.—The sensitivity of Model 1 was 65%, and the specificity was 84%. The sensitivity of Model 2 was 69%, and the specificity was 74%.

TABLE 3.—Cost Efficiency of Screening Strategies for Hepatitis C

Screening Strategy	Cases Detected/100 Screened	Cost/100 Screened	Average Cost/Case Detected	Marginal Cost/Case Detected*
Model 1	4.4	$1571	$ 357	Dominates†
Model 2	4.6	$2020	$ 439	$285
Model 3	3.5	$1706	$ 487	Base case
Model 4	4.1	$4292	$1047	$4310

*This incremental analysis starts with the least expensive strategy (Model 3) and computes the incremental cost to find 1 additional case using alternative strategies.

†Model 1 is both more effective and less expensive than Model 3 (i.e., dominates).

(Reprinted by permission of the publisher from Lapane KL, Jakiche AF, Sugano D, et al: Hepatitis C infection risk analysis: Who should be screened? Comparison of multiple screening strategies based on the National Hepatitis Surveillance Program. *Am J Gastroenterol* 93:591-596. Copyright 1998 from Elsevier Science Inc.)

The sensitivity of Model 3 was 53%, and the specificity was 77%. The sensitivity of Model 4 was 63% and the specificity was 92% (Tables 1 and 2). The cost per case was $357 for Model 1, $439 for Model 2, $487 for Model 3, and $1,047 for Model 4 (Table 3).

Conclusions.—The cost of screening for HCV compares favorably with accepted screening practices for other diseases. Screening with the Model 2 that was presented by this article seems appropriate for most medical settings, but screening directly with the HCV enzyme-linked immunosorbant assay is the most cost-effective method. Screening with Models 1 or 3 may be appropriate in some circumstances.

► The authors of this article rely on advanced statistical modeling and information from a selected database to determine who should be screened for HCV and how that screening should be performed. Their analysis reveals some important HCV risk factors and elucidates some principles of screening. This article will be part of the larger bank of studies that will be required to adequately address this issue, because it has grown into a worldwide health dilemma. Unfortunately, the scope of the problem and the diverse populations that it affects prevent any isolated study from answering all pertinent questions regarding screening for HCV.

M.J. Bernstein, M.D.

Ibuprofen-induced Hepatotoxicity in Patients With Chronic Hepatitis C: A Case Series

Riley TR III, Smith JP (Pennsylvania State Univ, Hershey)

Am J Gastroenterol 93:1563-1565, 1998 6–12

Background.—Nonsteroidal anti-inflammatory drugs (NSAIDs) are among the most frequently prescribed medications. Patients with hepatitis C virus (HCV) infection often complain of arthralgias, and frequently use NSAIDs to deal with this pain. NSAID-induced hepatitis flare-ups in 3 patients with chronic hepatitis were reported.

> *Care Report.*—White man, 33, was discovered to have abnormal liver transaminase levels during evaluation for infertility. Serum levels of HCV-RNA were 2,400,000 copies/mL. Percutaneous liver biopsy revealed chronic active hepatitis, with a Knodell score of 6 of 22. Baseline liver transaminase values were aspartate aminotransferase (AST) 63 U/L, and alanine aminotransferase (ALT) 212 U/L. A sudden increase in AST/ALT to 459/1,209 U/L was detected after the patient ingested 800 mg of ibuprofen. Levels returned to baseline within 3 months. Six months later, after the patient again ingested 800 mg ibuprofen, there was another increase in AST/ALT to 524/1285. Three months after discontinuation of ibuprofen, transaminase levels had returned to baseline again.

Conclusions.—This report describes 3 patients with chronic HCV infection who developed a greater than 5-fold elevation of liver transaminase levels after ingestion of ibuprofen. All transaminase levels returned to baseline within 3 months after discontinuation of ibuprofen. One patient demonstrated a second temporary increase in transaminase levels after a rechallenge with ibuprofen. Based on these findings, it is recommended that patients with chronic HCV infection should not use NSAIDs and should instead use acetaminophen, at a dose of no more than 2 g/24 hr, when necessary. If NSAIDs are necessary, careful monitoring of liver function should accompany use. Further study with a larger group of patients with chronic HCV is required to develop a rational approach to NSAID use in this population.

▶ Many physicians are reluctant to prescribe acetaminophen to patients with chronic hepatitis who are in need of low-potency analgesics. Their fears stem from the risk of severe hepatic injury that can be caused by significant, usually intentional, acetaminophen overdose. These fears are augmented by the recognition of the "therapeutic misadventure" that is hepatotoxicity from relatively unimpressive acetaminophen consumption by patients who are predisposed to this toxicity because of malnutrition and/or alcohol consumption.

NSAIDs, including ibuprofen, might seem to be a good alternative to acetaminophen when treating patients who have chronic hepatitis C. However, ibuprofen (even in standard doses) is associated with gastrointestinal injury, renal toxicity, and, as the authors demonstrate in this case series, marked hepatotoxicity. In their discussion, Drs Riley and Smith remind us that acetaminophen, especially in doses of less than 2 g over 24 hours, can be safely administered to patients with liver disease.

M.J. Bernstein, M.D.

Liver Transplantation

Outcome of Hepatitis C Patients With and Without Hepatocellular Carcinoma Undergoing Liver Transplant

Min AD, Saxena R, Thung SN, et al (Mount Sinai Med Ctr, New York)
Am J Gastroenterol 93:2148-2153, 1998 6–13

Purpose.—Infection with hepatitis C virus (HCV) has been linked to hepatocellular carcinoma (HCC). End-stage HCV cirrhosis is the major indication for liver transplantation, a therapy thought to have poor results in patients with HCC. The clinical characteristics and outcomes of liver transplantation were compared in patients with HCV cirrhosis who did and did not have HCC.

Patients.—The retrospective study included 55 patients undergoing transplantation for HCV cirrhosis in whom HCC was identified in the explanted liver. The group included 37 men and 18 women, mean age, 58 years. They were compared with 55 age- and sex-matched patients undergoing transplantation for HCV cirrhosis who did not have HCC. All

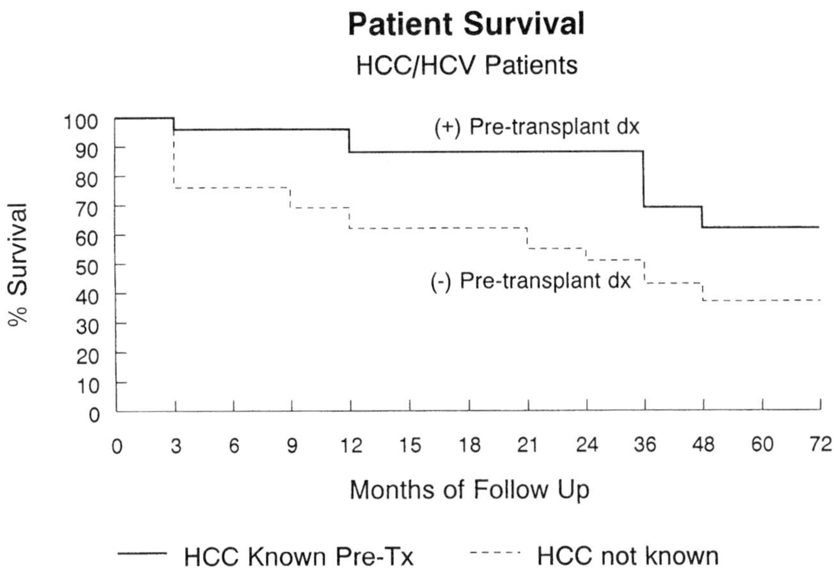

FIGURE 3.—Kaplan-Meier curves for patient survival after liver transplantation among patients with hepatocellular carcinoma (HCC) who were diagnosed with HCC before transplant (*solid line*) or who had incidental HCC on explants (*broken line*). The patient survival between the 2 groups was categorized according to the positive or negative pretransplant diagnosis of HCC was not significantly different by the log-rank test (p greater than 0.05). (Reprinted by permission of the publisher from Min AD, Saxena R, Thung SN, et al: Outcome of hepatitis C patients with and without hepatocellular carcinoma undergoing liver transplant. *Am J Gastroenterol* 93:2148-2153. Copyright 1998 by Elsevier Science Inc.)

patients had no history of alcohol abuse and were negative for hepatitis B surface antigen.

Findings.—The 2 groups were similar in terms of Child's class and United Network for Organ Sharing status when they received their transplants. In 45% of the HCC group, the presence of HCC was suspected before transplantation. A single focus of HCC was found in 46% of patients. Previous interferon therapy had been given in 14% of the HCC group and 12% of the non-HCC group. All interferon therapy was given within 5 years of liver transplantation and lasted 1 to 9 months. Two thirds of the HCC group were either IV drug users or had a history of transplantation. A history of parental exposure was also found in 58% of the non-HCC group. Patient survival and graft survival were comparable for patients with and without HCC (Fig 3).

Conclusions.—In about half of HCC cases accompanying HCV cirrhosis, the presence of HCC is not suspected before liver transplantation. Transplant patients with and without HCC are similar in terms of mode of HCV transmission, clinical status at transplant time, and results of transplantation. With careful patient selection, the presence of HCC should not be regarded as a contraindication to liver transplant for HCV cirrhosis.

▶ HCC is a known complication of many diseases that can lead to liver failure, including hepatitis C. Immunosuppression, required for the success of an organ transplant, could facilitate the progression of a malignant neoplasm. Therefore, in many circumstances, the presence of a malignancy or even recent history of a resected tumor is an absolute contraindication to transplantation. Nonetheless, liver transplantation has been performed on patients with HCC and respectable outcomes have been reported. While this study, researched from clinical data obtained at the Mount Sinai Medical Center, lacks the statistical power to prove that HCC does not compromise outcome after liver transplant, it does suggest that, when carefully selected, patients with HCC can benefit from liver transplantation.

M.J. Bernstein, M.D.

Outcomes Analysis in 100 Liver Transplantation Patients

Geevarghese SK, Bradley AE, Wright JK, et al (Vanderbilt Univ, Nashville, Tenn)

Am J Surg 175:348-353, 1998 6–14

Background.—Today's medical payors demand to know that what they are paying for is worth it. Thus, outcomes analysis is becoming increasingly important. These authors reviewed outcomes in patients undergoing liver transplantation, assessing clinical, surgical, and quality-of-life outcomes in light of cost-containment measures.

Methods.—Between February 1991 and March 1996, 100 patients (68 men and 32 women; mean age, 46 years) underwent liver transplantation. Standard patient protocols were used to provide evaluation, perioperative hospital care, and long-term follow-up care. Halfway through enrollment, the protocols were revised to improve quality and cost-effectiveness, thus allowing comparison of the effects of the cost containment measures during the second half of the study. Clinical and surgical outcomes were gathered from medical records and follow-up visits. Quality of life was measured objectively by the Karnofsky Performance Index (a scale of 0 to 100, with 100 representing normal function) and subjectively by the Psychosocial Adjustment to Illness Scale (a 46-item questionnaire covering 7 domains of psychosocial adjustment) at regular intervals up to 6 years after treatment. Costs were calculated from billing records.

Findings.—Kaplan-Meier actuarial survival at 1 and 6 months and 1, 2, and 3 to 5 years was 92%, 86%, 84%, 83%, and 78%. Survival of the first 50 patients did not differ significantly from that of the last 50 patients. Rates of complications (including 10 cases of graft failure, 26 cases of biliary complications, and 12 cases of renal failure) and episodes of rejection (46 cases) also did not differ between the first and last 50 patients. Objective measures of quality of life before surgery reflected the patients' poor performance status, with a mean Karnofsky score of 53 ± 2. After surgery, however, performance status improved quickly and significantly, with scores of 72 ± 2 at 3 months, 90 ± 1 at 1 year, and 97 ± 1 at 5 years. Furthermore, mean Karnofsky scores were significantly higher in the first 50 patients at 1 and 2 years (which is the extent of follow-up so far).

Subjective measures of quality of life also indicated significant improvement after surgery, particularly in sexual relationships and the domestic environment. Subjective measures did not differ between the first and last 50 patients. However, the median length of hospital stay declined significantly for the last 50 patients (19 vs. 11 days), as did the median hospital charges ($105,000 vs. $90,000).

Conclusions.—Liver transplantation significantly improves the patient's quality of life, with good 5-year survival rates. Cost-effectiveness can be achieved by establishing patient care protocols to improve quality while containing costs.

► More than anything else, this investigation demonstrates the importance of using medical data in developing guidelines for clinical care. For their purposes, the authors use their experience with liver transplantation as the study model. They showed that their successful outcome record was preserved, even when the study population faced more severe illness before transplantation. Furthermore, many costs were contained and even reduced by the implementation of well-thought-out clinical protocols.

The shortage of donor organs complicates liver transplantation by forcing caregivers to manage patients with liver failure for longer periods of time before transplantation. This forces transplant teams to operate on patients with ever more compromised clinical status. Skyrocketing medical costs only add to the difficulties. The collaborative liver transplantation team at Vanderbilt serves as a positive example of how, with diligent care, liver transplantation can remain a useful and practical treatment option in the management of end-stage liver disease.

M.J. Bernstein, M.D.

Colon Carcinoma in Patients Undergoing Liver Transplantation

Fabia R, Levy MF, Testa G, et al (Baylor Univ Med Ctr, Dallas)
Am J Surg 176:265-269, 1998 6–15

Background.—The risk for colon carcinoma may be especially high in organ transplant recipients with ulcerative colitis (UC). The incidence and pattern of colon carcinoma development in such patients were compared with those in transplant recipients without UC.

Methods and Findings.—Data on 1,085 liver transplant recipients were analyzed retrospectively. In the 1,022 patients without UC, adenocarcinoma developed in a colonic polyp in only 1 patient, for an incidence of less than 0.1%, 46 months after transplantation. By contrast, colon adenocarcinoma developed in 8% of liver recipients with UC, 22 to 66 months after liver transplantation. Two of the 5 patients with UC and colon adenocarcinoma died.

Conclusion.—Coexistent UC in patients needing liver transplantation appears to constitute a high risk for the development of colonic cancer, which develops late after transplantation. Such patients need to be followed closely, with frequent colonoscopic and histologic screening of the colon.

▶ UC and primary sclerosing cholangitis are major reasons for orthotopic liver transplantation. The consequences of colon carcinoma in an individual after liver transplantation are disastrous if the tumor is not identified at an early stage. Screening patients with UC using colonoscopy is difficult, even in the era of dysplasia, because the cancer found in UC is normally a flat, endophytic, spreading, poorly differentiated tumor.

The article from Dallas, reveals an 8% to 11% incidence of colon cancer in patients with longstanding UC who underwent orthotopic liver transplantation. An aggressive pretransplant screening of all patients with UC is essential. In fact, in a patient with dysplasia who is anticipating a transplant, it is reasonable to proceed with a colectomy. Patients who have UC, but no dysplasia who undergo liver transplantation also deserve frequent colonoscopic follow-up and screening to detect dysplasia or the occurrence of cancer.

This is a very controversial area and there are no concrete recommendations for the management of these individuals. The long-term consequences, however, are disastrous if an aggressive tumor develops and metastasizes. The policy of aggressive pretransplant screening and follow-up colonoscopy is, therefore, warranted.

J.W. Fleshman, Jr., M.D.

Quality of Life of Patients After Intestinal Transplantation

Rovera GM, DiMartini A, Schoen RE, et al (Univ of Pittsburgh Med Ctr, Pa)

Transplantation 66:1141-1145, 1998 6–16

Objective.—The quality of life (QOL) of patients who underwent intestinal transplantation (ITx) and patients receiving home parenteral nutrition (HPN) was compared in a cross-sectional analysis.

Methods.—The Quality of Life Inventory was self-administered by 10 surviving adult ITx patients, (average age, 34.2 years) with functioning grafts and 10 adult HPN patients (average age, 36.4 years), with irreversible intestinal failure. The longitudinal change in QOL was evaluated over an average of 1.3 to 2.7 years in 4 HPN and 4 ITx patients, respectively.

Results.—ITx patients were evaluated an average of 2.8 years after transplantation and an average of 5.1 years after intestinal failure. HPN patients were evaluated an average of 5.3 years after intestinal failure. QOL assessments differed significantly in only 2 of 25 domains—drug use and medical compliance. ITx patients reported significantly more drug use (sleep medication) and significantly less medical compliance (more difficulty taking medication on schedule, less likely to see a physician for physical problems, and less likely to report physical or emotional changes) than HPN patients. ITx patients reported significantly less anxiety, significantly improved sleep, and significantly less impulsiveness after transplantation.

Conclusion.—QOL was similar for ITx and HPN patients. QOL for ITx patients improved as they reported less anxiety, improved sleep, and less impulsiveness after surgery.

▶ This is an interesting paper in that it compares QOL after intestinal transplantation with total parenteral nutrition. The important finding is that very few of the patients who have undergone ITx reenter the work world. In fact, more patients receiving TPN actually return to work than those who have had ITx. Whereas both groups' QOL improved with time on their respective methods of treatment, there does seem to be some difference if fewer transplant patients return to work. Medical compliance was also lower in the transplant groups, which probably reflects the desire of these individuals to return to normal and the hope that they would no longer have to take immune suppressants, etc. One issue that does not enter this discussion but should eventually influence choice is the overall cost of each treatment. Certainly, studies have shown complication and survival rates as comparable, but the cost may actually determine the selection of the treatment in the future.

J.W. Fleshman, Jr., M.D.

Cirrhosis

Parenteral Antibiotic Prophylaxis of Bacterial Infections Does Not Improve Cost-Efficacy of Oral Norfloxacin in Cirrhotic Patients With Gastrointestinal Bleeding

Sàbat M, Kolle L, Soriano G, et al (Hospital de la Santa Creu i Sant Pau, Barcelona)

Am J Gastroenterol 93:2457-2462, 1998 6–17

Purpose.—Patients with cirrhosis and gastrointestinal (GI) bleeding are at high risk for nosocomial bacterial infection. Selective intestinal decontamination can reduce the risk with the use of norfloxacin. However, this prophylactic strategy may be ineffective in bleeding cirrhotic patients with ascites, encephalopathy, or shock. This randomized trial evaluated the efficacy of a short course of systemic ceftriaxone, in addition to oral norfloxacin, to prevent bacterial infections in cirrhotic patients with GI bleeding at high risk of infection.

Methods.—Of 140 cirrhotic patients with GI bleeding, 56 were identified at high risk of infection because of ascites, hepatic encephalopathy, or hypovolemic shock. All patients received oral norfloxacin, 400 mg every 12 hours for 7 days. In addition, 1 group received IV ceftriaxone, 2 g per day for the first 3 hospital days. The 2 treatments were compared for efficacy of selective intestinal decontamination, with close monitoring for bacterial infections and drug side effects.

Results.—The final analysis included 46 patients with 10 excluded because of community-acquired pneumonia, surgery, or death within 24 hours of admission. The rate of bacterial infections during hospitalization was not significantly different: 18.1% in the norfloxacin-only group and 12.5% in the norfloxacin plus ceftriaxone group. The rate of severe infections (i.e., spontaneous bacterial peritonitis, bacteremia, or pneumonia) was also similar: 9% and 8.3%, respectively. The higher cost of antibiotic therapy in the norfloxacin plus ceftriaxone group was not justified by any reduction in length of hospital stay or mortality.

Conclusions.—In cirrhotic patients with GI hemorrhage, adding IV ceftriaxone to oral norfloxacin does not improve the prophylactic efficacy of norfloxacin alone. There is no advantage in terms of the incidence of infections or severe infections, hospitalization duration, or mortality. Future studies might identify a subgroup of patients who could benefit from parenteral antibiotics.

► Infections, especially pneumonia and spontaneous bacterial peritonitis, can lead to further decompensation for patients with end-stage liver disease. Cirrhotic patients admitted to the hospital with GI bleeding are at high risk of infection. Instrumentation, especially injection sclerotherapy of esophageal varices, can lead to transient bacteremia. Antibiotic prophylaxis seems appealing in theory, but the benefits vs. the cost and the risk of selecting resistant organisms remain unproven. This study demonstrates no readily identified advantage to antibiotic prophylaxis with parenteral ceftriaxone and oral norfloxacin over norfloxacin alone. The authors refer to previous work to suggest an advantage to norfloxacin therapy over no prophylaxis; yet the routine use of antibiotic prophylaxis after a variceal hemorrhage has not been universally accepted.

M.J. Bernstein, M.D.

Does Transjugular Intrahepatic Portosystemic Shunt (TIPS) Resolve Thrombocytopenia Associated With Cirrhosis?

Jabbour N, Zajko A, Orons P, et al (Univ of Pittsburgh, Pa; Univ of Southern California, Los Angeles)

Dig Dis Sci 43:2459-2462, 1998 6–18

Background.—Thrombocytopenia is a common complication of liver cirrhosis, and it is believed to result from splenic congestion caused by portal hypertension. The transjugular intrahepatic portosystemic shunt (TIPS) has been introduced as a means of managing cirrhosis complicated by variceal bleeding or intractable ascites. The effect of the portal decompression of a TIPS on thrombocytopenia in patients with cirrhosis was evaluated.

Study Design.—The study group consisted of 22 female and 40 male patients with an average age of 54 years and who survived more than 1 month after a TIPS without requiring orthotopic liver transplantation. Indications for a TIPS were acute or uncontrollable recurrent variceal bleeding. Before the TIPS, all patients were examined by upper endoscopy

TABLE 3.—Follow-Up of Platelet Count After TIPS in Relation to Pre-TIPS Thrombocytopenia and Degree of Portal Decompression by TIPS

	Pre-TIPS Thrombocytopenia		No pre-TIPS Thrombocytopenia	
	Post-TIPS PSG < 12 mm Hg	Post-TIPs PSG ≥ 12 mm Hg	Post-TIPS PSG < 12 mm Hg	Post-TIPS PSG ≥ 12 mm Hg
Patients (*N*)	20	10	18	14
Mean PSG pre-TIPS	24.7 ± 6.2	30.8 ± 4.3	22.8 ± 4.3	27.3 ± 4.1
Mean PSG post-TIPS	7.9 ± 2.3	14.7 ± 2.9	7.6 ± 2.5	13.8 ± 2.5
Mean PL pre-TIPS	68 ± 21	75 ± 14	134 ± 38	176 ± 71
Mean PL at 1 month	85 ± 20	82 ± 18	173 ± 65	142 ± 32
Mean PL at 6 months	74 ± 28	65 ± 11	148 ± 54	146 ± 43
Mean PL at 12 months	71 ± 31	86 ± 12	142 ± 46	161 ± 49

PL, platelet count; *PSG*, portosystemic gradient.

(Courtesy of Jabbour N, Zajko A, Orons P, et al: Does transjugular intrahepatic portosystemic shunt (TIPS) resolve thrombocytopenia associated with cirrhosis? *Dig Dis Sci* 43:2459-2462, 1998. Plenum Publishing Corporation.)

and Doppler ultrasound, and their platelet counts were obtained. Portosystemic pressure gradient was assessed before and after the TIPS was in place. Patients were followed-up with physical examination, laboratory tests, and liver ultrasound with Doppler studies at 1 week, and 1 month and then at 3-month intervals.

Results.—The prevalence of thrombocytopenia in the study group was 49% before the TIPS. The patients with and without thrombocytopenia had similar demographics, degree of liver disease, portosystemic gradient, and clinical status. The TIPS had no effect on thrombocytopenia, even when the portosystemic gradient was reduced to less than 12 mm Hg (Table 3).

Conclusions.—Thrombocytopenia in patients with end-stage liver disease did not respond to the portal decompression induced by a TIPS. This indicates that the pathogenesis of thrombocytopenia in these patients is not completely explained by splenic congestion that occurs secondary to portal hypertension.

► TIPS has evolved into an established therapy in the management of portal hypertension-related esophagogastric variceal bleeding and ascites. Although, the technique has gained acceptance, it is not without risks. The greatest risk that there is about a 25% chance of further hepatic decompensation, which often manifests as new or more severe metabolic encephalopathy. Furthermore, maintaining the patency of a TIPS can be difficult and expensive, sometimes necessitating repeated or follow-up procedures.

Thrombocytopenia is a frequent complication of cirrhosis. It is commonly felt to be the result of portal hypertension and the subsequent splenic sequestration of platelets. Superficially, it would seem that by decreasing portal hypertension with a TIPS, physicians would be able to correct the underlying pathogenesis, which is described above, and improve the low platelet counts seen in patients with cirrhosis.

This study demonstrates that a TIPS procedure performed for the management of variceal hemorrhage is not an adequate treatment of thrombocytopenia that develops as a result of cirrhosis. If patients had undergone elective TIPS procedures solely for the management of low platelet counts (rather than for variceal hemorrhage), it seems possible—but unlikely—that the results would have been different. On the basis of available data, the TIPS cannot be routinely recommended for the management of thrombocytopenia. Furthermore, the pathogenesis of cirrhosis-associated thrombocytopenia seems more complex that the simplistic model outlined above.

M.J. Bernstein, M.D.

Hepatocellular Cancer

Risk Factors for Hepatocellular Carcinoma and Its Incidence After Interferon Treatment in Patients With Chronic Hepatitis C

Kasahara A, and the Osaka Liver Disease Study Group (Osaka Univ, Japan; et al)

Hepatology 27:1394-1402, 1998 6–19

Background.—Hepatocellular carcinoma (HCC) is a common malignancy in Southeast Asia. Chronic hepatitis C virus (HCV) infection has been linked to liver cirrhosis and HCC. In Japan, patients with chronic HCV infection are treated with interferon therapy to reduce serum alanine aminotransferase levels, HCV RNA levels, and cirrhosis. Between 15% and 35% of these patients are long-term responders to interferon therapy. The relationship between response to interferon therapy and the development of HCC among Japanese patients with chronic HCV infection was investigated.

Study Design.—The study group included 1,022 patients from 11 Japanese hospitals who had elevated serum alanine aminotransferase levels and histologically proven chronic hepatitis and who had undergone interferon treatment. The patients were categorized by response to interferon therapy into the following 3 groups: sustained responders, transient responders, and nonresponders. Patients were followed-up with ultrasonography and liver biopsy for a minimum of 13 months after interferon therapy.

Findings.—Of the 1,022 patients with chronic HCV patients in this study group, 313 had a sustained response, 304 had a transient response, and 405 had no response to interferon therapy. Of the 46 patients who developed HCC, 5 were sustained responders, 9 were transient responders, and 32 were nonresponders. The cumulative incidence of HCC was significantly higher in nonresponders than in either sustained or transient responders. There was no significant difference in the cumulative incidence of HCC among patients with different subtypes of HCV. Patients older than 55 years and male patients were at greater risk for developing HCC. The presence and degree of liver fibrosis were not significant risk factors for HCC.

Conclusions.—Patients with chronic HCV infections who respond to interferon treatment are at a significantly lower risk of developing HCC than nonresponders are, even if HCV is not eliminated. Patients with chronic HCV who are at particularly high risk for the development of HCC are older male patients who do not respond to interferon therapy, even transiently. These patients should be carefully monitored so that HCC may be detected as early as possible.

Retrospective Analysis of the Effect of Interferon Therapy on the Clinical Outcome of Patients With Viral Cirrhosis

Benvegnù L, Chemello L, Noventa F, et al (Univ of Padova, Italy; Univ of Verona, Italy)

Cancer 83:901-909, 1998 6–20

Background.—Liver cirrhosis is a risk factor for the development of hepatocellular carcinoma (HCC), especially when it is associated with chronic hepatitis. Interferon (IFN) treatment was shown to reduce viremia in a subset of patients with chronic hepatitis. The effect of IFN treatment on liver cirrhosis was retrospectively examined in patients with chronic hepatitis who were followed from 1986 to 1993.

Study Design.—The study group included 122 male and 67 female patients with biopsy-proven Child's stage A liver cirrhosis and ongoing hepatitis B or C infection. The average age of participants was 58.2 years and the average cirrhosis duration was 2.1 years at study entry. Of the 189 participants, 88 were treated with IFN. Patients were followed-up at 6-month intervals with abdominal ultrasound and laboratory tests. The average duration of follow-up was 71.5 months.

Findings.—Of the 88 treated patients, 8% experienced disease progression during follow-up, and of the 101 untreated patients, 22% experienced disease progression during follow-up. HCC developed in 6% of treated and 27% of untreated participants. During follow-up, 3% of treated and 20% of untreated patients died of their liver disease or had orthotopic liver transplants. With the use of the Cox regression analysis, it was found that no IFN treatment, high bilirubin levels, high alkaline phosphatase levels, low leukocyte counts, and low prothrombin (PT) activity were associated with increased liver cirrhosis. No treatment with IFN, long-term disease, low albumin and PT levels, and high γ-glutamyl transpeptidase levels were associated with HCC development. No IFN treatment, low albumin and PT levels, and high γ-glutamyl transpeptidase and alkaline phosphatase levels were significantly associated with survival reduction. Multivariate analysis indicated that IFN treatment was associated with significantly reduced disease progression in patients with hepatitis C.

Conclusions.—According to this retrospective analysis of a large cohort of patients with Child's Stage A liver cirrhosis, IFN treatment was associated with a reduced risk of disease progression and HCC development in patients with HCV. These conclusions need to be confirmed by large prospective clinical trials.

Relation of Interferon Therapy and Hepatocellular Carcinoma in Patients With Chronic Hepatitis C

Imai Y, for the Osaka Hepatocellular Carcinoma Prevention Study Group (Osaka Univ, Japan)

Ann Intern Med 129:94-99, 1998 6–21

Background.—Previous trials have shown that in patients with hepatitis C virus (HCV), interferon therapy can improve histologic findings, normalize serum alanine aminotransferase (ALT) levels, and eliminate serum HCV RNA. Whether interferon affects the incidence of hepatocellular cancer in patients with HCV was examined.

Methods.—The participants were 144 controls with chronic HCV or cirrhosis, who were not treated with interferon, and 419 patients with chronic HCV, who received interferon therapy for 6 months (median total interferon dose, 480 mU). All patients underwent liver biopsies for histologic staging. Abdominal ultrasonography or CT (to identify hepatocellular carcinomas) and measurements of ALT levels (to monitor the response to interferon) were performed regularly throughout follow-up, a median of 46.8 months for the controls and 47.6 months for the interferon group. A patient with a normal serum ALT level after interferon therapy that increased abnormally after therapy ended was said to have had a relapse.

Findings.—Of the 419 patients in the interferon group, there were 151 (36%) who had sustained responses, 120 (29%) who had relapses, and 148 (35%) who did not respond to therapy. During follow-up, hepatocellular carcinomas were significantly more common in the controls (19 patients, or 13.2%) than in the patients treated with interferon (28, or 6.6%) (Fig 2). Regression analysis indicated 4 independent risk factors for the development of hepatocellular carcinomas: interferon therapy, older

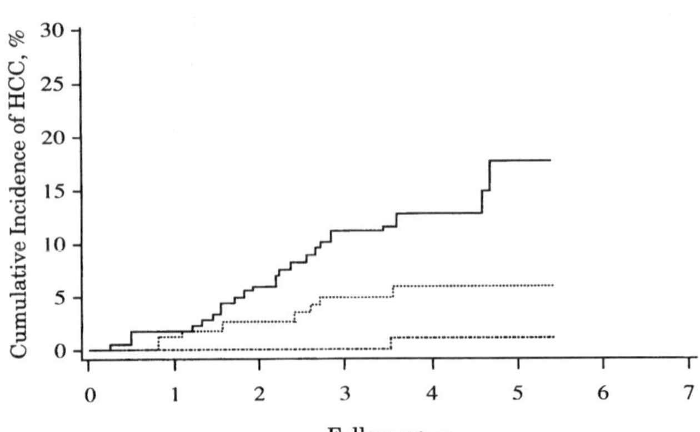

FIGURE 2.—Cumulative incidence of hepatocellular carcinoma (*HCC*) in interferon-treated patients with chronic hepatitis C categorized by sustained response (*dashed line*), relapse (*dotted line*), and nonresponse (*solid line*). A log-rank test of the 3 curves showed a significant difference among these groups (*P* less than 0.001). (Courtesy of Imai Y, for the Osaka Hepatocellular Carcinoma Prevention Study Group: Relation of interferon therapy and hepatocellular carcinoma in patients with chronic hepatitis C. *Ann Intern Med* 129:94-99, 1998.)

age, higher histologic activity, and worse histologic stage. Only 1 patient in the interferon group who showed a response later had a hepatocellular carcinoma develop; the majority of patients in the interferon group who had cancer develop did not have a response to therapy (n = 20) or were patients who had experienced relapses (n = 7). Compared with controls, patients who responded to interferon had a significantly lower risk for hepatocellular carcinomas (relative risk, 0.06); risks in patients who relapsed (0.51) and in those who did not show a response (0.95) were lower than in controls but not significantly so.

Conclusions.—Patients treated with interferon had a significantly lower risk of hepatocellular carcinoma developing than untreated controls did. Furthermore, patients treated with interferon who sustained their response to therapy had a significantly lower risk of hepatocellular carcinomas than patients who did not respond to interferon therapy or who experienced relapses. In patients with HCV, interferon therapy appears to lower the risk for hepatocellular carcinomas.

▶ These studies (Abstracts 6–19 to 6–21) are among a group that may receive a larger share of attention than any single investigation deserves. This statement is not meant to detract from the authors and their accomplishments. Rather, it reflects the difficulties that are at the root of interferon therapy. Physicians who treat hepatitis C-infected patients with interferon cannot help but be frustrated by the limited response rate. Hepatologists may be disheartened when patients who initially responded to interferon with normalization of ALT and clearance of detectable viremia subsequently relapse once therapy is discontinued. Therefore, there exists an eagerness to grasp for evidence that suggests that interferon therapy has previously unrecognized long-term benefits.

Specifically, these studies evaluate the impact that interferon therapy for hepatitis C has on the risk of hepatoma. The *Cancer* article (Abstract 6–20) is intriguing in that the study population was selected for patients with biopsy-proven cirrhosis, a group known to have a poorer response rate to interferon therapy; its retrospective design was its biggest liability. Still, interferon therapy seemed to decrease the risk of hepatocellular cancer. The *Annals of Internal Medicine* article (Abstract 6–21) and the *Hepatology* article (Abstract 6–19), both from Osaka, suggest a decreased risk of hepatoma, especially in patients who had a sustained response to therapy, but also, albeit to a lesser degree, in patients who had an initial response but subsequent relapse. Of these latter 2 studies, the *Annals* article was more limited because of the size of the study population, its retrospective design, and its shorter follow-up period. Both studies from Osaka overlap in their drawbacks of an unavailable control arm and reliance upon historical controls. Still, some will find these problems more apparent than real, and optimistics will cling to these results and conclusions. Certainly, the potential, previously unappreciated, long-term benefits of interferon therapy for hepatitis C will remain an area of intense investigation into the next millenium.

M.J. Bernstein, M.D.

Hepatocellular Carcinoma Outcomes Based on Indicated Treatment Strategy

Rose AT, Rose DM, Pinson CW, et al (Vanderbilt Univ Med Ctr, Nashville, Tenn)

Am Surg 64:1128-1135, 1998 6–22

Objective.—Because resection of tumors in patients with advanced-stage hepatocellular carcinoma (HCC) is frequently not possible, other treatment strategies have been developed. One institution's 7-years of experience with the presentation, stratification, treatment strategies, and outcomes is presented.

Methods.—Between January 1991 and January 1998, 117 patients (86 males), aged 16 to 85 years, were evaluated for treatment of HCC.

Results.—There were 69 patients (59.0%) with cirrhosis, which was caused by hepatitis C in 27 patients (39.1%); 39 patients with liver disease, which was caused by alcohol abuse in 24 (34.8%), hepatitis B in 12 (17.4%), and hemochromatosis in 3 (4.3%); and 16 patients (23.2%) with no identifiable cause. Treatment consisted of resection for 22 patients (19%), including 5 (22.7%) with cirrhosis; orthotopic liver transplantation for 8 patients (7%), including 7 (88%) with cirrhosis and 1 with unresectable multifocal fibrolamellar hepatoma; chemoembolization with or without systemic chemotherapy for 40 patients (35.0%), including 26 with cirrhosis (65%); systemic therapy for 16 (12.8%); and supportive care for 31 (27%). Only 2 untreated patients were alive at 1 year. In the transplant group, 1-, 2-, and 3-year survival rates were 87%, 87%, and 58%, respectively. Patients undergoing surgical resection had 1-, 2-, and 3-year survival rates of 69%, 52%, and 43%, respectively. Patients undergoing chemoembolization had 1-, 2-, and 3-year survival rates of 35%, 20%, and 11%, respectively. Patients receiving systemic chemotherapy had 1- and 2-year survival rates of 30% and 15%. Patients without cirrhosis had significantly better survival rates than patients with cirrhosis (47% vs. 29%). There was no difference in survival between patients aged 55 years and younger and patients older than 55 years.

Conclusion.—Patients whose hepatocellular carcinoma was treated with surgery had better survival rates.

▶ This retrospective review of the experience with hepatocellular carcinoma at Vanderbilt University illustrates several issues. First, a multimodality method of treating hepatocellular carcinoma is now required. Surgical treatment is still the best method for patients who are selected. However, other methods of treatment will avoid an operation if poor outcome is suspected. Survival after surgical therapy, either liver transplantation or hepatic resection, can be expected to be favorable if patients are selected very carefully. Second, this is the first use of the FDG-PET scan for selection of treatment methods for patients with hepatocellular carcinoma. About half of hepatocellular carcinomas will be visible on PET scanning. The discovery of extrahepatic disease can help select patients who are not good candidates for surgical treatment and who should be treated with other modalities.

Clearly, hepatocellular carcinoma is a tumor that requires more study to determine the best mode of therapy. Advances are being made, but there is room for continued improvement.

J.W. Fleshman, Jr., M.D.

Miscellaneous

Transjugular Intrahepatic Portosystemic Shunt (TIPS) for Variceal Bleeding in Portal Hypertension: Comparison of Emergency and Elective Interventions

Gerbes AL, Gülberg V, Waggershauser T, et al (Univ of Munich, Germany)
Dig Dis Sci 43:2463-2469, 1998 6–23

Background.—Transjugular intrahepatic portosystemic shunting (TIPS) has become a popular, nonsurgical approach to reducing portal hypertension for the prevention of rebleeding from esophageal varices. However, there are few data on the benefits of emergency TIPS for patients with acute variceal bleeding that does not respond to endoscopy and medical therapy. This study compared the effects and complications of emergency vs. cirrhotic TIPS for patients with cirrhosis.

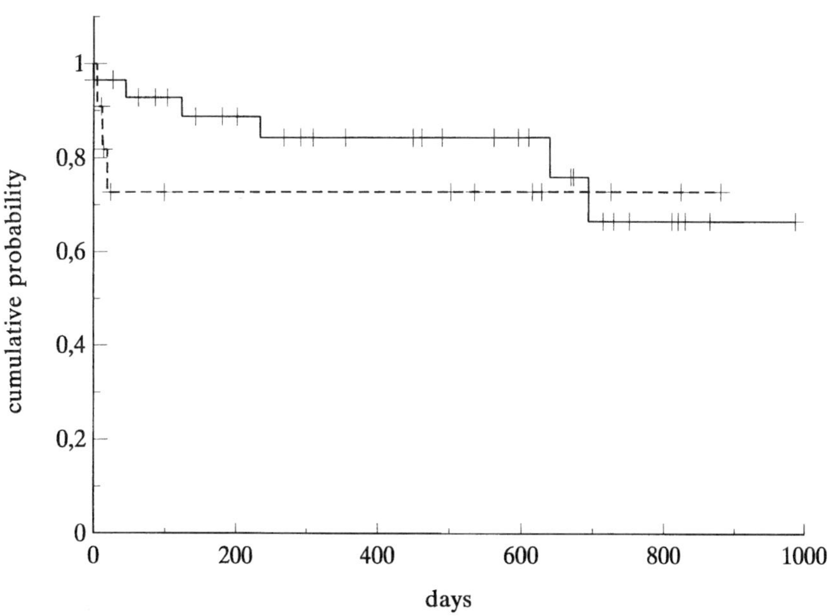

FIGURE 1.—Survival is not different in patients with emergency TIPS for refractory variceal bleeding (*solid line*) and patients who received TIPS for prevention of rebleeding (*dashed line*); (Kaplan-Meier plot; $P = 0.44$, log-rank test). (Courtesy of Gerbes AL, Gülberg V, Waggershauser T, et al: Transjugular intrahepatic portosystemic shunt (TIPS) for variceal bleeding in portal hypertension: Comparison of emergency and elective interventions. *Dig Dis Sci* 43:2463-2469, 1998, Plenum Publishing Corporation.)

Methods.—The emergency TIPS group comprised 11 patients undergoing TIPS as salvage therapy for refractory variceal hemorrhage (8 men and 3 women; mean age, 46 years) compared with 22 patients undergoing elective TIPS for prevention of variceal rebleeding (18 men and 4 women; mean age, 52 years). All patients were in stable condition when elective TIPS was performed. Follow-up, performed at intervals up to 3 months after TIPS, included clinical examination, blood sampling, Doppler assessment of TIPS flow, and upper gastrointestinal endoscopy. The patients were followed up for a median of 536 days in the emergency TIPS group and 580 days in the elective TIPS group.

Results.—Emergency TIPS controlled bleeding in 91% of patients. Kaplan-Meier probability of survival at 1 year was 0.73 in the emergency TIPS group and 0.84 in the elective TIPS group, a nonsignificant difference (Fig 1). Twenty-seven percent of patients in the emergency TIPS group had rebleeding within 2 weeks of the procedure, compared with none of the elective TIPS group. The rate of late rebleeding was not significantly different. Although the emergency group was more likely to have occlusion of TIPS, there was no difference in the rate of TIPS stenosis. The 2 groups were similar in their incidence of hepatic encephalopathy.

Conclusions.—Emergency TIPS is highly effective in the management of variceal bleeding that does not respond to medical treatment. For the more than two thirds of patients who survive the acute episode of bleeding, long-term survival is similar to that after elective TIPS. Emergency TIPS carries a greater risk of early rebleeding and stent occlusion than elective TIPS. However, the rates of stent occlusion, late rebleeding, long-term survival shunt stenosis, or hepatic encephalopathy do not differ.

▶ Gerbes and his associates have reaffirmed the usefulness of TIPS for the emergency management of variceal hemorrhage. Many of their findings are not surprising. Previous studies have demonstrated that emergency TIPS, while often effective in stopping variceal bleeding, is associated with a high incidence of short-term morbidity and mortality.

The unique nature of this study (in relation to other studies that have compared emergency and elective TIPS) is the duration of follow-up. Patients who underwent either elective or emergency TIPS were evaluated with a median follow-up duration of about 1½ years. Although the sample size was small, the results indicated that the incidence of late mortality associated with emergency TIPS was no different than with elective procedures.

M.J. Bernstein, M.D.

Effect of Ursodeoxycholic Acid Therapy on Hepatic Function in Children With Intrahepatic Cholestatic Liver Disease

Narkewicz MR, Smith D, Gregory C, et al (Univ of Colorado, Denver)
J Pediatr Gastroenterol Nutr 26:49-55, 1998 6–24

Background.—Children with chronic intrahepatic cholestatic hepatobiliary disease can progress to cirrhosis or liver failure. In adults with this disorder, ursodeoxycholic acid (UDCA) reduces pruritus and serum levels of alanine aminotransferase (ALT), bilirubin, and cholesterol. Results of controlled trials in children with this disorder suggest that UDCA can also improve symptoms and biochemical parameters of cholestasis, but there is no evidence to indicate that UDCA changes the prognosis of patients with liver disease. Thus, these authors examined the effectiveness of long-term UDCA therapy on clinical, biochemical, and hepatic parameters in children with chronic intrahepatic cholestasis.

Methods.—The subjects were 13 patients, ages 2 to 27 years (mean age, 13.1 years) with chronic intrahepatic cholestasis due to cystic fibrosis (6 patients), Alagille syndrome (4 patients), familial inheritance (2 patients), and nonsyndromic intrahepatic paucity of bile ducts (1 patient). No patient was taking cholestyramine or phenobarbital during the trial. Patients received UDCA (15 to 20 mg/kg/day) according to a schedule of 12 months on, 6 months off, 12 months on. At baseline and every 3 months thereafter, clinical symptoms were evaluated and biochemical tests were performed, including measurements of alanine ALT, aspartate aminotransferase (AST), and γ-glutamyl transpeptidase (GGT). Assessment of hepatic function every 6 months included hepatic scintigraphy and calculation of the elimination $t_{1/2}$ of galactose and caffeine.

Findings.—All patients completed 12 months or more of UDCA therapy. Among the 6 patients who had pruritus at baseline, symptoms improved with UDCA therapy. At 12 months, levels of ALT and GGT had decreased significantly (from 83 ± 33 to 45 ± 10 IU/L for ALT and from 263 ± 114 to 77 ± 32 IU/L for GGT). Similar significant decreases were also seen in plasma levels of copper (from 185 ± 17 to 169 ± 17 µg/dL) and manganese (from 2.2 ± 0.4 to 1.7 ± 0.4 ng/mL). However, galactose $t_{1/2}$ significantly worsened, from 17.3 ± 7.7 to 24.5 ± 17.3 minutes. UDCA therapy was discontinued after 12 months but had to be restarted within 1 month in 9 patients because of a doubling of the ALT (6 patients) or worsening pruritus (3 patients). Ten patients completed 24 months of therapy. At 24 months, ALT, AST, GGT, and copper levels were decreased from baseline, but not significantly so. The manganese level was significantly decreased (to 1.7 ± 0.6 ng/mL) at 24 months, and the galactose $t_{1/2}$ was slightly (but not significantly) worse (16.1 ± 2.1 ng/mL). Throughout the study, neither bilirubin nor cholylglycine levels, caffeine elimination, nor scintigraphic results changed significantly.

Conclusions.—UDCA therapy did improve pruritus and reduce levels of ALT and GGT. However, it had little effect on hepatic function in these patients. Thus, UDCA is unlikely to alter the prognosis for patients with intrahepatic cholestatic liver disease.

► Cystic fibrosis–related liver disease will become an increasing problem. As the survival rate improves, more patients will be at risk of cholestasis that can be complicated by progressive biliary cirrhosis. In theory, drugs that improve bile flow might prevent the progression of liver disease; however, this remains unclear. Other inherited cholestatic disorders, such as Alagille's syndrome, can be complicated by symptoms of pruritus and dysfunctional cholesterol metabolism. Both Alagille's syndrome and cystic fibrosis are associated with median survivals that make them a problem encountered not only by pediatricians but also by internists caring for older patients.

Ten of the thirteen patients examined for this paper had either Alagille's syndrome or cystic fibrosis–related liver disease. The response of these cholestatic processes (as assessed by blood tests, symptom scores, and scintigraphic measurements of bile flow) to treatment with UDCA has been inconsistent. That UDCA might have an impact on mortality remains unestablished. Still, the overall impression is that there seems to be some benefit and that adverse effects tend to be a minor issue. This impression is further supported by Narkewicz and his associates. Until better therapies are developed, it seems inevitable that UDCA will continue to be prescribed in the management of cholestatic disorders.

M.J. Bernstein, M.D.

Correlation Between Serum-Ascites Albumin Concentration Gradient and Endoscopic Parameters of Portal Hypertension

Torres E, Barros P, Calmet F (Universidad Peruana Cayetano Heredia, Hosp Nacional Cayetano Heredia, Lima, Peru)

Am J Gastroenterol 93:2172-2178, 1998 6–25

Introduction.—In patients with ascites, various measurements performed in ascitic fluid have been used to classify the ascites as transudative or exudative. Recent studies have shown the serum-ascites albumin concentration gradient (SAAG) to be superior in the discrimination of ascitic fluid. The minimally invasive SAAG technique offers a way of classifying ascitic fluids according to the absence or presence of portal hypertension (PHTN). The relationship between SAAG level and complications of PHTN—particularly esophageal varices (EV)—was assessed.

Methods.—The prospective, observational study included 31 patients with an ultrasound-confirmed diagnosis of ascites. All patients underwent measurement of SAAG and endoscopic assessment of the presence and size of EV. The study definition of high SAAG was 1.1 g/dL or greater. The association between SAAG and the presence and grade of EV was evaluated.

Results.—The SAAG was high in 81% of patients and low in 19%. Sixty-eight percent of the high-SAAG group had EV, compared with none of the low-SAAG group. All patients with alcoholic liver disease, compared with 27% of those without, had EV. Patients with a more advanced Child-Pugh score were more likely to have EV. Within the high-SAAG group, rates of EV were 40% at SAAG values of 1.10 to 1.49 g/dL, 67% in those with values of 1.50 to 1.99 g/dL, and 100% of those with values of 2.0 g/dL or greater. However, the SAAG level among high-SAAG patients was not significantly related to the size of the EV. On receiver operating characteristic curve analysis, an SAAG value of 1.435 or greater had a positive predictive value of 87.5% and a negative predictive value of 66.7% for the presence of EV.

Conclusions.—Among patients with ascites, those with high SAAG, as defined in this study, are more likely to have EV. Among patients with ascites and high SAAG, higher SAAG values are related to the likelihood of EV, but not to the size of EV. Useful predictors of the presence of EV in patients with ascites are a SAAG value of 1.435 or higher and the presence of alcoholic liver disease. Corroborative studies are needed.

▶ This article by Drs Torres, Barros, and Calmet serves as a reaffirmation that the SAAG can be used to distinguish ascites as a result of liver disease/portal hypertension from other causes of peritoneal fluid accumulation. Furthermore, other complication of portal hypertension—specifically in this article, esophageal varices—can be correlated with a high SAAG.

M.J. Bernstein, M.D.

Mesenteric Arterioportal Shunt After Hepatic Artery Interruption

Iseki J, Noie T, Touyama K, et al (Shizuoka Gen Hosp, Japan; Tokyo Univ)

Surgery 123:58-66, 1998 6–26

Background.—Extended pancreatobiliary operation with excision and reconstruction of either the hepatic artery (HA) or the portal vein can result in hepatic necrosis after thrombotic obstruction of the reconstructed HA or by proximal HA ligation. To prevent this fatal complication, the mesenteric arterioportal operative shunt was developed. This report describes 6 patients who underwent a procedure to receive this type of shunt.

Study Design.—Of 98 patients who had pancreatic or hepatic resection for pancreatobiliary carcinoma from 1989 though 1995, 6 were treated with mesenteric arterioportal shunt placement. The indication for this procedure was that the patient had postoperative hepatic arterial occlusion or main HA excision without reconstruction. Postoperative clinical and hemodynamic analyses were performed.

Findings.—Four of these 6 patients had good arterioportal shunt patency and favorable clinical courses. Fatal hepatic necrosis occurred in 1 patient, and shunt occlusion occurred in the remaining patient.

Conclusions.—During or after extended pancreatobiliary operation, a mesenteric arterioportal shunt appears to be useful for the prevention of the fatal complication of hepatic necrosis. The shunt is safe and effective, and it can be safely closed by transarterial embolization when it is no longer needed.

▶ For a patient with normal anatomy, the liver and the biliary tree are not at risk from hepatic artery occlusion. The proximal bile ducts, which receive blood from the hepatic artery, can easily be supplied by collateral circulation from the duodenum. The portal vein-not the hepatic artery—is responsible for supplying the majority of the liver parenchyma with their oxygen and nutrient needs. Extensive hepatopancreaticobiliary surgery alters duodenal and portal blood flow. Therefore, such surgery may compromise the perfusion reserve that is usually afforded to the liver; the liver can then be at risk for substantial ischemic injury.

Surgical reconstruction of the hepatic artery is difficult and often produces unsatisfactory results; these circumstances pose problems for surgeons when hepatopancreaticobiliary resections require or result in hepatic artery ligation. The authors of this article conceived a clever technique for increasing portal vein flow and improving the oxygen tension of portal blood. They hypothesized that doing these things might protect the liver from ischemia. The method they proposed involved constructing a shunt between a small mesenteric artery branch and a corresponding vein that drains into the portal circulation. The authors tested their technique in 6 patients and obtained good results. However, follow-up was limited because one of the 6 patients died perioperatively, and 3 others died within a year because of tumor recurrence.

The design, size, and duration of follow-up are 2 of this study's most obvious limitations. The described technique seems relatively straightforward, but theoretical risks include portal hypertension and bowel ischemia. Until it is more formally studied, the mesenteric arterioportal shunt after hepatic artery interruption should retain its status as a curiosity. It should be applied only in extraordinary circumstances rather than be considered a widely applicable surgical tool.

M.J. Bernstein, M.D.

Tamoxifen-induced Fatty Liver in Patients With Breast Cancer

Ogawa Y, Murata Y, Nishioka A, et al (Kochi Med School, Japan)

Lancet 351:725, 1998 6–27

Background.—Tamoxifen is widely used as adjuvant therapy to treat breast cancer. However, it can disrupt lipid metabolism, and severe tamoxifen-induced lipemia has been reported. The development of fatty liver related to long-term tamoxifen use in patients with breast cancer is described.

Methods.—During the past 8 years, 66 patients with breast cancer (mean age, 49.6 years) who have been taking tamoxifen have been followed up with annual abdominal CT scans. The mean daily dose of oral tamoxifen is 40 mg, and patients have taken the drug for 3 to 5 years. CT scans were evaluated for evidence of fatty liver.

Findings.—Of the 66 patients studied, 24 patients (36.4%) had evidence of fatty liver on annual CT scans. In most of these 24 patients, the fatty changes usually began focally, then progressed diffusely. After tamoxifen therapy was discontinued, the fatty changes disappeared from 1 to 14 months later. Abnormalities appeared on CT before they were detectable by laboratory tests. Nine of these 24 patients had no laboratory abnormalities, but 11 had increased liver enzyme levels and 4 had increased total cholesterol levels. Only 2 of the 24 patients had a dramatic increase in weight (more than 10 kg) after beginning tamoxifen therapy.

Conclusions.—Fatty liver developed in more than one third of these women with breast cancer who were taking long-term oral tamoxifen. This finding could be mistaken as a breast cancer metastasis to the liver. Also, fatty liver is associated with liver cirrhosis. Thus, patients with breast cancer who are taking oral tamoxifen should be monitored regularly with CT and/or ultrasonography to identify and monitor areas of fatty change in the liver.

▶ This short case series emphasizes the need for us to think of fatty liver, in patients who present with right upper quadrant abdominal pain and elevation of alkaline phosphatase, as a complication of tamoxifen. When studying breast cancer patients who are on tamoxifen, these findings obviously suggest metastases, and we may not think that it resulted from tamoxifen.

The development of liver filling defect from fatty liver occurred in one third of the patients of Ogawa and colleagues at an average of 18 months after starting tamoxifen (range, 1 to 44 months). Gilbert and Sullivan were once again proven correct: "Things are seldom what they seem, skim milk masquerades as cream."

J.S. Barkin, M.D.

A Prognostic Model for Patients With End-Stage Liver Disease

Cooper GS, Bellamy P, Dawson NV, et al (Case Western Reserve Univ, Cleveland, Ohio; Univ of California, Los Angeles; Marshfield Clinic, Wis; et al)

Gastroenterology 113:1278-1288, 1997 6–28

Introduction.—Survival of patients with end-stage liver disease is difficult to predict. A 2-stage, prospective cohort investigation was undertaken at 5 teaching hospitals to develop and analyze a model for prediction of death in patients with end-stage liver disease. Phase I and phase II patients were enrolled from June 1989 to June 1991 and January 1992 to January 1994, respectively.

Methods.—Data from 538 patients hospitalized with end-stage liver disease and 2 or more signs of decompensation were abstracted from medical charts from trial day 3 regarding the following: hospital discharge, each hospitalization during the next 6 months at the same facility, demographics, cause of liver disease, reason for admission, co-morbid illnesses, physical findings, laboratory indices of liver function, the Glasgow coma score, and severity of illness.

Results.—The cumulative incidence of death at 30 days and 6 months were 30% and 50%, respectively. The time to death in 295 patients in phase I was independently associated with 5 factors examined on day 3: renal insufficiency, cognitive dysfunction, ventilatory insufficiency, age 65 years or older, and prothrombin time of 16 seconds or more. These risk factors were used to stratify the 243 patients in phase II into low-, middle-, and high-risk groups. The cumulative incidences of death in the model created from phase I disease at 30 days were 12%, 40%, and 74%, respectively, for low-, middle-, and high-risk groups. Integration of this prognostic model with physicians' predictions improved estimates of the probability of death. Transplantation after trial entry was independently correlated with enhanced survival; intensity of other acute therapies was not correlated with enhanced survival.

Conclusion.—The risk of death in patients with end-stage liver disease could be calculated using 5 independent risk factors. These data provide a quantitative basis for supplementing physicians' prognostic estimates.

▶ Over the past year, I have been involved as a preceptor in the care of several patients with end-stage liver disease. Having had this study available would have been most useful. Decisions regarding transplantation, quality of life, and end of life entered into almost every office visit and, certainly, each hospitalization. Desiring, but often lacking, prognostic information, the patient, family, and physician struggle with these decisions. The information presented here will not guide treatment recommendations per se, but it will certainly inform the discussion with the patient and family.

W.W. Dexter, M.D.

7 Gallbladder and Biliary Tract

Cholecystectomy

ERCP and Sphincterotomy in the Context of Laparoscopic Cholecystectomy: Academic and Community Practice Patterns and Results

Davis WZ, Cotton PB, Arias R, et al (Duke Univ Med Ctr, Durham, NC; Med Univ of South Carolina, Charleston; Pinehurst Med Clinic, NC)

Am J Gastroenterol 92:597-601, 1997 7–1

Introduction.—Laparoscopic techniques for removing stones from the bile duct are usually well developed in specialist centers. They are used infrequently in community practices. Most series evaluating the technical success and complications of endoscopic retrograde cholangiopancreatography (ERCP) are published from academic centers. Little is known concerning the practice patterns and results of community-based gastroenterologists who perform perioperative ERCP. The use of ERCP in relation to laparoscopic cholecystectomy (LC) was compared in community and academic settings.

Methods.—Data were prospectively collected from 780 ERCPs performed before or after laparoscopic cholecystectomy. Fourteen "expert" biliary endoscopists from 4 academic centers and 33 community-based gastroenterologists with varying degrees of experience completed a comprehensive survey that addressed location of practice, size of referral base, proximity of a biliary expert, and in-training and lifetime number of ERCPs and sphincterotomies performed. Patient data forms were used to gather information regarding symptoms at initial evaluation, results of liver function tests, radiologic data, ERCP findings, endoscopic therapy performed, and any ERCP-related complications.

Results.—Indications for perioperative ERCP were similar in both academic centers and community practices. Academic centers performed a significantly higher proportion of postoperative procedures. All participants had high success rates. The least experienced group of community-based gastroenterologists had a significantly lower rate of success with sphincterotomy than their more experienced counterparts. Complication rates were similar for all participants.

Conclusion.—Experienced community-based gastroenterologists are able to perform ERCP and sphincterotomy in the context of LC with outcomes comparable to those of experts in the academic setting. Gastroenterologists with a lifetime experience of fewer than 200 ERCPs have lower success rates for sphincterotomy than more experienced practitioners in either practice setting.

► Common bile duct stones occur in up to 15% of patients with gallbladder stones. Laparoscopic cholecystectomy has become the standard of practice for removal of the gallbladder because of its easy performance in community practice and its good results. For patients with bile duct stones, laparoscopic bile duct exploration and choledochoscopy might become the standard of practice for management of bile duct stones in the same setting as cholecystectomy. Until these methods become more widespread, ERCP will remain an important adjunct to laparoscopic cholecystectomy to provide safe and effective management of common bile duct stones. This study evaluates success and complication rates for ERCP in both academic and community settings. The results were reassuring; success rates were high and complication rates were lower than expected in both academic and community centers, provided that the endoscopists had performed a suitable number of ERCPs. In fact, gastroenterologists who had performed fewer than 200 ERCPs had lower success rates for sphincterotomy than their more experienced counterparts. ERCP was more likely to be performed preoperatively in the community setting than in the expert center. This difference might reflect the reluctance in community practices to manage stones postoperatively, when failure might necessitate a second ERCP or an operation.

G. Aliperti, M.D.

Follow-up of More Than 10 Years After Endoscopic Sphincterotomy for Choledocholithiasis in Young Patients

Sugiyama M, Atomi Y (Kyorin Univ, Tokyo)

Br J Surg 85:917-921, 1998 7–2

Background.—The introduction of laparoscopic cholecystectomy has extended the indications for endoscopic sphincterotomy (ES) to younger patients with choledocholithiasis. However, the long-term outcomes of ES in this population have not been well documented.

Methods.—One hundred fifteen patients younger than age 60 years of age underwent ES for choledocholithiasis between 1977 and 1986. These patients' records were reviewed to classify stones and analyze the early and late outcomes of ES.

Findings.—Early complications developed in 7.8% of the patients. None of the patients died. In 110 patients, ES and stone clearance were judged to be successful. Long-term follow-up data were available for 103 patients. Mean follow-up was 14.2 years. Late complications, including stone recurrence or cholangitis and acute cholecystitis, developed in 9.7% of these patients. Choledochal complications occurred in 7 of 65 patients with calcium bilirubinate stones at ES and in 2 of 38 patients with cholesterol stones. Choledochal complications could be managed endoscopically.

Conclusions.—About 10% of patients younger than age 60 years have late complications after endoscopic sphincterotomy for choledocholithiasis. However, repeat endoscopic treatment is effective and safe. Thus, ES is a viable treatment modality for choledocholithiasis in younger persons.

▶ A number of studies have followed up patients for a prolonged time after sphincterotomy. This particular one concentrates on younger patients, defined as patients younger than 60 years. The indication for sphincterotomy was choledocholithiasis in all patients. This study finds long-term complications—defined as recurrence of stones, cholangitis, and acute cholecystitis—in 10% of the subjects. Recurrent disease occurred more commonly in patients with calcium bilirubinate stones than in those with cholesterol stones. Recurrent disease might be a better definition than "complications," which incriminates sphincterotomy as the primary reason for stone recurrences. As in all other long-term follow-up studies after sphincterotomy, whose incidence of recurrent disease might be as high as 24% after 20 years, all recurrent stones and cholangitis were safely treated by a second ERCP.

G. Aliperti, M.D.

Outcome After Laparoscopic Cholecystectomy for Chronic Acalculous Cholecystitis

Adams DB, Tarnasky PR, Hawes RH, et al (Med Univ of South Carolina, Charleston)

Am Surg 64:1-4, 1998 7–3

Objective.—Patients with biliary dyskinesia and biliary pain, without gallstones, may benefit from cholecystectomy. Outcome after laparoscopic cholecystectomy for presumed acalculous cholecystitis and the predictive value of cholecystokinin-stimulated hepatobiliary scintigraphy (CCK-HBS) were retrospectively assessed.

Methods.—Between 1991 and 1996, laparoscopic cholecystectomy was performed on 50 patients (8 men), average age 43 years, with chronic acalculous cholecystitis. All patients underwent preoperative CCK-HBS with technetium-99m mebrofenin. Patients were monitored for an average of 30 months.

Results.—CCK-HBS results were abnormal in 45 patients (ejection fraction range 0% to 35%), whereas intraoperative cholangiograms were normal in all patients. All patients showed evidence of chronic cholecystitis. No patient died, and no patient required conversion to an open procedure. One patient experienced urinary retention requiring catheterization. At follow-up, 78% of patients were pain free, including 35 of 45 patients with abnormal CCK-HBS values and 4 of 5 patients with normal CCK-HBS values. The positive and negative likelihoods for CCK-HBS were 0.99 and 1.13, respectively. Of the 11 patients with no improvement, 3 had abnormal ductography, 7 had abnormal biliary or pancreatic sphincter pressures, and 1 had unsuccessful biliary manometry. Six patients improved after biliary or biliary and pancreatic sphincterotomy.

Conclusion.—Most patients with chronic acalculous cholecystitis can benefit from laparoscopic cholecystectomy. Those with residual symptoms may be helped by biliary or biliary and pancreatic sphincterotomy.

▶ This article examines outcomes among patients undergoing cholecystectomy following a diagnosis of chronic acalculous cholecystitis. This is a relatively recently defined syndrome in which patients have typical symptoms of biliary colic yet have no evidence of gallstones on ultrasound. Biliary scintigraphy may demonstrate an abnormal ejection fraction, or bile analysis may demonstrate the presence of microcrystals. However, neither of these are absolutely diagnostic, and the syndrome is somewhat incompletely defined. In this series, the majority of patients undergoing cholecystectomy were pain free following laparoscopic cholecystectomy. The majority of patients not benefiting from laparoscopic cholecystectomy underwent endoscopic retrograde cholangiopancreatography with sphincter of Oddi manometry and were found to have abnormal sphincter of Oddi pressures and became pain free following endoscopic sphincterotomy. This article is important in several regards. First, it demonstrates that even patients with normal biliary scintigraphy but having typical symptoms have a high likelihood of being rendered pain free by laparoscopic cholecystectomy. Furthermore, not all patients with abnormal biliary scintigraphy will benefit from the procedure. In addition, it appears that most patients failing to benefit from this will, in fact, benefit from endoscopic retrograde cholangiopancreatography with sphincterotomy. It is also appropriately stressed in this manuscript that exclusion of acid-peptic disease is critical in identifying patients who will benefit from interventional approaches to the biliary tract. It is apparent that a significant fraction of patients fulfill the criteria for acalculous cholecystitis and, in fact, in the series presented here, roughly one sixth of laparoscopic cholecystectomy performed at a busy center was carried out for this diagnosis. While the removal of a stone-free gallbladder would have seemed heretical 20 years ago, it is difficult to argue with the clinical outcomes and results being shown by articles such as this.

J.A. Drebin, M.D., Ph.D.

Bile Duct

Common Bile Duct Stenting for Choledocholithiasis: A District General Hospital Experience

Bowrey DJ, Fligelstone LJ, Solomon A, et al (Royal Gwent Hosp, Newport, Wales)

Postgrad Med J 74:358-360, 1998 7–4

Introduction.—Retained stones in the common bile duct after an initial endoscopic procedure are associated with a 3-fold rise in complications. Management of patients in whom duct clearance is not possible is controversial. The outcome of patients stented for common bile duct stones is reported retrospectively.

Methods.—Information from a computerized database was reviewed to identify patients who underwent stenting for choledocholithiasis between January 1992 and November 1994. Patients were followed up in the outpatient clinic for a minimum of 6 months.

Results.—During the 2-year evaluation period, 204 endoscopic retrograde cholangiopancreatographic examinations for choledocholithiasis were performed. Duct clearance was realized at the initial procedure in 165 patients (81%). A stent was deployed in 39 patients in whom duct clearance was not possible. Of 36 patients for whom complete data were available, 14 were men and 22 were women. Median age was 73 years (range, 23-89 years). Fifteen patients were over the age of 75 years. Median follow-up was 12.5 months (range, 0.5 to 36 months). Stents remained in situ for a median of 5 months (range, 0.5 to 36 months). In patients stents were placed as a temporary measure, and in 18 patients considered unsuitable for surgery stents were deployed as definitive therapy (Table 1). There were 3 treatment-related deaths—2 from cholangitis and 1 from pancreatitis. All 3 patients were over age 75 years. There were 4 deaths of unrelated causes. There were no deaths in patients in whom stents were placed as a temporizing measure.

TABLE 1.—Patient Characteristics by Intention of Stenting

Intention of stenting:	Temporising (*n*=18)	Definitive (*n*=18)	
Male:female	11:7	3:15	p<0.05
Median age in years (range)	66 (23-83)	81 (70-89)	p<0.05
Prior cholecystectomy	5 (28%)	4 (22%)	p=0.70
Duct clearance achieved	10 (56%)	0 (0%)	p<0.05
Surgery undertaken	15 (83%)	0 (0%)	p<0.05
Treatment-related morbidity	5 (28%)	4 (22%)	p=0.70
Treatment-related mortality	0 (0%)	3 (17%)	p=0.07
Unrelated causes mortality	0 (0%)	4 (22%)	p<0.05
Median duration of stenting (months) (range)	2.5 (1-26)	10.5 (0.5-36)	p<0.05
Median duration of follow-up (months) (range)	20 (6-34)	10.5 (0.5-36)	p=0.36

(Courtesy of Bowrey DJ, Fligelstone LJ, Solomon A, et al: Common bile duct stenting for choledocholithiasis: A district general hospital experience. *Postgrad Med J* 74:358-360, 1998.)

Conclusion.—Endobiliary stents may be used with an acceptable complication rate. It is recommended that in patients under the age of 75 stents be placed only as a temporizing measure; patients over 75 and those considered unfit on physiologic grounds should be stented on a long-term basis as definitive treatment.

▶ Retained common bile duct stones after endoscopic sphincterotomy are associated with unacceptably high complication rates, in the neighborhood of 3-fold excess. For this reason, the dilated common bile ducts should be cleared of stones at the time of the initial procedure. Unfortunately, complete common bile duct clearance is not achieved in 15% to 20% of patients, although the failure rate is considerably reduced in expert centers. As an alternative in the subgroup of patients with retained bile duct stones who are not fit for surgical exploration, interim or permanent stenting of the common bile duct is utilized as a means of nonsurgical management. In the cases in which repeat endoscopic therapy is planned, the stent functions as a transient means of drainage. In the case of some elderly and debilitated patients in whom even repeat endoscopic therapy might be risky, or where the availability of advanced endoscopic intervention is lacking, permanent stenting has been used to facilitate bile drainage around the stones. Endoscopic stents are thought to fragment bile duct stones into smaller ones, but endoscopic stents do occlude over time. Additionally, in patients with gallbladder in situ, further passage of stones from the gallbladder might increase the common duct burden. As a consequence, the subgroup of patients with permanent, indwelling stents will develop further complications of their disease. The current study suggests that permanent stenting can be employed with an acceptable complication rate in patients with scant alternatives.

G. Aliperti, M.D.

Effect of Endoscopic Sphincterotomy on Gall Bladder Bile Lithogenicity and Motility

Sharma BC, Agarwal DK, Baijal SS, et al (Sanjay Gandhi Postgraduate Inst of Med Sciences, Lucknow, India)

Gut 42:288-292, 1998 7–5

Introduction.—Endoscopic sphincterotomy (ES) is commonly used for extraction of common bile duct (CBD) stones in patients who have undergone cholecystectomy and those with intact gallbladders. It is possible that sphincterotomy diminishes stone formation by inhibiting the effects of lithogenic bile on gallbladder muscle contraction and by enhancing the ability of the muscle to empty the lithogenic bile. Alterations in bile composition, nucleation time, and gallbladder motility after ES were assessed in 20 patients who underwent ES for CBD stones.

Methods.—Median patient age was 55 years (range, 40 to 60). Twelve patients had gallbladder calculi, and 8 had chronic gallbladder inflammation. Ten of 20 age- and sex-matched controls had gallstone disease with an intact sphincter of Oddi and no stones, and 10 had diseased gallbladders without gallbladder calculi. Ultrasonography was used to determine gallbladder motility. Duodenal bile collected by nasogastric tube after gallbladder stimulation by intravenous ceruletid infusion was examined for cholesterol, phospholipid, and bile acid concentrations, cholesterol saturation index, and nucleation time.

Results.—Significant reductions were observed in mean fasting volume and residual volume in patients who underwent ES. Significant increases were observed in mean ejection fraction and rate constant of gallbladder emptying. Median nucleation time was 17 days in treated patients and 6 days in controls, a significant difference. There were significant decreases in total mean lipid concentrations, cholesterol, and cholesterol saturation index (CSI). There were no significant changes in mean phospholipid and bile acid concentrations.

Conclusion.—Endoscopic sphincterotomy significantly extended nucleation time, reduced cholesterol and total lipid concentration, and did not influence phospholipid and bile acid concentrations. Gallbladder motility was enhanced by ES in diseased gallbladders.

▶ This is an important physiologic study, performed in patients with diseased gallbladders, either with gallstones, or with chronic inflammation alone, after sphincterotomy. The study reveals that there is enhanced contractility of the gallbladder after sphincterotomy. Bile lithogenicity, assessed both as nucleation time and as CSI, is decreased after sphincterotomy, as compared with before sphincterotomy, in the same patients. Together, these findings explain the reduced incidence of gallbladder calculi after ES. The prognostic value of these results might affect management planning in the ever-growing number of patients with a retained gallbladder who undergo sphincterotomy for treatment of sphincter of Oddi dysfunction. Confirmation of these results with prolonged follow-up in patients with biliary symptoms and without gallstones (ie, patients with primary sphincter of Oddi disease or microlithiasis) may lead to deferral of cholecystectomy in lieu of sphincterotomy in this difficult patient population. This well-reported article will be useful to the interested reader, as the discussion includes a lucid review of the literature on this subject.

G. Aliperti, M.D.

Towards T-Tube Free Laparoscopic Bile Duct Exploration: A Methodologic Evolution During 300 Consecutive Procedures

Martin IJ, Bailey IS, Rhodes M, et al (Royal Brisbane and Wesley Hosps, Queensland, Australia)

Ann Surg 228:29-34, 1998 7–6

Objective.—Various methods of laparoscopic common bile duct exploration (CBDE) have been developed for treating bile duct stones. Data from 300 CBDE procedures were reviewed retrospectively for 100 and prospectively for 200 procedures to determine safety and reproducibility of the procedure.

Methods.—Between August 1991 and January 1993, operative cholangiography was performed using a transcystic approach in 173 patients and with choledochotomy for bile ducts greater than 7 mm in diameter in 127 patients. Outcome measures were morbidity and mortality.

Results.—The overall clearance rate was 90%. The clearance rates were 73% for flushing, 92% for transcystic exploration, 84% for choledochotomy and T-tube insertion, 98% for choledochotomy and primary duct closure, and 100% for choledochoduodenostomy. Complications during surgery were an impacted Dormia basket requiring endoscopic manipulation in 1 patient, a split in the cystic duct at the junction resulting in a 5-day leak in 1 patient, a perforated right hemidiaphragm requiring laparoscopic repair, and a perforated bile duct. Postoperative complications included 1 death (0.3%), T-tube complications in 10 (16.4%) of 61 patients, 3 bile leaks, 2 patients who required resuturing, 2 patients with worsening jaundice, and 11 repeat procedures. Only 2 patients had unsuccessful stone clearance.

Conclusion.—Laparoscopic CBDE is safe, effective, and reproducible.

▶ This article provides a large, single-institution experience with laparoscopic CBDE. The authors treated 300 patients using a laparoscopic approach and were able to successfully remove stones in 90% of these patients. The majority of successful stone extractions were performed using a transcystic approach, but 40% required choledochotomy. The incidence of complications in this series was significant, with 16% of the patients undergoing T-tube closure after choledochotomy and 10% of the patients undergoing primary bile duct closure after choledochotomy experiencing leaks or other complications that required surgery or endoscopic procedures. This is somewhat higher than the rate that would be seen with open CBDE. However, it is important to appreciate that the majority of patients indeed had successful clearance of stones via laparoscopic approaches. This article serves to reiterate that (1), in many cases stones can be extracted laparoscopically, particularly via transcystic approach with minimal complications, and (2), that performance of laparoscopic choledochotomy, regardless of whether T-tube or primary duct closure is used, is associated with a higher incidence of complications and requires advanced laparoscopic skills and thus is not something that should be done on a casual basis. The authors point out that in their last series of 100, there was a 98% success rate with fewer complications, again pointing to a learning curve for laparoscopic CBDE. Because the need for this technique is not great, most surgeons will not perform the numbers necessary to become facile with formal laparoscopic choledochotomy and the transcystic approach probably ought to be the limit of laparoscopic management of stones for most surgeons.

J.A. Drebin, M.D., Ph.D.

Cholangitis

The Role of Surveillance Endoscopic Retrograde Cholangiopancreatography in Preventing Episodic Cholangitis in Patients With Recurrent Common Bile Duct Stones

Geenen DJ, Geenen JE, Jafri FM, et al (St Luke's Med Ctr, Milwaukee, Wis)
Endoscopy 30:18-20, 1998 7–7

Introduction.—The rate of recurrence of common bile duct stones is 2% to 7% in patients who have undergone previous bile duct clearance with either endoscopic or surgical extraction. Some patients have multiple recurrences, with repeated episodes of life-threatening, ascending cholangitis. The incidence, clinical presentation, and objective findings among patients with recurrent disease were examined.

Methods.—A retrospective review of 2,096 patients who underwent endoscopic retrograde cholangiopancreatography (ERCP) for cholelithiasis identified 45 patients with recurrent common bile duct stones within 1 year of the initial ERCP. Thirteen of the 45 patients with recurrent disease had 2 or more recurrences without any obvious predisposing factors. The mean age of patients with recurrent stones was 57 years. Medical records were reviewed for information regarding sphincterotomy size, liver function tests, and contrast drainage time.

Results.—All 13 patients with recurrent stones had ascending cholangitis with stones that were soft, golden-brown, and accompanied by a large amount of sludge. The common bile duct in all 13 patients was dilated and had notable, widely patent sphincterotomies. Significant delayed drainage was detected in 77% of the patients. With yearly surveillance ERCPs, the rate of acute cholangitis episodes per patient decreased from 2 episodes to 0.6 episode during a 4-year follow-up.

Conclusion.—Annual surveillance ERCP with stone removal diminished the rate of recurrent episodes of ascending cholangitis, with its associated morbidity and mortality in patients with multiple recurrences of common bile duct stones.

▶ This study, by one of the larger pancreaticobiliary units in the United States, assesses the subpopulation with choledocholithiasis presenting with recurrent cholangitis associated with formation of new common bile duct stones. The authors report endoscopic surveillance at early intervals as a successful method of reducing the incidence of cholangitis in this patient subgroup. The authors reserved their annual surveillance for elderly patients, in whom cholangitis could have been lethal. This option becomes even more palatable when one considers that this group of elderly patients is rarely fit for surgical drainage.

G. Aliperti, M.D.

Cancer

Endoscopic Retrograde Cholangiopancreatography and Endoscopic Endoprosthesis Insertion in Patients With Klatskin Tumors

Liu C, Lo C, Lai ECS, et al (Univ of Hong Kong, China; Queen Mary Hosp, Hong Kong, China)

Arch Surg 133:293-296, 1998 7–8

Background.—Endoscopic retrograde cholangiopancreatography (ERCP) is commonly used to treat patients with malignant hilar biliary obstruction that includes Klatskin tumor. Endoscopic endoprosthesis insertion is also often performed for preoperative drainage in patients with resectable disease or as palliative treatment in those who do not have resectable disease. Reports of endoscopic endoprosthesis insertion as palliative treatment include a high rate of drainage success in patients with malignant hilar biliary obstruction, but it is not known whether such results can be obtained in patients with Klatskin tumor only. The value and associated morbidity of ERCP and endoscopic endoprosthesis insertion were determined in patients with Klatskin tumors.

Methods.—In a retrospective study, 55 consecutive patients with Klatskin tumors that had been diagnosed on the basis of typical cholangiographic and CT findings were studied. The median patient age was 68 years. Standard ERCP with endoscopic stenting was used. After cholangiogram confirmed the diagnosis of Klatskin tumor, endoscopic stenting was carried out to bypass the stricture. When necessary, multiple stents were inserted to ensure adequate biliary drainage. The success rates of ERCP, of endoscopic endoprosthesis insertion, and of drainage were determined, as well as early complications of the endoscopic procedure, procedure-related mortality rates, and the long-term outcome of endoprosthesis.

Results.—Cholangiography was performed in 53 of the 55 patients. Endoscopic stenting was attempted in 49 patients. The procedure was successful on the first attempt in 28 patients and on the second attempt in 8 patients; the cumulative success rate was 73%. Of these patients, only 20 had satisfactory biliary drainage, resulting in an overall drainage success rate of 41%. Early complications were seen in 25% of the patients and included acute cholangitis, acute pancreatitis, and postpapillotomy bleeding. There were 3 deaths from procedure-related complications. Median patency of the first endoprosthesis inserted was 1 week, and the mortality rate at 30 days was 18%.

Discussion.—These results indicate that in patients with Klatskin tumors, ERCP and endoscopic endoprosthesis insertion are associated with a low drainage success rate, high morbidity, a high procedure-related mortality rate, and limited long-term palliation. It is concluded that ERCP and endoscopic endoprosthesis insertion have limited value in the treatment of patients with Klatskin tumors.

► This retrospective study investigates the outcome of endoscopic stenting in patients with proximal cholangiocarcinoma. This study documents low success rates, high morbidity, and high procedure-related mortality rates in patients with Klatskin tumors. In contrast to patients with distal bile duct obstruction, who can usually be adequately palliated with endoscopic stents, patients with proximal tumors often have segmental bile duct involvement, and complete biliary drainage is often impossible, despite the insertion of multiple stents. Ineffective drainage of segmental ducts may result in sepsis, especially after opacification with contrast during endoscopy. Even when adequate drainage is initially achieved, progressive tumor growth can occur, resulting in segregation of segmental ducts. These results reflect the experience accrued worldwide with endoscopic stenting of proximal cholangiocarcinoma and reflect the location of the disease more than the sophistication of the operators. It should be kept in mind that the alternatives are equally unsatisfactory, as the overwhelming majority of patients with Klatskin tumors are considered unsuitable or unfit for curative surgical resection because of advanced disease or concomitant illness. Surgical palliation is associated with an equally high morbidity and mortality rate in these patients. With morbidity and mortality rates approaching 35% and 30%, respectively, even in the best hands, percutaneous drainage is also largely unsatisfactory because its adequacy reflects placement of a different drain in each segment and quality of life is significantly hindered by the presence of multiple indwelling percutaneous catheters.

These tumors, which are generally poorly sensitive to chemotherapy, are often sensitive to radiation therapy. However, tenacious stricturing of bile ducts often results, leading again to segregation of liver segments with associated morbidity. In regard to this particular study, one should also keep in mind the well-known fact that the incidence of cholangitis is unusually high in the region where the study was carried out.

G. Aliperti, M.D.

Miscellaneous

The Relation of Physical Activity to Risk for Symptomatic Gallstone Disease in Men

Leitzmann MF, Giovannucci EL, Rimm EB, et al (Harvard School of Public Health, Boston; Harvard Med School, Boston)

Ann Intern Med 128:417-425, 1998 7–9

Background.—Gallstone disease is a major source of morbidity in the United States. The effect of physical activity on the risk of development of symptomatic gallstone disease was examined in a large cohort of male health professionals in the United States.

Study Design.—The Health Professionals Follow-up Study is a longitudinal study involving 51,529 American male health professionals who were between the ages of 40 and 75 years in 1986. Participants complete a detailed health questionnaire every 2 years. For this analysis, the sample was composed of 45,813 men who had never had gallstone disease and

TABLE 2.—Relative Risk for Symptomatic Gallstone Disease in Relation to Total, Vigorous, and Nonvigorous Physical Activity Among U.S. Men in the Health Professionals Follow-up Study, 1986-1994*

Variable	Cases	Person-Years	RR in Multivariate Analysis (95% CI)†	RR in Multivariate Analysis with BMI (95% CI)‡
Total physical activity, *MET hours/wk*				
0-2.7	209	63 108	1.00	1.00
2.8-7.7	182	62 240	0.88 (0.72-1.08)	0.90 (0.74-1.10)
7.8-16.5	170	64 522	0.83 (0.68-1.02)	0.89 (0.73-1.09)
16.6-32.5	145	65 945	0.72 (0.58-0.89)	0.78 (0.64-0.98)
≥32.6	122	66 541	0.63 (0.51-0.79)	0.72 (0.58-0.90)
P value for trend§			<0.001	0.003
Vigorous activity, *MET hours/wk*‖				
0	386	116 842	1.00	1.00
0.1-3.5	134	54 608	0.82 (0.67-1.00)	0.84 (0.69-1.03)
3.6-10.5	126	48 893	0.89 (0.73-1.10)	0.95 (0.77-1.16)
10.6-25.0	109	51 162	0.82 (0.66-1.02)	0.89 (0.72-1.12)
≥25.1	73	50 851	0.58 (0.45-0.75)	0.65 (0.50-0.85)
P value for trend§			<0.001	0.004
Nonvigorous activity, *MET hours/wk*¶				
0-0.8	179	72 476	1.00	1.00
0.9-2.3	154	59 553	1.02 (0.82-1.27)	1.01 (0.81-1.25)
2.4-4.9	166	64 376	0.97 (0.78-1.19)	0.97 (0.78-1.20)
5.0-11.3	160	63 648	0.94 (0.76-1.16)	0.94 (0.76-1.17)
≥11.4	169	62 302	0.93 (0.75-1.15)	0.97 (0.78-1.19)
P value for trend§			0.12	>0.2

*BMI = body mass index; MET = metabolic equivalent; RR = relative risk.

†Controlled for age (5-year categories); history of diabetes mellitus (two categories); smoking (three categories); and intake of cholesterol-lowering drugs (two categories), thiazide diuretics (two categories), nonsteroidal anti-inflammatory drugs (two categories), alcohol (quintiles), energy-adjusted dietary fiber (quintiles), and energy-adjusted carbohydrates (quintiles).

‡Controlled for body mass index at 21 years of age (quintiles), body mass index in 1986 (quintiles), and all covariates controlled for in the multivariate analysis without body mass index.

§Based on modeling the continuous variable.

‖Also controlled for nonvigorous activity (quintiles).

¶Also controlled for vigorous activity (quintiles).

(Courtesy of Leitzmann MF, Giovannucci EL, Rimm EB, et al: The relation of physical activity to risk for symptomatic gallstone disease in men. *Ann Intern Med* 128:417-425, 1998.)

who were studied from 1986 to 1994. Physical activity was scored as metabolic equivalents, with activities requiring more than 6 metabolic equivalents per hour considered vigorous. A weekly physical inactivity score based on hours spent watching television was calculated separately. Men under the age of 65 years were compared with older men.

Results.—During the 324,263 person-years of this study, there were 828 documented cases of symptomatic gallstones, of which 661 required cholecystectomy. After adjustment for multiple confounding variables, increased physical activity was inversely related to the risk for symptomatic gallstone disease (Table 2). This association was stronger for men under the age of 65 years (Table 3 and Table 4). Sedentary behavior was positively related to risk for symptomatic gallstone disease. Men who watched television more than 40 hours per week had a significantly higher risk for symptomatic gallstone disease than those who watched less than 6 hours per week. Increasing exercise to 30 minutes of endurance training 5 times

TABLE 3.—Relative Risk for Symptomatic Gallstone Disease in Relation to Total, Vigorous, and Nonvigorous Physical Activity in Younger and Older U.S. Men in the Health Professionals Follow-up Study, 1986-1994*

Variable	Men 40-64 Years of Age (*n* = 524) Cases *n*	Multivariate RR (95% CI)†	Men ≥65 Years of Age (*n* = 304) Cases *n*	Multivariate RR (95% CI)†
Total physical activity, *MET hours/week*				
0-2.7	135	1.00	74	1.00
2.8-7.7	114	0.89 (0.69-1.15)	68	0.87 (0.62-1.21)
7.8-16.5	113	0.87 (0.67-1.11)	57	0.79 (0.56-1.13)
16.6-32.5	87	0.67 (0.51-0.88)	58	0.83 (0.59-1.19)
≥32.6	75	0.58 (0.44-0.78)	47	0.75 (0.52-1.09)
P value for trend‡		<0.001		0.09
Vigorous activity, *MET hours/week*§				
0	218	1.00	168	1.00
0.1-3.5	88	0.84 (0.66-1.08)	46	0.79 (0.57-1.09)
3.6-10.5	89	0.96 (0.75-1.23)	37	0.80 (0.56-1.15)
10.6-25.0	79	0.82 (0.63-1.06)	30	0.85 (0.57-1.26)
≥25.1	50	0.52 (0.38-0.72)	23	0.81 (0.52-1.26)
P value for trend‡		<0.001		>0.2
Nonvigorous activity, *MET hours/wk*‖				
0-0.8	126	1.00	53	1.00
0.9-2.3	100	0.94 (0.73-1.23)	54	1.21 (0.82-1.77)
2.4-4.9	109	0.99 (0.77-1.29)	57	0.94 (0.65-1.38)
5.0-11.3	101	0.95 (0.73-1.23)	59	0.95 (0.65-1.38)
≥11.4	88	0.94 (0.72-1.24)	81	0.94 (0.66-1.34)
P value for trend‡		>0.2		>0.2

*MET = metabolic equivalent; RR = relative risk.
†Controlled for age (5-year categories); history of diabetes mellitus (two categories); smoking (three categories); and intake of cholesterol-lowering drugs (two categories), thiazide diuretics (two categories), nonsteroidal anti-inflammatory drugs (two categories), alcohol (quintiles), energy-adjusted dietary fiber (quintiles), and energy-adjusted carbohydrates (quintiles).
‡Based on modeling the continuous variable.
§Also controlled for nonvigorous activity (quintiles).
‖Also controlled for vigorous activity (quintiles).
(Courtesy of Leitzmann MF, Giovannucci EL, Rimm EB, et al: The relation of physical activity to risk for symptomatic gallstone disease in men. *Ann Intern Med* 128:417-425, 1998.)

a week could prevent 34% of cases of symptomatic gallstone disease in men.

Conclusion.—Physical activity may be important in the prevention of symptomatic gallstone disease in men. These results can be generalized to American men over the age of 40 years but may not apply to other at-risk populations. Further research is needed to expand these findings to other groups, especially women, who are at higher risk for gallstones.

▶ This article supports the hypothesis that physical activity decreases the incidence of newly symptomatic gallstone disease in men. Moderate but constant activity appears to reduce the risk for this disease by 20% to 40%. The effects were more striking in men younger than 65, perhaps because of the increased level of vigorous activity in younger men. The focus of the study is not formation of gallstones but symptoms of known gallstones. In fact, all participants had gallstones, and the results aimed at the clinical relevance of symptomatic gallstones.

G. Aliperti, M.D.

TABLE 4.—Relative Risk for Symptomatic Gallstone Disease in Relation to Specific Types of Exercise in Younger and Older U.S. Men in the Health Professionals Follow-up Study, 1986-1994*

Variable	Men 40-64 Years of Age (n = 524) Cases n	RR (95% CI)†	*P* Value for Trend‡	Men ≥65 Years of Age (n = 304) Cases n	RR (95% CI)†	*P* Value for Trend‡
Jogging and running, *MET hours/wk*§						
0	218	1.00		168	1.00	
0.1-24.9	83	0.70 (0.54-0.92)		15	0.62 (0.36-1.06)	
≥25.0	21	0.57 (0.35-0.90)	0.049	1	0.23 (0.03-1.65)	0.07
Racquet sports, *MET hours/wk*§						
0	218	1.00		168	1.00	
0.1-12.9	45	0.81 (0.59-1.11)		9	0.77 (0.39-1.49)	
≥13.0	33	0.66 (0.46-0.94)	0.08	8	0.48 (0.23-0.96)	0.02
Rowing and calisthenics, *MET hours/wk*§						
0	218	1.00		168	1.00	
0.1-6.0	88	0.73 (0.57-0.94)		38	0.71 (0.50-1.02)	
≥6.1	33	0.85 (0.58-1.23)	>0.2	18	1.01 (0.62-1.66)	>0.2
Cycling, *MET hours/wk*§						
0	218	1.00		168	1.00	
0.1-6.9	118	0.89 (0.70-1.12)		48	0.78 (0.57-1.08)	
≥7.0	39	0.88 (0.62-1.25)	>0.2	32	1.28 (0.87-1.89)	0.13
Swimming, *MET hours/wk*§						
0	218	1.00		168	1.00	
0.1-3.5	35	0.73 (0.51-1.05)		18	0.81 (0.49-1.33)	
≥3.6	16	0.71 (0.42-1.18)	>0.2	14	0.94 (0.54-1.64)	>0.2
Stair climbing, *MET hours/wk*‖						
0-0.19	227	1.00		150	1.00	
0.2-0.7	221	1.01 (0.84-1.22)		118	1.03 (0.81-1.32)	
≥0.8	76	1.08 (0.83-1.40)	>0.2	36	0.81 (0.56-1.17)	>0.2
Walking and hiking, *MET hours/wk*‖						
0-1.4	186	1.00		75	1.00	
1.5-14.9	262	1.00 (0.83-1.21)		156	1.08 (0.82-1.43)	
≥15.0	76	0.92 (0.69-1.20)	>0.2	73	0.95 (0.69-1.32)	>0.2
Walking pace, *mph*						
<2	39	1.00		40	1.00	
2.0-2.9	263	0.84 (0.59-1.17)		174	1.02 (0.72-1.45)	
≥3	222	0.69 (0.49-0.97)	0.03	90	0.75 (0.51-1.10)	0.02

*MET = metabolic equivalent; RR = relative risk.

†Controlled for age (5-year categories); history of diabetes mellitus (two categories); smoking (three categories); and intake of cholesterol-lowering drugs (two categories), thiazide diuretics (two categories), nonsteroidal anti-inflammatory drugs (two categories), alcohol (quintiles), energy-adjusted dietary fiber (quintiles), and energy-adjusted carbohydrates (quintiles).

‡Based on modeling the continuous variable.

§The reference group for vigorous activities is defined as men obtaining 0 MET hours per week from all sources of vigorous exercise.

‖The reference group for nonvigorous activities is defined as the lowest tertile of MET hours per week for each activity.

(Courtesy of Leitzmann MF, Giovannucci EL, Rimm EB, et al: The relation of physical activity to risk for symptomatic gallstone disease in men. *Ann Intern Med* 128:417-425, 1998.)

Ursodeoxycholic Acid Delays the Onset of Esophageal Varices in Primary Biliary Cirrhosis

Lindor KD, Jorgensen RA, Therneau TM, et al (Mayo Clinic, Rochester, Minn)

Mayo Clin Proc 72:1137-1140, 1997 7–10

Introduction.—Earlier trials have shown that ursodeoxycholic acid (UDCA) treatment in patients with primary biliary cirrhosis (PBC) provides biochemical improvement, delays time until treatment failure, and prolongs time until liver transplantation or death. The effect of UDCA on the development of varices has not been determined, therefore the effect of UDCA therapy on the development of esophageal varices was prospectively assessed in 180 patients with PBC.

Methods.—Patients were randomized to up to 4 years of treatment with either UDCA, 13-15 mg/kg daily, or placebo. All patients underwent endoscopy every 2 years or as clinically necessary. All patients in the placebo group were offered UDCA at completion of the 4-year assessment period. The risk of the development of endoscopically confirmed varices was calculated.

Results.—At trial entry, esophagogastroduodenoscopy revealed that of 180 patients, 139 had no esophageal varices and 41 had varices. At completion of the 4-year treatment, the risk of new development of endoscopically confirmed varices was significantly less for the UDCA group than for the placebo group (16% vs. 58%). Treatment with UDCA was correlated with a significantly lower risk of varices development in patients with PBC.

Conclusion.—Treatment with UDCA reduces the risk of the development of esophageal varices in patients with PBC. These findings support the growing evidence that UDCA is an effective therapy for patients with this disease.

► The last line of the article is really the bottom line: "The results of the current study further support the growing evidence that UDCA is an effective treatment for patients with PBC." The reduction in varices in this placebo-controlled trial is just one of a number of positive results from this medication. Interestingly, the incidence of variceal bleeding actually increased. The explanation, that UDCA treatment increases time to transplant, allowing more time to have a bleed, is certainly plausible. In any case, I included this article as a reminder that UDCA is effective therapy for PBC.

W.W. Dexter, M.D.

8 The Pancreas

Pancreatitis

Pancreatic Stenting Prevents Pancreatitis After Biliary Sphincterotomy in Patients With Sphincter of Oddi Dysfunction

Tarnasky PR, Palesch YY, Cunningham JT, et al (Med Univ of Southern Carolina, Charleston, SC)

Gastroenterology 115:1518-1524, 1998 8–1

Background.—The risk of pancreatitis developing after endoscopic biliary sphincterotomy is high in patients with sphincter of Oddi dysfunction, most likely because of impaired pancreatic drainage caused by pancreatic sphincter hypertension. A study was undertaken to determine whether ductal drainage with pancreatic stenting protects against pancreatitis after biliary sphincterotomy in patients with pancreatic sphincter hypertension.

Methods.—Eighty patients with pancreatic sphincter hypertension were included in the prospective, randomized, controlled study. Forty-one were assigned to pancreatic duct stents and 39 to no stents after biliary sphincterotomy.

Findings.—Pancreatic stenting significantly reduced the risk of pancreatitis from 26% to 7%. Pancreatitis developed after sphincterotomy in 1 patient in the stent group. In another 2 patients, pancreatitis developed at the time of stent extraction. Patients who did not receive stents were 10 times more likely to have pancreatitis immediately after sphincterotomy than patients who received stents.

Conclusions.—In patients with pancreatic sphincter hypertension undergoing biliary sphincterotomy, pancreatic duct stenting significantly protects against pancreatitis after endoscopic retrograde cholangiopancreatography (ERCP). Pancreatic duct stenting should be considered after biliary sphincterotomy for sphincter of Oddi dysfunction. Manometry can identify which patients may benefit from pancreatic stenting.

► Pancreatitis is the most common complication of biliary sphincterotomy during ERCP. This complication occurs in approximately 5% of cases over all and is substantially higher in patients undergoing sphincterotomy for sphincter of Oddi dysfunction. In fact, pancreatitis is reported in up to one fourth of patients with this disease. The current study, in addition to offering considerable aid to the clinician managing this type of patient, also supports a disease mechanism that has been hypothesized but is still somewhat controversial. Spasm arising at the time of sphincterotomy in patients with primary pancreatic sphincter hypertension may be the mechanism of post-ERCP pancreatitis in this subgroup of patients, impairing pancreatic drainage.

In an attempt to determine the cost savings of treating patients with stents to prevent pancreatitis, the authors applied an elegant financial cost model. If 50 cases of moderate pancreatitis were prevented by insertion of a stent at the time of biliary sphincterotomy, the cost savings would result in more that $150,000. Thus, substantial cost savings would be achieved and, most, important, the morbidity of pancreatitis would be reduced.

G. Aliperti, M.D.

Endoscopic Drainage in Benign Pancreatic Disease: Immediate and Medium Term Outcome

Hammarström L-E, Stridbeck H, Ihse I (Univ Hosp, Lund, Sweden)

Eur J Surg 163:577-589, 1997 8–2

Background.—The benefits of endoscopic drainage procedures in the management of benign pancreatic diseases have been questioned. The current study reports the immediate and medium-term results of endoscopic drainage in patients with benign pancreatic disease.

Methods.—One hundred thirty-six of 319 patients undergoing endoscopic retrograde cholangiopancreatography (ERCP) for known or suspected pancreatic disease with abnormal findings on duodenoscopy or ductography were included in the retrospective analysis. In 28 patients, endoscopic treatment was indicated by recurrent acute pancreatitis, chronic pancreatitis, pancreatic pain syndrome, pancreatic fistula with ascites, pseudocyst, or appreciable biliary obstruction from chronic pancreatitis. Pancreatic duct drainage, attempted in 18 patients, was successful in 13. Endoscopic sphincterotomy (EST) alone was performed in 7 of 13 patients, and an endoprosthesis was placed in 6. Bile duct drainage was successful in all 10 patients in whom it was attempted by EST and dilation, with or without simultaneous stent placement. Patients were assessed within 30 days of treatment and were followed up for a median of 48 months.

Findings.—Immediately after treatment and at the last follow-up, the outcome of pancreatic duct drainage was excellent in 62% and good in 67%. The complication rate of the endoscopic procedure was 31%. One patient had infection with abscess formation, 1 had repeated stent clogging, and 2 had stent migration. Three patients needed subsequent surgery because of intra-abdominal abscess, recurrent pain, or lack of pain relief. Medium-term outcome of biliary drainage indicated liver function tests within the reference ranges in 70% of the patients. Two patients needed subsequent biliodigestive shunts at 7 and 13 months after EST.

Conclusions.—Endoscopic drainage appears to be effective and safe for relieving pain and biliary obstruction in selected patients with benign pancreatic disease. The immediate and medium-term outcomes of this procedure were favorable in the current series.

► Chronic pancreatitis is a clinically silent disease until structural changes of the pancreas occur, often after 1 to 2 decades. Obstructive structural changes are at the basis of recurrent attacks and pain syndromes. Endoscopic management of the obstruction in benign pancreatic diseases has been introduced in recent years. The beneficial effects are difficult to assess because of the subtle course of the disease itself, spontaneous remissions that may occur without intervention, and continuation of the principal insult, often alcohol in western countries. Psychological factors, such as the frequent substitution of alcohol addiction with addiction to narcotic analgesics and, at times, the transference of alcohol dependence to a state of dependence on medical care also play a role in the difficulties encountered in assessing outcomes of therapy.

This paper assesses response to endoscopic intervention in terms of recurrent attacks of pancreatitis and pain. The authors find drainage a safe and effective method for temporary and medium-term amelioration of symptoms. The major difficulty that the authors encountered is the same as in many other studies of a similar nature—the difficulty of establishing a priori which patient will respond most effectively to drainage. In our experience, patients with continued alcohol intake, those with "small-duct disease," and patients with rapid recurrence of an obstructing stricture are the ones with less favorable results. Pancreatic sphincterotomy and removal of pancreatic stones in patients who remain abstinent as well as drainage of obstructing pseudocysts are techniques with the most favorable outcomes.

G. Aliperti, M.D.

Enteral Nutrition Is Superior to Parenteral Nutrition in Severe Acute Pancreatitis: Results of a Randomized Prospective Trial

Kalfarentzos F, Kehagias J, Mead N, et al (Univ of Patras, Greece)

Br J Surg 84:1665-1669, 1997 8–3

Background.—Early aggressive nutritional support is essential in severe acute pancreatitis. The standard method of providing exogenous nutrients to these patients has been total parenteral nutrition (TPN). The usefulness, tolerance, clinical outcome, and cost of TPN were compared with enteral feeding (EF) for nutritional support of patients with severe acute pancreatitis in a prospective, randomized clinical trial.

Methods.—Between July 1990 and December 1995, 326 patients with acute pancreatitis participated in this study. All patients were intensively monitored for 72 hours and given fluid replacement and respiratory support as needed. Patients were randomized to EF through a nasoenteric feeding tube with a peptide-based formula (18 patients) or standard TPN through a subclavian catheter (20 patients). Patient records were reviewed for complications, ICU stay, hospital stay, ventilator days, number of days of nutritional support, antibiotics, and average cost.

Results.—Enteral feedings was well tolerated by patients with severe acute pancreatitis and were as efficacious as TPN. The EF patients had fewer complications and had a lower risk of sepsis development, compared with the TPN patients. The cost of TPN support was 3 times higher than the cost of EF support for these patients.

Conclusion.—Enteral support was safe, well-tolerated, and effective and was associated with fewer complications and fewer infections than TPN. The results of this prospective, randomized trial suggest that EF should be the preferred method of nutritional support for patients with severe acute pancreatitis.

▶ "Nothing by mouth" has been a standard order written for patients with acute pancreatitis. This study challenges this dogma while supporting a lesson I learned during my surgical rotations as a medical student: If the gut works, use it. This was a small study of patients who were quite ill. Enteral feedings proved less costly, were effective and safe, and led to few complications.

This population probably does not represent the typical pancreatitis patient a family physician might manage. One wonders if this approach would work as well for patients with less severe disease. Note that the patients in this study all received nothing by mouth during the first 3 days of treatment, about the length of time it takes to "quiet down" someone with moderate disease.

Thus, I am not ready to change my practice just yet. I would like to see a larger study that also looks at more moderate disease and earlier feeding. For severe disease, these results are very intriguing, and early EF is worth discussing with your consultants as you manage these patients.

W.W. Dexter, M.D.

Débridement and Closed Packing for the Treatment of Necrotizing Pancreatitis

Fernández-del Castillo C, Rattner DW, Makary MA, et al (Harvard Med School, Boston)

Ann Surg 228:676-684, 1998 8–4

Objective.—Management of necrotizing pancreatitis is controversial. Débridement followed by closed packing and drainage was studied to determine whether this technique increases patient survival and reduces complications.

Methods.—Between February 1990 and November 1996, 64 consecutive patients (21 women), aged 30 to 81, with necrotizing pancreatitis were treated with blunt débridement of the lesser sac via an incision in the mesocolon. Cavities were packed with Penrose drains stuffed with gauze and fitted with closed-suction drains that were removed one at a time 6 to 10 days after surgery.

Results.—Nineteen patients required blood transfusions, 20 underwent cholecystectomy, 9 had gastrostomy, 3 received cholecystostomy or choledochostomy, 2 had jejunostomy, 2 had splenectomy, 3 received colectomy, and 1 had small-bowel resection. The median number of drains used was 6. Infection or necrosis was found in 36 (56%) patients. The mortality rate was 6.2%. There were 90 complications including 10 patients with enteric fistulas, 34 with a pancreatic fistula, and 9 with a wound infection. Diabetes mellitus developed in 6 patients and exocrine insufficiency in 16. The average hospital stay was 41 days, and patients took an average of 4.9 months to return to regular activities. There were no significant differences in mortality, reintervention, and complication rates in patients who had early rather than delayed débridement. Mortality rates were similar for patients with infected vs. sterile necrosis. Eleven patients required a second procedure, and 13 needed percutaneous drainage. Patients with a longer duration of pancreatitis had a significantly poorer outcome. Sequential group comparison of the timing of surgery showed that there was no benefit to delaying surgery beyond day 27.

Conclusion.—Débridement and closed packing for the treatment of necrotizing pancreatitis carries low mortality and complication rates. The reintervention rate is only 17%. Delayed intervention for patients with symptomatic necrosis beyond day 27 is not merited.

▶ This article addresses one of the two methods of managing necrotizing pancreatitis. This single-institution series reports 64 consecutive patients who were treated with débridement followed by abdominal closure over drains. Patients undergoing surgery had a 56% incidence of infected necrosis with the remainder of patients being operated on for persistent discomfort, metabolic decompensation, or failure to tolerate a diet. The overall mortality in this series was a remarkably low 6.6%, and only 17% required a second surgical procedure after the initial débridement although an additional 15% needed placement of percutaneous drains. The incidence of enteric fistulas was 16%, which is significantly lower than that seen with open packing techniques but indicates this still remains a problem in a sizable fraction of patients with necrotizing pancreatitis. Hospital stay after surgery was also remarkably good in the series, but the patients still needed approximately 5 months in order to be well enough to return to work. This paper shows the best results yet described for management of necrotizing pancreatitis with débridement and closure over drains. It is important to emphasize, however, that only half of these patients had infected necrosis and, thus, some would suggest that the remaining patients might have been able to have been managed without surgery. The authors also provide a description of their operative approach, which involves entering the lesser sac via the transverse mesocolon rather than an approach via the gastrocolic omentum, which may have significant merit in the setting of a dense inflammation of the stomach to the transverse colon. This study emphasizes the excellent results that can be obtained in high-volume pancreatic surgery centers for this difficult clinical problem and supports advocates of mandatory débridement for patients with necrotizing pancreatitis.

J.A. Drebin, M.D., Ph.D.

Pancreatic Cancer

Prognostic Value of CA 19-9 Levels in Patients With Carcinoma of the Pancreas Treated With Radiotherapy

Katz A, Hanlon A, Lanciano R, et al (Fox Chase Cancer Ctr, Philadelphia)
Int J Radiat Oncol Biol Phys 41:393-396, 1998 8–5

Objective.—Carbohydrate antigen (CA) 19-9, a tumor marker, has a sensitivity of 81% and a specificity of 90% for detecting pancreatic cancer. Patients with lower levels of CA 19-9 survive longer than patients with high levels of the marker. The usefulness of CA 19-9 in patients treated with external beam radiotherapy, resection, and chemotherapy was reviewed retrospectively.

Methods.—The 104 patients (48 women) treated for pancreatic cancer at Fox Chase Cancer Center between 1980 and 1994 were divided into group I (n = 25), planned preoperative radiotherapy and resection; group II (n = 35), planned preoperative radiotherapy without successful resection; group III (n = 21), postoperative radiotherapy; and group IV (n = 23), radiotherapy without resection. For groups I to III, the median dose for external beam radiotherapy was 50.4 Gy. The median dose for group IV was 55.8 Gy. In Groups I to III, 97% of the patients were treated with 5-fluorouracil. In group IV, 61% were treated with 5-fluorouracil. Baseline and posttreatment CA 19-9 levels were available for 69 patients.

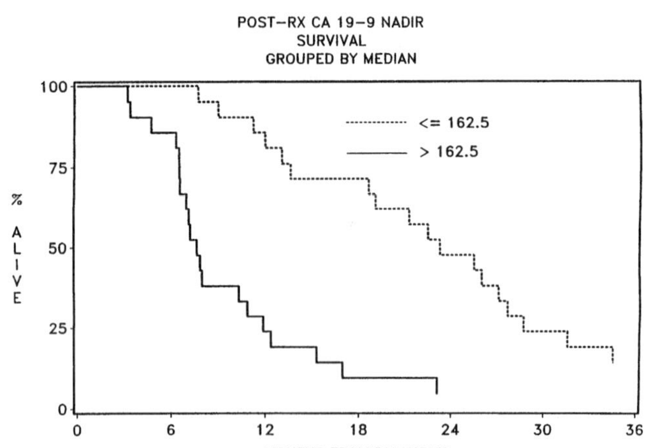

FIGURE 2.—Patients with posttreatment CA 19-9 nadirs less than or equal to the median value of 162.5 U/mL (n = 21) had improved survival when compared with those with nadirs above the median (n = 21). (Courtesy of Katz A, Hanlon A, Laciano R, et al: Prognostic value of CA 19-9 levels in patients with carcinoma of the pancreas treated with radiotherapy. *Int J Radiat Oncol Biol Phys* 41:393-396. Copyright 1998, with permission from Elsevier Science.)

Results.—Median survival time was 10 months, and there were significant differences among groups of 22 months for group I, 10 months for group II, 17 months for group III (Fig 2), and 12 months for group IV. Patients who underwent resection survived significantly longer than patients who did not (19 vs. 11 months, respectively). According to multivariate analysis, pretreatment CA 19-9 level was the only significant predictor of survival.

Conclusion.—Pretreatment CA 19-9 level was a significant predictor of survival in patients with pancreatic cancer who underwent radiotherapy.

▶ Pancreatic carcinoma is a relatively common and almost universally fatal neoplasm. Unfortunately, there has been little progress in treating this disease, and current treatment strategies involve complex, expensive, and highly toxic interventions. It is essential that patients be given an accurate assessment of their likelihood of benefiting from treatment. The traditional predictive tools, such as clinical staging, have proved to be of little benefit in this regard. According to the results of this study, CA 19-9 has predictable clinical usefulness in prognosticating outcomes and perhaps in directing treatment of patients with pancreatic cancer who undergo combined treatment modalities. Posttreatment nadir of CA19-9 reflects response to treatment and also appears to predict survival.

G. Aliperti, M.D.

Standard Versus Extended Lymphadenectomy Associated With Pancreatoduodenectomy in the Surgical Treatment of Adenocarcinoma of the Head of the Pancreas: A Multicenter, Prospective, Randomized Study

Pedrazzoli S, and the "Lymphadenectomy Study Group" (Univ of Padova, Milano, Italy; et al)

Ann Surg 228:508-517, 1998 8–6

Objective.—The regional pancreatectomy procedure with extended lymph node dissection was developed to improve long-term survival rates in patients with adenocarcinoma of the pancreas. The validity of the extended lymph node dissection for extending survival of patients with adenocarcinoma of the pancreas was investigated in a multicenter, prospective, randomized study.

Methods.—Between March 1991 and March 1994, 81 patients with potentially curable ductal adenocarcinoma of the head of the pancreas were randomly allocated to standard (n = 40) or extended (n = 41) lymphadenectomy and soft-tissue removal. Patients were examined every 3 months, if possible. Cause and date of death were recorded.

Results.—Demographic and histopathologic characteristics and postoperative morbidity and mortality were similar for both groups. Lymph node retrieval was significantly higher in the extended group than in the standard group (19.8 vs. 13.3). Actual survival rates at 1, 2, 3, and 4 years were 50.6%, 22.2%, 8.6%, and 7.4%, respectively. Overall survival rates were similar for both groups, but node-positive patients with extended lymphadenectomy had a significantly better survival rate than did their counterparts having the standard procedure. The extent of procedure did not affect survival of node-negative patients.

Conclusion.—The extended procedure did not increase morbidity and overall mortality of patients with adenocarcinoma of the pancreas, but node-positive patients undergoing the extended procedure had a significantly better survival rate than did their counterparts having the standard procedure.

▶ This article addresses the role of lymphatic clearance in patients undergoing resection of the pancreatic head for pancreatic carcinoma. This was a multi-institutional study done in a randomized, prospective fashion in which patients received either a standard pancreaticoduodenectomy or more extensive lymphadenectomy. The study appears to be well done overall in the sense that the 2 groups were comparable with regard to known risk factors. The patients undergoing the extended lymphadenectomy required a bit more operative time and had a bit more blood loss, although these were not significant differences. There was no significant difference in mortality or major morbidity and perhaps most reassuringly, a greater number of lymph nodes were removed in the patients undergoing extended lymphadenectomy than in standard lymphadenectomy. The overall survival curves of patients randomized to the two treatment modalities did not appear significantly different. This study reiterates previous findings, namely that patients with tumors less than 2 cm do significantly better than patients with tumors greater than 2 cm. In addition, patients with well-differentiated cancer do better than patients with poorly differentiated cancer, and the lymph node status is a major predictor of outcome. The power of this study to detect small differences was not very great because there were only approximately 40 patients in each treatment arm. However, there is an interesting trend toward patients with lymph-node–positive disease who underwent extended lymphadenectomy appearing to do a bit better than patients with positive lymph nodes who had the standard lymphadenectomy. In fact, the patients with positive lymph nodes who had the extended resection have survival curves that are superimposable on lymph-node–negative outcomes. This suggests that there may, in fact, be some small benefit of an extended lymphadenectomy, although it would take a larger study to demonstrate this. It is also notable that the patient in this study did not have adjuvant therapy of any sort. Thus, it is possible that postoperative therapy might improve results a bit, although this should not benefit one group over the other. The American College of Surgeons Clinical Trials Group is currently attempting to organize a multi-institutional prospective, randomized study of lymphadenectomy to specifically address the questions raised by this intriguing but limited study.

J.A. Drebin, M.D., Ph.D.

Statewide Regionalization of Pancreaticoduodenectomy and Its Effect on In-hospital Mortality

Gordon TA, Bowman HM, Tielsch JM, et al (Johns Hopkins Univ, Baltimore, Md)

Ann Surg 228:71-78, 1998 8–7

Objective.—The mortality rate for pancreaticoduodenectomy at high-volume hospitals is 4% or less. One hospital in Maryland increased the number of such procedures until it performed more than 50% of pancreaticoduodenectomies in the state. The effect of regionalization on the decrease in mortality was evaluated over a 12-year period.

Methods.—The 52 nonfederal acute care hospitals in the state performing pancreaticoduodenectomies for state residents were classified as high volume (≥20/y for 6 of the 12 years and an average volume of ≥20/y) or low volume. Trends in volumes, percentages of market share, and in-hospital mortality rates were analyzed by provider group.

Results.—There were 795 pancreaticoduodenectomies performed in 43 hospitals. One hospital was considered high volume. During the study period, annual state volume increased from 29 in 1984 to 123 in 1995, from 6 (20.7%) to 72 (58.5%) in the high-volume provider, and from 23 to 51 in the low-volume providers. During this period, statewide mortality from this procedure declined from 17.2% to 4.9%, from 3.2% to 1% in the high-volume provider, and from 19.5% to 12.4% in the low-volume providers. Regionalization was estimated to reduce mortality by 60.8%.

Conclusion.—Regionalization of pancreaticoduodenectomies improved survival.

► This article is the latest in a series of articles documenting the excellent outcome seen in patients undergoing pancreaticoduodenectomy at the Johns Hopkins Hospital. This is one of several high-volume surgery centers that has shown a really striking improvement in outcomes with this procedure over the past several decades. This study demonstrates that improvements resulting from the concentration of such procedures in high-volume centers can actually have striking effects on overall statewide mortality, and an increase in the total volume of such procedures carried out could result. There are now abundant data that surgeon and institutional experience directly affect outcomes for a variety of complex procedures including pancreaticoduodenectomy, hepatectomy, and esophagectomy, and that concentration of these procedures in high-volume centers will serve to decrease overall morbidity and mortality.

J.A. Drebin, M.D., Ph.D.

Lack of Survival Benefit of Extended Lymph Node Dissection for Ductal Adenocarcinoma of the Head of the Pancreas: Retrospective Multi-institutional Analysis in Japan

Mukaiya M, Hirata K, Satoh T, et al (Sapporo Med Univ, Japan)
World J Surg 22:248-253, 1998 8–8

Background.—Mortality rates for ductal adenocarcinoma of the head of the pancreas approach 100%. Five-year survival after surgical resection is dismal (< 10%), and some authors have suggested that excision of lymph nodes and lymphatic vessels can improve survival. These authors examined data from patients with ductal adenocarcinoma of the head of the pancreas and compared the survival rates of those who did and did not receive extended lymph node dissection.

Methods.—From 1991 through 1994, 501 patients (316 men, 185 women; mean age, 64 years) with ductal adenocarcinoma of the head of the pancreas underwent surgical resection at 1 of 77 medical facilities in Japan. Based on the TNM staging system, 90 of the patients had stage I disease, 82 had stage II, 327 had stage III, and 2 had stage IV. Based on histology, 40 patients had papillary adenocarcinoma, and 40 had poorly differentiated, 268 had moderately differentiated, and 117 had well-differentiated adenocarcinoma. Three categories were used to classify the extent of the resection: microscopically curative resection, macroscopically curative resection, and noncurative resection. Three categories were used to classify lymph node dissection: palliative (no resection; n = 41), standard (resection of the peripancreatic lymph nodes; n = 167), and extended (resection of the para-aortic lymph nodes from above the celiac axis to below the inferior mesenteric artery; n = 293). Extended resection was used for 38 patients with stage I disease, 42 with stage II, 206 with stage III, and 1 patient with stage IV. Survival rates at 1 and 3 years were calculated by Kaplan-Meier analysis.

Findings.—Eighteen patients (3.6%) died within 30 days; overall median survival was 355 days. Three-year survival rates for patients with stage I, II, III, or IV disease were 32.0%, 8.3%, 5.8%, and 0% ($P < .05$ for stage I vs stages II or III disease). Three-year survival for patients with papillary adenocarcinoma, and well-, moderately, and poorly differentiated adenocarcinomas were 32.0%, 12.6%, 6.2%, and 4.1% ($P < .05$ for papillary vs moderately or poorly differentiated adenocarcinomas). Three-year survival rates for patients with microscopically curative, macroscopically curative, or noncurative resections were 29%, 14%, and 6% ($P < .001$ curative vs noncurative resections). Of the 94 patients who underwent microscopic resection, mean survival of the patients without lymph node metastasis did not differ significantly between those who underwent extended (848 ± 96.4 days) or standard (767 ± 10.1 days) lymph node excision. Furthermore, survival of the patients with lymph node metastasis who underwent extended lymph node excision was significantly worse (mean survival, 352 ± 52.6 days). For all patients, extended lymph node dissection did not improve survival significantly over that seen with standard or palliative lymph node dissection.

Conclusions.—Regardless of the patient's stage of disease, extended lymph node dissection did not improve survival of patients with ductal adenocarcinoma of the head of the pancreas.

▶ This article addresses the outcome of patients undergoing pancreaticoduodenectomy for carcinoma of the pancreatic head. This is a summary of multi-institutional experience over 3 years at 77 facilities in Japan. A total of 501 patients are included in this series. The authors examined a variety of factors and evaluated them for their ability to predict outcomes as in previous studies from other institutions. Lymph node status and tumor differentiation both proved to be predictors of outcome as did margin-negative resection. However, when an attempt was made to evaluate the extent of lymphadenectomy, there was no evidence of a benefit in patients undergoing a more extended dissection than in patients undergoing standard pancreaticoduodenectomy—admittedly, a relatively radical procedure. This study suffers from the limitations of multi-institutional studies, namely that surgical procedures were not standardized across the multiple institutions surveyed. What was considered an "extended lymph node dissection" was not entirely homogeneous across multiple institutions. Nevertheless, the results suggest that major factors in pancreatic cancer outcome are the underlying tumor biology, as reflected in tumor differentiation by the presence of nodal metastases, and achieving a negative margin of resection. A more extensive lymphadenectomy is of modest, if any, benefit. These results also suggest that although survival may be extended by performing pancreaticoduodenectomy in pancreatic cancer patients with more advanced localized tumors or lymph node metastases, such patients are rarely, if ever, cured. The only patients with any significant chance of long-term survival are those patients with small, lymph-node negative tumors.

J.A. Drebin, M.D., Ph.D.

Cystadenomas of the Pancreas: Is Enucleation an Adequate Operation?

Talamini MA, Moesinger R, Yeo CJ, et al (Johns Hopkins Univ, Baltimore, Md; Med College of Wisconsin, Milwaukee)

Ann Surg 227:896-903, 1998 — 8–9

Background.—Mucinous cystadenoma of the pancreas is difficult to distinguish from pseudocysts or simple pancreatic cysts. Enucleation is often used for benign lesions, such as hepatic cysts and hemangiomas. These authors sought to determine whether enucleation could be used safely and effectively to extirpate mucinous cystadenoma of the pancreas.

Methods.—The subjects were 36 patients with mucinous cystadenoma of the pancreas. Twenty-six patients (9 men and 17 women; mean age, 53 years) underwent tumor resection by means of distal pancreatectomy (73%) or pancreatoduodenectomy (27%), and 10 patients (6 men and 4 women; mean age, 63 years) underwent enucleation. Additional procedures included splenectomy in 54% of the patients undergoing distal pancreatectomy and combined procedures (including cholecystectomy, gastric fundoplication, longitudinal pancreaticojejunostomy, or pancreatoduodenectomy for adenocarcinoma of the head of the pancreas) in 40% of the patients undergoing enucleation. CT was used preoperatively to characterize the cysts and postoperatively for follow-up (average 48.6 months for the resection group and 42.9 months for the enucleation group).

Findings.—Two patients in the resection group died (of cerebrovascular accident or sepsis), but no patient in the enucleation group died. Enucleation was associated with a shorter operative time (272 vs. 313 minutes) and significantly less blood loss (209 vs. 511 mL). However, enucleation was also associated with significantly more pancreatic fistula (50% vs. 12%) than was resection. This complication responded to conservative management but did significantly extend the hospital stay of the enucleation group (19.5 vs. 10 days). Other complications occurred with a similar frequency in the resection and enucleation groups. During follow-up, none of the patients who underwent enucleation had late sequelae or recurrence of the cystic lesion, but diabetes developed in 10% of the patients who underwent resection.

Conclusions.—Simple operative cyst enucleation can be safely and effectively performed in patients with mucinous cystadenoma of the pancreas. In one half of the patients who underwent enucleation a pancreatic fistula developed, but this complication resolved with conservative management, and overall morbidity was similar between the enucleation and resection groups.

▶ This article addresses the appropriate management of mucinous cystadenomas of the pancreas. These are premalignant lesions, which must be distinguished from benign pseudocysts and serous cystadenomas as well as from cystadenocarcinomas and from adenocarcinomas with a cystic degeneration. The authors of this study present a 7-year experience from a major pancreatic center in which a total of 36 such tumors were presented. Twenty-six of these were managed with resection, and 10 were managed with enucleation. Patients undergoing enucleation had somewhat smaller tumors, but the tumors were distributed throughout the pancreas and the difference in size was not statistically significant. Of note, blood loss appeared to be less in patients undergoing enucleation, but the complication of pancreatic fistula was significantly higher in the enucleation group than in the resection group. As a result of this, the hospital stay was also longer in the enucleation group. Although the authors convincingly demonstrate that enucleation can be carried out safely and that the postoperative complications of enucleation can be adequately managed, the suggestion that this is a worthwhile approach to these lesions is not entirely convincing. Specifically, the issue of distinguishing nonmalignant from malignant cystic tumors of the pancreas is a difficult clinical problem for which no combination of laboratory tests and radiologic studies is 100% accurate. Clearly, enucleation is less likely to be a satisfactory approach to a malignant neoplasm, and the risk of spilling a cyst containing malignant cells must give the surgeon pause. In addition, the possibility of performing an enucleation, having a postoperative pancreatic fistula with resulting inflammation, and then obtaining a final pathology report on the resected specimens showing a focus of carcinoma requiring reoperation would present a clinical nightmare. I think that, given these limitations, it is difficult to present enucleation as a general strategy for management of mucinous cystic tumors of the pancreas. Clearly, however, in selected cases, particularly in patients who may not tolerate prolonged surgery, this approach may have some utility.

J.A. Drebin, M.D., Ph.D.

Pancreaticoduodenectomy

Results of a Technique of Pancreaticojejunostomy That Optimizes Blood Supply to the Pancreas

Strasberg SM, McNevin MS (Washington Univ, St Louis)
J Am Coll Surg 187:591-596, 1998 — 8–10

Background.—Anastomotic failure after pancreaticojejunostomy continues to be a problem, with no reduction in failure rates seen in the past 30 years. Previous attempts to decrease anastomotic failure at pancreaticojejunostomy have not addressed pancreatic blood supply. Whether pancreaticojejunostomy performed by a technique that optimized blood supply to the pancreas would reduce the anastomotic failure rate was investigated.

Methods.—Forty patients undergoing pancreaticojejunostomy, 39 undergoing pancreaticoduodenectomy, and 1 with traumatic transection of the pancreatic neck were studied prospectively. Blood supply to the pancreatic neck was assessed clinically and by Doppler methods. When blood supply was judged to be marginal, the pancreas was resected again 1.5 to 2 cm to the left, away from the vascular watershed.

Findings.—The blood supply at the cut margin of the pancreas was determined to be brisk in 24 patients and marginal in 16. Resection of a pancreatic section in the latter group resulted in brisk bleeding from the new cut margin in all patients but one, who had an anomalous artery that had to be sacrificed for oncologic reasons. This patient had the only fistula in the series. No intra-abdominal abscesses occurred.

Conclusions.—Relative ischemia of the pancreatic transection margin appears to contribute to anastomotic failure after pancreaticojejunostomy with local leakage and abscess or fistula. Methods that ensure a good blood supply at the cut margin may help decrease the incidence of these complications. In some patients, preserving good arterial supply may not be possible because of oncologic considerations. In such patients, the surgeon must decide whether to resect the remaining pancreas or to accept a greater risk of anastomotic failure.

► Pancreatic fistula is a very common complication of pancreaticoduodenectomy. The results of this operation have been linked to the experience of the operator and to meticulous technical performance. The observation by Dr. Strasberg that an ischemic transection might contribute to anastomotic failure after pancreaticojejunostomy with local leakage and an abscess or fistula is an important one. The technique that he proposes to ensure good blood supply at the resected margin appears to be beneficial in reducing the incidence of these complications. The general perception that only surgeons who perform adequate numbers of this operation should continue their performance for better results remains a valid one.

G. Aliperti, M.D.

Obesity

Biliopancreatic Diversion

Scopinaro N, Adami GF, Marinari GM, et al (Univ of Genoa, Italy)
World J Surg 22:936-946, 1998 8–11

Background.—These authors described their 21-year experience using biliopancreatic diversion (BPD) to treat obesity.

Methods.—The authors have performed BPD in 2,241 obese patients (mean excess weight, 69 kg) over 21 years. In the past 15 years (1,356 patients), they have combined BPD with a reduction in gastric volume based on the patient's individual characteristics (e.g., age, expected degree of compliance, nutritional risk).

Findings.—On average, about 75% of the initial excess weight has been lost, and this loss has been maintained. Although patients eat about 1.5 times as much food by 1 year after BPD as they did before surgery, they can absorb little fat and starch. This reduction in energy intake seems to be responsible for maintenance of the weight loss. Furthermore, in the patients with hyperglycemia or type 2 diabetes, serum glucose and cholesterol levels normalized without the use of medications and while following an unrestricted diet. Other beneficial effects include the resolution of somnolence and gout in 100% of the patients with these complaints, and the resolution of hypertension, fatty liver, and hyperuricemia in more than 80% of the patients with these complaints. As for complications, dumping syndrome and diarrhea are absent after BPD, and patients typically have 2 to 4 soft bowel movements each day. Operative mortality is less than 1%, about 1% of patients have intestinal obstruction, and about 10% have incisional hernia. Other significant complications include anemia (reduced to less than 5% after iron supplementation), stomal ulcer (reduced to less than 4% after oral H_2-blocker therapy), bone demineralization (peaks at 4 years after surgery, improves thereafter; requires calcium and vitamin D supplementation), and peripheral neuropathy and Wernicke's encephalopathy (prevented by administering thiamine to at-risk patients). Protein malnutrition is the most serious, late, specific complication of BPD, and these patients generally require parenteral feeding. The occurrence of protein malnutrition is reduced to a minimum of 3% by adapting the volume of the remaining stomach and the length of the alimentary limb of the BPD to the patient's initial excess weight. For recurrent protein malnutrition, surgical revision of the BPD is required. Other more minor complications such as hemorrhoids, anal rhagades, perianal abscess, acne, inguinoperineal furunculosis, and night blindness occur in less than 5% of patients.

Conclusions.—BPD is a flexible procedure that can achieve permanent weight loss in obese patients. The best results occur when the operation is adapted to the patient's characteristics, aiming for higher weight loss in patients at little nutritional risk and less weight loss in patients at greater risk for nutritional problems.

▶ This article addresses one successful approach to bariatric surgery. There are a variety of operative approaches to the problem of obesity, which can be divided into those that attempt to restrict the volume of the stomach, leading to early satiety and limited caloric intake on this basis, or those that attempt to divert the intestinal stream, resulting in malabsorption with resulting weight loss, regardless of caloric intake. In this latter group, jejunolileal bypass developed a deserved bad reputation for failing to adequately control weight and also for a variety of unpleasant side effects, particularly hepatic failure. In contrast, BPD creates 2 parallel small-bowel tracts in the abdomen, one running from the bile duct and pancreas and joining the other that comes down from the stomach to the terminal ileum. Thus, the biliary and pancreatic secretions mix with the gastrointestinal secretions, but only over the last 50 or so centimeters. In this fashion, there is absence of digestion of fats and protein, except in the last 50 cm. In addition, BPD can be combined with a hemigastrectomy to reduce the volume of the stomach and to alter the caloric intake. The authors have extensive experience with this combined procedure, having carried it out in well over 1,000 patients over more than 10 years. The complication rate with this combined procedure is quite satisfactory, with an operative mortality of less than 1%, a wound infection rate of less than 1%, and an incisional hernia rate of approximately 10%. The relatively unique morbidity of BPD is the possibility of creating pancreatitis as a result of adhesions obstructing the biliopancreatic limb. Fortunately, this appears to be an uncommon problem in this patient series. The major complication of the procedure, which has required its reversal in a small fraction of patients, is protein malnutrition. The authors discuss specific factors such as the length of the alimentary limb of the diversion as well as the size of the gastric remnant that may alter the development of protein malnutrition. Overall, this is an interesting article that documents an extensive experience with a technique, which—while not widely adapted in the United States—certainly appears to be effective as an approach to bariatric surgery.

J.A. Drebin, M.D., Ph.D.

9 Acquired Immune Deficiency Syndrome

Crohn's Disease Stable Remission After Human Immunodeficiency Virus Infection

Pospai D, René E, Fiasse R, et al (Bichat Claude-Bernard Univ, Paris; Saint Luc Univ, Brussels, Belgium; Rothschild Univ, Paris; et al)

Dig Dis Sci 43:412-419, 1998 9–1

Introduction.—Immune mechanisms are thought to play an important role in the development of Crohn's disease (CD). The involvement of CD4 T cells may account for the response of CD to cyclosporin A treatment. It has been suggested that CD may go into clinical remission after HIV infection as a result of a reduction in mucosal T lymphocytes of the helper-inducer phenotype. Four cases of longstanding CD that went into remission after the patients became infected with HIV are reported.

Patients.—The patients were 3 men and 1 woman, all with long histories of CD. Age at diagnosis of CD was 14 to 20 years; the disease had been present for 4 to 21 years, with 4 to 15 relapses. All patients went into stable remission of CD symptoms. Four months to 5 years later, HIV infection was diagnosed. Three patients remained in remission for 5 to 8 years before dying of AIDS-related disease. The remaining patient was alive and still in remission 7 years after HIV infection was diagnosed. The onset of HIV infection was not followed by opportunistic infection-related diarrhea or by a change in the quantity of ileal effluent in ileostomy patients.

Discussion.—This experience supports previous reports of clinical remission in CD patients who become infected with HIV. The integrity of the immune response, and especially of CD4 T cells, appears to play a key role in the mechanism of tissue injury in Crohn's disease. Further research into the immune mechanisms in the gut may lend insight into the pathogenesis of nonspecific inflammatory bowel disease.

► The interaction between HIV and inflammatory bowel disease has not been well characterized. This interesting case study concerns 4 patients with frequent relapses of active CD whose extended remission coincides with the presumed time of infection with HIV. The case study further supports, at least in part, the extensive literature reinforcing the critical role of CD4 T cells, in the pathophysiology of CD. However, the overall picture of both diseases is certainly far more complex. While CD4 T cells are unquestionably central in both diseases, perturbations of the CD4 T cell have ramifications in other aspects of the immune system. A case of CD has been reported, which developed in an HIV infected patient as well as which suggests other alterations in the immune system may be responsible for the development and progression of CD. Nevertheless, this report suggests additional targets for disease control in CD.

G. Aliperti, M.D.

10 Miscellaneous

Impairment of Health and Quality of Life in People With Large Waist Circumference

Lean MEJ, Han TS, Seidell JC (Univ of Glasgow, Scotland; Natl Inst of Public Health and the Environment, Bilthoven, The Netherlands)

Lancet 351:853-856, 1998 10–1

Objective.—The number of overweight individuals is increasing. Waist circumference has been related to increased health risks. The range of health outcomes according to waist circumference was investigated in men and women in The Netherlands.

Methods.—Anthropomorphic measurements were made in 5,887 men and 7,018 women, aged 20 to 59 years, from the general population. Body mass indices and waist-to-hip ratios were used to determine action levels (men: action level less than 1, less than 94.0 cm; action levels 1 to 2, 94.0 to 101.9 cm; action level 2, 102.0 cm or greater and women: action level less than 1, less than 80.0 cm; action levels 1 to 2, 80.0 to 87.9 cm; action level 2, 88.0 cm or greater). Respiratory insufficiency, low back pain, degree of physical function, presence of non–insulin-dependent diabetes mellitus, and cardiovascular risk factors were assessed.

Results.—Age-adjusted risks and symptoms increased with increasing waist size in both men and women. Shortness of breath when walking uphill increased significantly with increasing waist circumference in men and women smokers. Significantly more women with waist circumferences greater than action level 2 than women with waist circumference less than action level 1 had low back pain. Significantly more men with waist circumferences greater than action level 2 lost jobs because of low back pain compared with men with waist circumferences less than action level 1.

Conclusion.—Individuals with waist circumferences exceeding action level 2 are at increased risk of health and quality-of-life problems. Strategies need to be developed to help individuals maintain lower waist circumferences as they age. Health planners need to be aware of the increased health problems that accrue to individuals with high waist circumferences.

Body Mass Index and Mortality in a General Population Sample of Men and Women: The Buffalo Health Study

Dorn JM, Schisterman EF, Winkelstein W Jr, et al (State Univ of New York, Buffalo; Univ of California, Berkeley)
Am J Epidemiol 146:919-931, 1997 10–2

Background.—Obesity is associated with a number of coronary heart disease (CHD) risk factors and other health risks. The long-term relationship between body mass index (BMI) and mortality from all causes and specific causes in the general population was investigated.

Methods.—Six hundred ninety-seven women and 611 men, aged 20 to 96 years, were included in the 29-year follow-up study. The research subjects were selected randomly from the population of Buffalo, New York, in 1960. Since study entry, 295 men and 281 women died.

Findings.—In a Cox proportional hazards model, BMI was significantly, linearly associated with all-cause mortality in men younger than 65 years at baseline, after adjustment for age, education, and cigarette smoking. This relationship was not found in women. In men aged 65 years and older, the association was quadratic, and the lowest risk occurred in the BMI range of 23 to 27. In women and younger men but not in older men, BMI was most strongly associated with cardiovascular disease (CVD) and CHD. BMI was not correlated with an increased risk of death from non-CVD or cancer in either sex.

Conclusions.—BMI is an important risk factor for CVD and CHD mortality in certain population groups. Most of the effect of BMI on overall mortality results from the strong relationship between relative weight and these specific causes of death.

▶ Unfortunately, the prevalence of overweight Americans is increasing. Obesity has been shown to be a risk factor for CHD. A long-term (almost 3 decades) follow-up study (Abstract 10–2) of white men and women confirmed this significant linear association between BMI and all cause mortality in men younger than 65 years but not in women. BMI was most strongly related to CVD and CHD mortality in women and men younger than 65 years.

Lean et al. (Abstract 10–1), in a cross-sectional study of approximately 13,000 individuals, found that waist circumferences greater than 41 inches in men and 35 inches in women are strongly associated with the development of hypertension, elevated cholesterol levels, and difficulties with daily activities. A slight waist reduction of 2 to 4 inches can result in improvements in several cardiovascular risk factors. Obesity accounts for use of excessive health care services and is risky for an individual and costly to society. We must, therefore, stress the importance of treatment.

J.S. Barkin, M.D.

Subject Index

A

C

D

F

G

I

M

N

O

P

Q

R

S

U

V

W

X

Author Index

A

B

C

D

E

F

Z